MW00379765

Specialty Topics in Pediatric Neuropsychology

More information about this series at http://www.springer.com/series/11701

Cynthia A. Riccio • Jeremy R. Sullivan
Editors

Pediatric Neurotoxicology

Academic and Psychosocial Outcomes

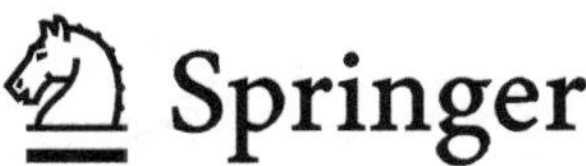

Editors
Cynthia A. Riccio
Department of Educational Psychology
and Institute of Neuroscience
Texas A&M University
College Station, TX, USA

Jeremy R. Sullivan
Department of Educational Psychology
University of Texas at San Antonio
San Antonio, TX, USA

Specialty Topics in Pediatric Neuropsychology
ISBN 978-3-319-32356-5 ISBN 978-3-319-32358-9 (eBook)
DOI 10.1007/978-3-319-32358-9

Library of Congress Control Number: 2016944372

Printed on acid-free paper

This Springer imprint is published by Springer Nature
The registered company is Springer International Publishing AG Switzerland

Dedicated to Amanda, Molly,
and Patrick—thanks for giving me the time
to work on this project (JRS).
Also to Jess for his continued support (CAR).

Preface

In 1931, Aldous Huxley wrote *Brave New World*, his satiric perspective on the future. Huxley envisioned extensive use of pharmaceuticals, both for medical and leisure purposes. Interestingly, in *Brave New World* both chemicals and conditioning techniques were used to shape children's cognitive and physical development, as a way to control their position in society. Thus, even in the context of science fiction, there has long been an appreciation for the potentially harmful effects of exposure to environmental toxins on children's development. In the years since then, many changes have occurred that impact the lives of all, most importantly, the youngest generation. With advances in medicine and technology, research examining environmental influences on child development has burgeoned, as have efforts of people to alter or change the environment and behavior.

Paralleling these changes, researchers question the potential effects, especially negative ones, that manifest with exposure to substances that are, in some contexts at least, toxic. As with much research, early studies considered adult exposure, for example, to pesticides or air pollution, with child-based research coming along a bit later. The available research is scattered among different disciplines, not easily available to those who work with children who have been exposed to neurotoxins or are currently exposed even in their classrooms. This edited collection is a compilation of the research on a variety of neurotoxins and their potential impact on children's academic and psychosocial function. The chapters reflect perspectives from medicine and public health, as well as from neuropsychology. We hope this book will serve as a helpful resource for practitioners such as school psychologists, neuropsychologists, and medical professionals who work with educational systems to enhance the developmental outcomes of children exposed to neurotoxins.

College Station, TX, USA — Cyndi A. Riccio
San Antonio, TX, USA — Jeremy R. Sullivan

Acknowledgements

We thank all of the contributors to this volume, as this project would not have been completed successfully without their expertise, timeliness, and enthusiasm for their work. We also want to thank Elaine Fletcher-Jantzen for developing this important series.

Contents

Contributors

Maria J. Castro, M.A. Department of Educational Psychology, The University of Texas at San Antonio, San Antonio, TX, USA

Genny Carrillo, M.D., Sc.D., M.P.H., M.S.P.H. Department of Environmental and Occupational Health, School of Public Health, Texas A&M Health Science Center, College Station, TX, USA

Morgan B. Drake, M.Ed. Department of Educational Psychology, Texas A&M University, College Station, TX, USA

Megan Galbally, M.B.B.S., F.R.A.N.Z.C.P., Ph.D. Foundation Chair in Perinatal Psychiatry, Murdoch University, University of Notre Dame and Fiona Stanley Hospital, Murdoch, WA, Australia

Elizabeth E. Gerard, M.D. Feinberg School of Medicine, Northwestern University, Chicago, IL, USA

Leila Glass, M.S. Center for Behavioral Teratology, Department of Psychology, San Diego State University, San Diego, CA, USA

Natalie M. Johnson, Ph.D. Department of Environmental and Occupational Health, School of Public Health, Texas A&M Health Science Center, College Station, TX, USA

Faculty Member of the Texas A&M Interdisciplinary Faculty of Toxicology, College Station, TX, USA

Adelaide Lang, Ph.D. Case Western Reserve University, Cleveland, OH, USA

Andrew Lewis, Ph.D. School of Psychology, Deakin University, Waurn Ponds, VIC, Australia

David W. Loring, Ph.D., A.B.P.P. Departments of Neurology and Pediatrics, Emory University, Atlanta, GA, USA

Sarah N. Mattson, Ph.D. Center for Behavioral Teratology, Department of Psychology, San Diego State University, San Diego, CA, USA

Kimford J. Meador, M.D. Department of Neurology & Neurological Sciences, Stanford University, Stanford, CA, USA

Ranjana K. Mehta, Ph.D., M.S. Department of Environmental and Occupational Health, School of Public Health, Texas A&M Health Science Center, College Station, TX, USA

Faculty of the Texas A&M Institute for Neuroscience, College Station, TX, USA

Meeyoung O. Min, Ph.D. Case Western Reserve University, Cleveland, OH, USA

Sonia Minnes, Ph.D. Case Western Reserve University, Cleveland, OH, USA

Leandra Parris, Ph.D. Department of Psychology, Illinois State University, Normal, IL, USA

Josephine Power, M.B.B.S., M.P.M., F.R.A.N.Z.C.P. Department of Perinatal Mental Health, Mercy Hospital for Women, Melbourne, VIC, Australia

General Hospital Mental Health, Austin Health, Melbourne, VIC, Australia

Cynthia A. Riccio, Ph.D. Department of Educational Psychology and Institute of Neuroscience, Texas A&M University, College Station, TX, USA

Lynn T. Singer, Ph.D. Case Western Reserve University, Cleveland, OH, USA

Jeremy R. Sullivan, Ph.D. Department of Educational Psychology, University of Texas at San Antonio, San Antonio, TX, USA

Victor Villarreal, Ph.D. Department of Educational Psychology, The University of Texas at San Antonio, San Antonio, TX, USA

Chapter 1
Neurotoxins and Neurodevelopment

Cynthia A. Riccio, Morgan B. Drake, and Jeremy R. Sullivan

Developmental perspectives for understanding how neurological factors relate to overall functioning and behavior across the life span are imperative. The leading cause of neonatal mortality is birth defects (McKenzie et al., 2014), in some cases the result of exposure to neurotoxins. Even when not resulting in death, damage or insult to the developing brain or nervous system from exposure to neurotoxins can result in ramifications that range from mild to severe and are lifelong (Gilbert, Miller, Martin, & Abulafia, 2010). Consistent with a developmental framework, models of pathology should be based on what is known about typical development and underlying neurological processes (Sonuga-Barke, 2014). Additionally, the neurodevelopmental timing of the deviation or damage is important with effects on the pathogenesis of disorders in children. Because their brains are still developing, children are particularly susceptible to the deleterious effects of neurotoxins (Dietrich et al., 2005; Gilbert et al., 2010; Konijnenberg & Melinder, 2011; Lidsky, Heaney, Schneider, & Rosen, 2007). Therefore, those who work with children, expectant mothers, or families should be knowledgeable about neurotoxins and

C.A. Riccio, Ph.D. (✉)
Department of Educational Psychology and Institute of Neuroscience,
Texas A&M University, 4225 TAMU, College Station, TX 77843-4225, USA
e-mail: criccio@tamu.edu

M.B. Drake, M.Ed.
Department of Educational Psychology, Texas A&M University,
4225 TAMU, College Station, TX 77843-4225, USA
e-mail: mbdrake13@email.tamu.edu

J.R. Sullivan, Ph.D.
Department of Educational Psychology, University of Texas at San Antonio,
501 W. Cesar E. Chavez Blvd., San Antonio, TX 78207, USA
e-mail: jeremy.sullivan@utsa.edu

C. Riccio, J. Sullivan (eds.), *Pediatric Neurotoxicology*, Specialty Topics in Pediatric Neuropsychology, DOI 10.1007/978-3-319-32358-9_1

their effects on child development in order to enhance prevention efforts, improve diagnosis, and formulate and implement research-based interventions. In each of the ensuing chapters the research specific to a class of neurotoxins is summarized, with a focus on the potential effects on neurocognitive and neurobehavioral domains.

What Are Neurotoxins?

Neurotoxins are harmful substances that damage or destroy neural tissue (Costa, Aschner, Vitalone, Syversen, & Porat-Soldin, 2004). Toxic exposure comprises contact with a large range of substances that ultimately are poisonous to one or more aspects of the neural system (Williams & Ross, 2007). Neurotoxins include environmental substances that naturally occur, manmade substances, prescribed medications, and recreational substances. Environmental and chemical teratogens, such as lead (see Chap. 8); mercury, manganese, arsenic, toluene, polychlorinated biphenyls (PCBs), and pesticides (see Chap. 7); and air pollution (see Chap. 9) can often be found in the child's environment and can be a serious threat to development (Gilbert et al., 2010; Landrigan, Lambertini, & Birnbaum, 2012; Winneke, 2007). Proximity to sources of natural gas, for example, is associated with cardiac defects and neural tube defects (McKenzie et al., 2014). Issues related to toxic effects of environmental substances received increased attention following the passage of an executive order by President Bill Clinton acknowledging children's increased vulnerability to the harmful effects of environmental toxins and the need to protect them from these risks (Executive Order No. 13045, 1997). Healthy People 2010 also included environmental quality as an important health indicator, given the contributions of poor air quality and environmental toxins to preventable illnesses (U.S. Department of Health and Human Services, 2000).

Exposure to neurotoxins may be in the form of direct interaction, as in the case of a child who chews on a toy that has been finished with lead paint or was inadvertently contaminated with pesticides. Some research indicates that the majority of exposure to neurotoxic chemicals such as lead occurs postnatally, while most of the exposure to mercury and PCBs occur prenatally. It is important to note, however, that exposure has been found to occur across the life span and can have detrimental consequences to neurodevelopment and associated behaviors (Winneke, 2007).

Environmental toxins are not the only teratogens that can have an impact on neurodevelopmental functioning. From the time of conception, the developing fetal brain is exposed to the chemical and electrical environment of the mother. Studies consistently indicate that substance use and consumption of certain medications by pregnant women place their unborn children at risk. Effects on an unborn child are indirect and occur through maternal contact or ingestion of the toxin, including prescribed medications. Medications may be prescribed to address concerns with the maintenance of the pregnancy (e.g., diethylstilbestrol [DES], thalidomide) or to address the medical status of the mother (e.g., seizure control, diabetes). A wide range of medications have been identified as disturbing the normal developmental process in utero (Pillard et al., 1993; Titus-Ernstoff et al., 2003). With medical treatment, however, where both maternal health and child health are of concern, determining appropriate protocols and potential effects is ongoing (see Chap. 5 on antiepileptic drug effects; Chap. 6 on other psychotropic medications). A final consideration is the use of recreational and addictive substances during pregnancy, such as alcohol (see Chap. 2), stimulants including nicotine and cocaine (see Chap. 3), and opiates and marijuana (see Chap. 4). As detailed in these chapters, children who have been exposed to various recreational drugs by their mothers demonstrate increased risk for poor academic and social-emotional outcomes.

Mechanisms of Impact on the Developing Child

Any disruption in the extended process of central nervous system development can affect structures or functions of the nervous system, with associated negative consequences for later developing functions and behaviors (Gilbert et al., 2010). Moreover, brain and neural development occurs in stages, with some time periods accounting for more critical development of specific functional systems (Costa et al., 2004; Jian'an et al., 2015; Stiles & Jernigan, 2010). Thus, neurotoxin exposure during different periods of development may yield very different symptoms or alterations in developmental trajectory (Costa et al., 2004; Jian'an et al., 2015; Miodovnik, 2011; Richardson, Goldschmidt, Larkby, & Day, 2015). Given the importance of communication across areas of the brain, abnormal development (or an interruption in normal development) of any one area of the brain for any reason leads to associated abnormalities at levels of functioning and can potentially affect multiple systems (Zillmer, Spiers, & Culbertson, 2008). Even for in utero exposure, timing is important.

In Utero Exposure

Effects on the fetus are likely associated with neuronal rapid cell proliferation, synaptic pruning, suppression, and neuronal cell death (i.e., apoptosis) as a result of exposure (Gilbert et al., 2010). In the early developmental stages in utero, rapid cell proliferation, differentiation, migration, and apoptosis contribute to the formation of cognitive structures and brain area specialization (Gilbert et al., 2010; Stiles & Jernigan, 2010). The rapid changes in neuronal development make in utero development especially vulnerable to the adverse effects of neurotoxins (Konijnenberg & Melinder, 2011; Rice & Barone, 2000). Research documenting negative effects has led to some pesticides, for example, being banned in the USA (e.g., dichlorodiphenyldichloroethylene [DDE]), although it is still being used in Mexico and other countries with adverse effects (Osorio-Valencia et al., 2015). Moreover, the potential for harm caused by neurotoxin exposure in utero is increased because the blood–brain barrier is not fully developed until approximately 6 months of age, making the developmental periods before and immediately following birth especially vulnerable (Costa et al., 2004).

Childhood and Beyond

In addition to in utero exposure to neurotoxins, children and adults potentially are exposed to neurotoxins in the environment across the life span. Synaptic development, myelination, and pruning occur throughout the life span, but are especially prevalent in childhood and adolescence (Rice & Barone, 2000; Winneke, 2007). As such, children continue to be vulnerable to cognitive, behavioral, and emotional deficits that stem from neurotoxins. Disruption of synaptic pruning can adversely affect the amount of synaptic connections made and retained in the brain (Costa et al., 2004). Additionally, structural changes in grey and white matter continue into young adulthood and affect behavior (Stiles & Jernigan, 2010). Fine-tuning of neural functioning continues throughout the life span and is continuously affected by environmental contexts. It is the functioning of the neural system that sets the stage for behavior. As a result, neurotoxin exposure during these developmental periods can adversely affect brain development and manifest as various learning and developmental disorders (Rice & Barone, 2000). While there is minimal understanding of the long term effects of exposure, there is research to suggest impact on children, as well as adults.

Impact and Diagnostic Considerations

It is well established that various mechanisms can affect neural development negatively, and, as a result, alter the developmental trajectory of specific abilities, processes, and functions. Development of the brain and central nervous system starts in utero and continues through adolescence or early adulthood (Archer, Kostrzewa, Beninger, & Palomo, 2010). Individuals with neurodevelopmental disorders are those who have, or who are at risk for, limitations in some or all life activities as a result of impairments in the central nervous system (Mudrick, 2002; Spreen, Risser, & Edgell, 1995). The possible consequences and limitations range from mild to severe cognitive, sensory, motor, educational, and behavioral or psychological impairments (Mendola, Slevan, Gutter, & Rice, 2002), as well as physical effects. It is believed that developmental and learning disorders stem from disruption in brain development and function that results in negative effects on performance, ability, and achievement (Gilbert et al., 2010). Although some neural impairments may be apparent at birth, other effects are latent and do not appear until later in life or until a time where the effect is more noticeable, such as cognitive, attention, and emotional regulation deficits that become more conspicuous as the academic and behavioral demands placed on the child increase (Costa et al., 2004; Lanphear, Wright, & Dietrich, 2005; Rice & Barone, 2000; Trask & Kosofsky, 2000; Weiss, 2000).

As already noted, different manifestations of neurodevelopmental problems are dependent on the time in development when exposure occurs (Archer et al., 2010; Costa et al., 2004; Konijnenberg & Melinder, 2011; Miodovnik, 2011; Riley & McGee, 2005; Trask & Kosofsky, 2000; Vajda et al., 2010). For example, there is growing evidence that exposure to PCBs in utero has negative consequences on cognitive abilities, executive functioning, and behavior; however, exposure to PCBs via breast milk in infancy was not found to be associated with cognitive or attentional impairments (Ribas-Fito, Sala, Kogevinas, & Sunyer, 2001; Williams & Ross, 2007). This importance of timing applies regardless of the neurotoxin.

The effects of neurotoxin exposure can be diffuse and affect all areas of function as well as global neurocognitive and neurobehavioral outcomes. Alternatively, the effects may be more focal and affect only specific functional systems and outcomes. For example, exposure to toxic chemicals and environmental agents has been linked to decreased intelligence, psychomotor and language deficits, inattention, aggression, and hyperactivity (Henn et al., 2012; Lin et al., 2013; Perera et al., 2006; Rice & Barone, 2000; Winneke, 2007). Regardless of whether the substance is alcohol, opiates, cocaine, or nicotine, the associated deficits in self-regulation, attentional control, overreactivity, and excitability have been noted (Bandstra, Morrow, Anthony, Accornero, & Fried, 2001; Bard, Coles, Platzman, & Lynch, 2000; Molitor, Mayes, & Ward, 2003). Overall, it is estimated that at least 3 % of developmental disorders may stem from exposure to neurotoxins, while 25 % may be attributed to the interaction between neurotoxins and genetics (National Research Council, 2000).

Moderating Factors

Maturation theory posits that functional asymmetry of the cerebral hemispheres develops with age, beginning at conception, and is influenced by environmental events and stimulation (Boles, Barth, & Merrill, 2007). Sonuga-Barke (2014) posited the critical role of environment with an emphasis on stress exposure and the social-ecological context. Stress and risk in this context is generally considered the social sphere (i.e., family interactions, resources) in which the individual functions. Known risk factors include low socioeconomic status, family violence, and low parental intelligence (Williams & Ross, 2007). With some forms of exposure, males seem to be more susceptible to effects as compared to females (e.g., Evans et al., 2015). As such, overall functioning is not only the result of the integrity of brain function, but that brain function is influenced by (and influences) environmental/social contexts. Hence, the context in which the individual functions is of importance.

Genetic Contribution

Genetic contributions may serve as a predisposition or diathesis that can be altered or modified for better or worse by environmental stimulation or exposure (Asbury, Wachs, & Plomin, 2005; Pennington et al., 2009; Schmidt, Polak, & Spooner, 2005). Due to genetic variation, people vary in their susceptibility to damage after exposure to neurotoxins (Gilbert et al., 2010; Meador et al., 2013). A child who already has a genetic predisposition to low intellectual functioning may face even more substantial cognitive deficits if exposed to a neurotoxin, compared to another child without that genetic predisposition. For women taking various medications research suggests increased vulnerability as a function of genotype (Meador, Baker, Cohen, Gaily, & Westerveld, 2007). Additionally, neurotoxins have been found to alter gene expression (Gilbert et al., 2010; Landrigan et al., 2012). Specifically, these gene modifications can result in deficits in cognitive and developmental function (Gilbert et al., 2010). Furthermore, some evidence suggests that disorders such as autism, attention deficit hyperactivity disorder, and other developmental and behavioral disorders stem from a combination of genetic factors and environmental triggers, including neurotoxin exposure (Archer et al., 2010; Konijnenberg & Melinder, 2011; Landrigan et al., 2012; Riccio, Sullivan, & Cohen, 2010). Similar to the interactions seen between neurotoxins and environmental factors, genes can shape the likelihood and expression of neural damage.

Stimulation

While neuropsychology embraces the idea that the integrity of the neurological system determines behavior, there is evidence that environmental factors, including failure to stimulate particular areas of the brain, will impact functioning (Zillmer et al., 2008). Throughout childhood and adolescence, there are critical, specific windows of time where certain developmental events must occur to have the most impact (Mundkur, 2005). If the child is not exposed to the developmental experience during this time period, they may not develop normally or the critical experience will have a reduced effect. For example, if a child hears very little spoken language in the first few years of life, they may have underdeveloped language abilities, which they may be unable to recover from or improve upon (Mundkur, 2005).

Additionally, environmental factors can increase or diminish the scope of the damages caused by neurotoxin exposure (Cory-Slechta, 2005; Cory-Slechta et al., 2013; Gilbert et al., 2010; Weiss, 2000). For example, negative environmental experiences, such as stress associated with low socioeconomic status or abuse, have been found to exacerbate the effects of neurotoxin exposure (Cory-Slechta, 2005; Cory-Slechta et al., 2013; Konijnenberg & Melinder, 2011). On the other hand, positive experiences and environmental components, such as higher socioeconomic status, enrichment programs, and parental support can attenuate neurotoxic damage (Cory-Slechta et al., 2013). Humans may be exposed to neurotoxins across the life span, while the toxicity and manifestations of the exposure are determined by a variety of negative and positive environmental factors (Cory-Slechta, 2005; Trask & Kosofsky, 2000; Weiss, 2000). Overall, whether neurotoxin exposure occurs or not, stress and environmental factors play a large role in the development of a variety of cognitive and behavioral disorders. Thus, two different children exposed to the same neurotoxin may experience divergent outcomes based on the interactions among these genetic and environmental factors.

Considerations for Prevention and Intervention

When introduced prenatally, exposure may be time limited, yet these substances can have both indirect and direct effects on children across their lifetime. At the same time, there is continued risk across the life span of exposure. Research findings have led to some changes in environmental policy as well as health care. For example, many pesticides are no longer considered acceptable and modifications to air exchange systems are being made. With increased knowledge of the effects of drugs on the developing fetus, there is considerable caution exercised with regard to the use of medications of any type by pregnant women (Bercovici, 2005; Meador, 2002), as well as decreased exposure to environmental toxins of the mother.

Due to neuroplasticity, it is important that deficits due to neurotoxic exposure are detected early in life. Neuroplasticity refers to the brain's ability to change structurally and functionally in response to experience (Mundkur, 2005; Rice & Barone, 2000). Early experience can have a large impact on the development and pruning of synapses, which can affect memory, cognition, and behavior (Mundkur, 2005). Early detection of brain and nervous system deficits is imperative so that intervention effects can be maximized due to the high neuroplasticity of the child brain (Mundkur, 2005; Quattlebaum & O'Connor, 2012; Westrup, 2013). The sooner the interventions are implemented, the more the functional and behavioral gains made and sustained for a longer period of time (Quattlebaum & O'Connor, 2012; Westrup, 2013).

Early intervention is also essential due to the economic impact of developmental, cognitive, and behavioral disorders (Bales, Boyce, Heckman, & Rolnick, 2006; Quattlebaum & O'Connor, 2012; Weiss, 2000). According to a study by Landrigan, Schechter, Lipton, Fahs, and Schwartz (2002), the annual cost in the USA of lead poisoning induced cognitive impairments, intellectual disabilities, autism, and cerebral palsy stemming from environmental pollutants has been estimated to be $50 billion. These estimates do not even include the costs of neurotoxic exposure to drugs and medications or the annual expenditures for other deficits that stem from neurotoxin exposure (e.g., fetal alcohol syndrome). Cognitive and intellectual impairments can result in a reduced workforce, higher medical costs, and a greater need for enrichment programs in schools and communities, all of which can create an economic burden (Weiss, 2000). Additionally, behavioral and psychological deficits can increase crime and incarceration rates and medical expenditures (Weiss, 2000). These global economic costs do not even consider the individual monetary costs to the family or the emotional and psychological toll that neurodevelopmental, cognitive, and behavioral deficits can produce.

Conclusion

Levy (2015) argued that carbon monoxide pollution and associated effects on neurodevelopment constitute a public health concern. This continues to be the prevalent assertion across disciplines of psychology, medicine, and public health and reflects both increased awareness of neurotoxins and increased use of substances, prescribed and otherwise. In the past 30 years, there has been continued advancement in technology with increased ability to examine brain structures using multiple methods (Williams & Ross, 2007); however, what is known about the effects of toxic exposure is still limited. With advanced capability for functional imaging methods and consideration of the physical and chemical environment, there is hope for greater insight and information about the potential risks. At the same time, this increased technology will yield a better understanding of brain behavior in relation to neurodevelopmental disorders (Berkelhammer, 2008). Additionally, with hundreds of thousands of manmade and natural chemicals, future research must focus on identifying potential neurotoxins and their effects on development (Goldman et al., 2004; Miodovnik, 2011; Szpir, 2006; Trask & Kosofsky, 2000). Greater identification of neurotoxic chemicals may aid in decreasing the incidence of neurodevelopmental, behavioral, and psychological disorders that stem from neurotoxic exposure and reduce economic costs.

Another area for future research includes investigating the environmental and genetic factors that can either increase or ameliorate the effects of neurotoxin exposure (Trask & Kosofsky, 2000). These features can aid in intervention and maximize outcomes, as well as provide targets for preventive measures, such as parent training. Furthermore, as noted by Sonuga-Barke (2014), what continues to be evident is the lack of identified developmental pathways that lead to pathology or disorder. Greater knowledge about the specific effects of various neurotoxins on the developing brain can aid in the creation of targeted interventions (Trask & Kosofsky, 2000; Williams & Ross, 2007). Moreover, there is a need for research that centers on identifying evidence-based approaches for early intervention for children (or adults) exposed to toxins as opposed to waiting until the effects fully manifest. More targeted and effective interventions can reduce the economic costs of neurotoxin exposure and maximize human potential. Although research efforts move the fields of cognitive and social neuroscience forward, there is still a long way to go. The remainder of this volume explores the current state of knowledge regarding the academic and psychosocial outcomes associated with neurotoxin exposure, and highlights current gaps in the literature that will set the stage for future research.

References

Archer, T., Kostrzewa, R. M., Beninger, R. J., & Palomo, T. (2010). Staging perspectives in neurodevelopmental aspects of neuropsychiatry: Agents, phases and ages at expression. *Neurotoxic Research, 18*, 287–305.

Asbury, K., Wachs, T. D., & Plomin, R. (2005). Environmental moderators of genetic influence on verbal and nonverbal abilities in early childhood. *Intelligence, 33*, 643–661.

Bales, S. N., Boyce, W. T., Heckman, J., & Rolnick, A. J. (2006). Early exposure to toxic substances damages brain architecture. *National Scientific Council of the Developing Child, Working Paper, 4*, 1–16.

Bandstra, E. S., Morrow, C. E., Anthony, J. C., Accornero, V. H., & Fried, P. A. (2001). Longitudinal investigation of task persistence and sustained attention in children with prenatal cocaine exposure. *Neurotoxicology and Teratology, 23*, 545–559.

Bard, K. A., Coles, C. D., Platzman, K. A., & Lynch, M. E. (2000). The effects of prenatal drug exposure, term status, and caregiving on arousal and arousal modulation in 8-week-old infants. *Developmental Psychobiology, 36*, 194–212.

Bercovici, E. (2005). Prenatal and perinatal effects of psychotropic drugs on neuro-cognitive development in the fetus. *Journal on Developmental Disabilities, 11*(2), 1–20.

Berkelhammer, L. D. (2008). Pediatric neuropsychological evaluation. In M. Herson & A. M. Gross (Eds.), *Handbook of clinical psychology* (pp. 497–519). Hoboken, NJ: Wiley.

Boles, D. B., Barth, J. M., & Merrill, E. C. (2007). Asymmetry and performance: Toward a neurodevelopmental theory. *Brain and Cognition, 66*(2), 124–139.

Cory-Slechta, D. A. (2005). Studying toxicants as single chemicals: Does this strategy adequately identify neurotoxic risk? *NeuroToxicology, 26*, 491–510.

Cory-Slechta, D. A., Merchant-Borna, K., Allen, J. L., Liu, S., Weston, D., & Conrad, K. (2013). Variations in the nature of behavioral experience can differentially alter the consequences of developmental exposure to lead, prenatal stress, and the combination. *Journal of Toxicological Sciences, 13*, 194–205.

Costa, L. G., Aschner, M., Vitalone, A., Syversen, T., & Porat-Soldin, O. (2004). Developmental neuropathology of environment agents. *Annual Review of Pharmacology and Toxicology, 44*, 87–110.

National Research Council. (2000). *Scientific frontiers in developmental toxicology and risk assessment*. Washington, DC: National Academy Press.

Dietrich, K. N., Eskenazi, B., Schantz, S. L., Yolton, K., Rauh, V. A., Johnson, C. B., … Berman, R. F. (2005). Principles and practices of neurodevelopmental assessment in children: Lessons learned from the Centers for Children's Environmental Health and Disease Prevention Research. *Environmental Health Perspective, 113,* 1437–1446.

Evans, S. F., Kobrosly, R. W., Barrett, E. S., Thurston, S. W., Calafat, A. M., Weiss, B., … Swan, S. H. (2015). Prenatal bisphenol A exposure and maternally reported behavior in boys and girls. *NeuroToxicology, 45,* 91–99.

Executive Order No. 13045, 3 C.F.R. 198-201 (1997). *Protection of children from environmental health risks and safety risks*.

Gilbert, S. G., Miller, E., Martin, J., & Abulafia, L. (2010). Scientific and policy statements on environmental agents associated with neurodevelopmental disorders. *Journal of Intellectual and Developmental Disability, 35*, 121–128.

Goldman, L., Falk, H., Landrigan, P. J., Balk, S. J., Reigart, J. R., & Etzel, R. A. (2004). Environmental pediatrics and its impact on government health policy. *Journal of Pediatrics, 113*, 1146–1157.

Henn, B.C., Schnaas, L., Ettinger, A.S., Schwartz, J. Lamadrid-Figueroa, H., Hernandez-Avila, M., … Tellez-Rojo, M.M. (2012). Associations of early childhood manganese and lead coexposure with neurodevelopment. *Environmental Health Perspectives, 120,* 126–131.

Jian'an, L., Dingguo, G., Yuming, C., Jin, J., Qiansheng, H., & Yajun, C. (2015). Lead exposure at each stage of pregnancy and neurobehavioral development of neonates. *NeuroToxicology, 44*, 1–7.

Konijnenberg, C., & Melinder, A. (2011). Prenatal exposure to methadone and buprenorphine: A review of the potential effects on cognitive development. *Child Neuropsychology, 17*, 495–519.

Landrigan, P. J., Lambertini, L., & Birnbaum, L. S. (2012). Editorial: A research strategy to discover the environmental causes of autism and neurodevelopmental disabilities. *Environmental Health Perspectives, 120*, A258–A260.

Landrigan, P. J., Schechter, C. B., Lipton, J. M., Fahs, M. C., & Schwartz, J. (2002). Environmental pollutants and disease in American children: Estimates of morbidity, mortality, and costs for lead poisoning, asthma, cancer, and developmental disabilities. *Environmental Health Perspectives, 110*, 721–728.

Lanphear, B. P., Wright, R. O., & Dietrich, K. N. (2005). Environmental neurotoxins. *Pediatrics in Review, 26*, 191–198.

Levy, R. J. (2015). Carbon monoxide pollution and neurodevelopment: A public health concern. *Neurotoxicology and Teratology, 49*, 31–40.

Lidsky, T. I., Heaney, A. T., Schneider, J. S., & Rosen, J. F. (2007). Neurodevelopmental effects of childhood exposure to heavy metals: Lessons from pediatric lead poisoning. In M. M. M. Mazzocco & J. L. Ross (Eds.), *Neurogenetic developmental disorders: Variations in the manifestation in childhood* (pp. 335–363). Cambridge, MA: MIT Press.

Lin, C.C., Chen, Y.C., Su, F.C., Lin, C.M., Liao, H.F., Hwang, Y.H., … Chen, P.C. (2013). In utero exposure to environmental lead and manganese and neurodevelopment at 2 years of age. *Journal of Environmental Research, 123,* 52–57.

McKenzie, L. M., Guo, R., Witter, R. Z., Savitz, D. A., Newman, L. S., & Adgate, J. L. (2014). Birth outcomes and maternal residential proximity to natural gas development in rural Colorado. *Environmental Health Perspectives, 122*, 412–417.

Meador, K. J. (2002). Neurodevelopmental effects of antiepileptic drugs. *Current Neurology and Neuroscience Reports, 4*, 373–378.

Meador, K.J., Baker, G.A., Browning, N., Cohen, M.J., Bromley, R.L., Clayton-Smith, J., … Loring, D.W. (2013). Fetal antiepileptic drug exposure and cognitive outcomes at age of 6 years (NEAD study): A prospective observational study. *Lancet Neural, 12,* 244–252.

Meador, K. J., Baker, G., Cohen, M. J., Gaily, E., & Westerveld, M. (2007). Cognitive/behavioral teratogenetic effects of antiepileptic drugs. *Epilepsy & Behavior, 11*, 292–302.

Mendola, P., Slevan, S. G., Gutter, S., & Rice, D. (2002). Environmental factors associated with a spectrum of neurodevelopmental deficits. *Mental Retardation and Developmental Disabilities Research Reviews, 8*, 188–197.

Miodovnik, A. (2011). Environmental neurotoxicants and developing brain. *Mount Sinai Journal of Medicine, 78*, 58–77.

Molitor, A., Mayes, L. C., & Ward, A. (2003). Emotion regulation behavior during a separation procedure in 18-month-old children of mothers using cocaine and other drugs. *Development and Psychopathology, 15*, 39–54.

Mudrick, N. R. (2002). The prevalence of disability among children: Paradigms and estimates. *Physical Medical Rehabilitation Clinics of North America, 13*, 775–792.

Mundkur, N. (2005). Neuroplasticity in children. *Indian Journal of Pediatrics, 72*, 855–857.

Osorio-Valencia, E., Torres-Sánchez, L., López-Carrillo, L., Cebrián, M. E., Rothenberg, S. J., … Schnaas, L. (2015). Prenatal p,p′-DDE exposure and establishment of lateralization and spatial orientation in Mexican preschoolers. *NeuroToxicology, 47,* 1–7.

Pennington, B. F., McGrath, L. M., Rosenberg, J., Barnard, H., Smith, S. D., … Olson, R. K. (2009). Gene x environment interactions in reading disability and attention-deficit/hyperactivity disorder. *Developmental Psychology, 45,* 77–89.

Perera, F.P., Rauh, V., Whyatt, R.M., Tsai, W.Y., Tang, D., Diaz, D., … Kinney, P. (2006). Effect of prenatal exposure to airborne polycyclic aromatic hydrocarbons on neurodevelopment in the first 3 years of life among inner-city children. *Environmental Health Perspectives, 114,* 1287–1292.

Pillard, R. C., Rosen, L. R., Meyer-Bahlburg, H., Weinrich, J. D., Feldman, J. F., Gruen, R., et al. (1993). Psychopathology and social functioning in men prenatally exposed to diethylstilbestrol (DES). *Psychosomatic Medicine, 55*, 485–491.

Quattlebaum, J. L., & O'Connor, M. J. (2012). Higher functioning children with prenatal alcohol exposure: Is there a specific neurocognitive profile? *Child Neuropsychology: A Journal on Normal and Abnormal Development in Childhood and Adolescence, 19*, 561–578.

Ribas-Fito, N., Sala, M., Kogevinas, M., & Sunyer, J. (2001). Polychlorinated biphenyls (PCBs) and neurological development in children: A systematic review. *Journal of Epidemiol Community Health, 55*, 537–546.

Riccio, C. A., Sullivan, J. R., & Cohen, M. J. (2010). *Neuropsychological assessment and intervention for childhood and adolescent disorders*. Hoboken, NJ: Wiley.

Rice, D., & Barone, S., Jr. (2000). Critical periods of vulnerability for the developing nervous system: Evidence from human and animal models. *Environmental Health Perspectives, 108*, 511–533.

Richardson, G. A., Goldschmidt, L., Larkby, C., & Day, N. L. (2015). Effects of prenatal cocaine exposure on adolescent development. *Neurotoxicology and Teratology, 49*, 41–48.

Riley, E., & McGee, C. (2005). Fetal alcohol spectrum disorders: An overview with emphasis on changes in brain and behavior. *Experimental Biology and Medicine, 230*, 357–365.

Schmidt, L. A., Polak, C. P., & Spooner, A. L. (2005). Biological and environmental contributions to childhood shyness: A diathesis-stress model. In W. R. Crozier & L. E. Alden (Eds.), *The essential handbook of social anxiety for clinicians* (pp. 33–55). Hoboken, NJ: Wiley.

Sonuga-Barke, E. J. S. (2014). Editorial: Developmental foundations of mental health and disorder – moving beyond "Towards…". *Journal of Child Psychology and Psychiatry, 55*, 529–531.

Spreen, O., Risser, A. H., & Edgell, D. (1995). *Developmental neuropsychology*. London: Oxford University Press.

Stiles, J., & Jernigan, T. L. (2010). The basics of brain development. *Neuropsychology Review, 20*, 327–348.

Szpir, M. (2006). New thinking on neurodevelopment. *Environmental Health Perspectives, 114*, A100–A107.

Titus-Ernstoff, L., Perez, K., Hatch, E. F., Troisi, R., Palmer, J. W., Hartge, P., et al. (2003). Psychosocial characteristics of men and women exposed prenatally to diethylstilbestrol. *Epidemiology, 14*, 155–160.

Trask, C. L., & Kosofsky, B. E. (2000). Developmental considerations of neurotoxic exposures. *Journal of Clinical Neurobehavioral Toxicology, 18*, 541–561.

U.S. Department of Health and Human Services. (2000). *Healthy people 2010: Understanding and improving health* (2nd ed.). Washington, DC: U.S. Government Printing Office.

Vajda, F. J. E., Graham, J., Hitchcock, A. A., O'Brien, T. J., Lander, C. M., & Eadie, M. J. (2010). Foetal malformations after exposure to antiepileptic drugs in utero assessed at birth and 12 months later: Observations from the Australian pregnancy register. *Acta Neurologica Scandinavica, 124*(1), 9–12.

Weiss, B. (2000). Vulnerability of children and the developing brain to neurotoxic hazards. *Environmental Health Perspectives, 108*, 375–381.

Westrup, S. (2013). Foetal alcohol spectrum disorders: As prevalent as autism? *Educational Psychology in Practice: Theory, Research and Practice in Educational Psychology, 29*, 309–325.

Williams, J. H. G., & Ross, L. (2007). Consequences of prenatal toxin exposure for mental health in children and adolescents: A systematic review. *Journal of European Child and Adolescent Psychiatry, 16*, 243–253.

Winneke, G. (2007). Appraisal of neurobehavioral methods in environmental health research: The developing brain as a target for neurotoxic chemicals. *International Journal of Hygiene and Environmental Health, 210*, 601–609.

Zillmer, E. A., Spiers, M. V., & Culbertson, W. C. (2008). *Principles of neuropsychology*. Belmont, CA: Thomson Wadsworth.

Chapter 2
Fetal Alcohol Spectrum Disorders: Academic and Psychosocial Outcomes

Leila Glass and Sarah N. Mattson

Definitional Issues and Prevalence

Prenatal exposure to alcohol is the leading cause of preventable birth defects, developmental disorders, and intellectual disability (American Academy of Pediatrics Committee on Substance Abuse and Committee on Children with Disabilities, 2000). However, the precise nomenclature and criteria for diagnostic categories used to define the population of affected individuals remains contested. The effects of intrauterine alcohol exposure result in a continuum of behavioral, cognitive, neurological, and physical symptoms. As a consequence of the heterogeneity of clinical presentation, the categorization of affected children has been defined differently across a variety of classification systems (see Table 2.1).

Although some variability exists in the details, there is relative consensus regarding the medical diagnosis of fetal alcohol syndrome (FAS), which relies on a triad of symptoms: (1) evidence of two or more characteristic facial features, such as short palpebral fissures, smooth philtrum, and a thin vermillion border of upper lip; (2) evidence of prenatal or postnatal growth deficiency with a height or weight of below the 10th percentile at any point of the child's life (corrected for racial norms, if possible); and (3) evidence of deficient brain growth or abnormal morphogenesis (Astley, 2013; Hoyme et al., 2005; Jones et al., 2006). See Fig. 2.1. The third criterion can be satisfied by the presence of structural brain abnormalities or microcephaly (head circumference ≤10th percentile). Receiving a diagnosis of FAS is often recognized as a qualifying disorder to provide access to referrals and services (Bertrand et al., 2004). See Fig. 2.2.

L. Glass, M.S. • S.N. Mattson, Ph.D. (✉)
Center for Behavioral Teratology, Department of Psychology, San Diego State University, 6330 Alvarado Court, Suite 100, San Diego, CA 92120, USA
e-mail: lglass@mail.sdsu.edu; sarah.mattson@sdsu.edu

C. Riccio, J. Sullivan (eds.), *Pediatric Neurotoxicology*, Specialty Topics in Pediatric Neuropsychology, DOI 10.1007/978-3-319-32358-9_2

Table 2.1 Summary and comparison of the various diagnostic schemas for prenatal alcohol related disorders

	4-Digit Code	Revised Institute of Medicine	Canadian	National Task Force on FAS/FAE
FAS				
Facial characteristics	Simultaneous presentation of short palpebral fissures (≤2 SDs), thin vermillion border, smooth philtrum[a]	Two of the following: short palpebral fissures (≤10th percentile), thin vermillion border, smooth philtrum	Simultaneous presentation of short palpebral fissures (≤2 SDs), thin vermillion border, smooth philtrum	Simultaneous presentation of short palpebral fissures (≤10th percentile), thin vermillion border, smooth philtrum
Growth retardation	Height or weight ≤10th percentile	Height or weight ≤10th percentile	Height or weight or disproportionately low weight-to-height ratio (≤10th percentile)	Height or weight ≤10th percentile
Central nervous system (CNS) involvement	Head circumference (occipital-frontal circumference [OFC]) ≥2 SDs below norm or significant abnormalities in brain structure or evidence of hard neurological findings or significant impairment in three or more domains of brain function (≥2 SDs below the mean) as assessed by validated and standardized tools	Head circumference (OFC) ≤10th percentile or structural brain abnormality	Evidence of three or more impairments in the following CNS domains: hard and soft neurologic signs; brain structure; cognition; communication; academic achievement; memory; executive functioning and abstract reasoning; attention deficit/hyperactivity; adaptive behavior, social skills, social communication	Head circumference (OFC) ≤10th percentile or structural brain abnormality or neurological problems or other soft neurological signs outside normal limits or functional impairment as evidenced by global cognitive or intellectual deficits, below the 3rd percentile (2 SDs) below the mean or functional deficits below the 16th percentile (1 SD) below the mean in at least three domains: cognitive or developmental markers, executive functioning, motor, social skills, attention/hyperactivity, and other (i.e., sensory, memory, language)

Alcohol exposure	Confirmed or not confirmed	Confirmed or not confirmed	Confirmed or not confirmed	Confirmed or not confirmed
Partial FAS				Not proposed
Facial characteristics	Short palpebral fissures (≤2 SDs) and either a smooth philtrum or thin vermillion border, with the other being normal OR palpebral fissure (≤1 SD) and both a smooth philtrum and thin vermillion	Two or more of the following: short palpebral fissures (≤10th percentile), thin vermillion border, smooth philtrum	Two or more of the following: short palpebral fissures, thin vermillion border, smooth philtrum	Not applicable
Growth retardation	Not required	Either height or weight ≤10th percentile OR (see CNS involvement)	Not required	Not applicable
Central nervous system (CNS) involvement	Same as for FAS	Head circumference ≤10th percentile or structural brain abnormality or behavioral and cognitive abnormalities inconsistent with developmental level	Same as for FAS	Not applicable

(continued)

Table 2.1 (continued)

	4-Digit Code	Revised Institute of Medicine	Canadian	National Task Force on FAS/FAE
Alcohol exposure	Confirmed	Confirmed or not confirmed	Confirmed	Insufficient data to provide guidance for this diagnosis. Formed group to discuss
Alcohol-related neurodevelopmental disorder	Does not propose this diagnostic category, but rather has several categories assessing functional deficits			Not applicable
Central nervous system involvement	Same as for FAS	Either (1) structural brain anomaly or OFC ≤10th percentile or (2) evidence of a complex pattern of behavioral or cognitive abnormalities inconsistent with developmental level that cannot be explained by genetics, family background, or environment alone	Same as for FAS	Not applicable

Alcohol exposure	Confirmed	Confirmed	Confirmed	Not applicable
Notes	The 4-Digit Code provides an assessment of effects in four areas (growth, face, CNS, and alcohol exposure) that results in 256 different codes and 22 diagnostic categories A specific pattern or level of alcohol exposure is not required, just that alcohol exposure is confirmed or not	Alcohol exposure is defined as a pattern of excessive intake or heavy episodic drinking	Alcohol exposure is defined as a pattern of excessive intake or heavy episodic drinking A domain is considered "impaired" when on a standardized measure: Scores are ≥2 SDs below the mean, or there is a discrepancy of at least 1 SD between subdomains or there is a discrepancy of at least 1.5–2 SD among subtests on a measure	Alcohol exposure levels are not defined, but the authors cite evidence of alcohol exposure based upon clinical observation; self-report; reports of heavy alcohol use during pregnancy by a reliable informant; medical records documenting positive blood alcohol levels, or alcohol treatment; or other social, legal, or medical problems related to drinking during pregnancy

Table from Warren KR, Hewitt BG, Thomas JD (2011) Fetal alcohol spectrum disorders: Research challenges and opportunities. Alcohol Research and Health 34:4–14

All of the diagnostic schemes assume that genetic or medical causes have been ruled out and that appropriate norms are used when available

[a]For palpebral fissure norms, the 4-Digit Code uses Hall et al. 1989, Hoyme utilizes Thomas et al. 1987, and Chudley provides both the Thomas and Hall charts; the National Task Force guidelines do not mention which chart to use. Hall recently wrote that her charts underrepresented normal palpebral fissure length (Hall 2010) and should be replaced by those from Clarren et al. (2010)

[b]All of the diagnostic schemes use the University of Washington Lip-Philtrum Guide (http://depts.washington.edu/fasdpn/htmls/lip-philtrum-guides.htm), Astley (2004)

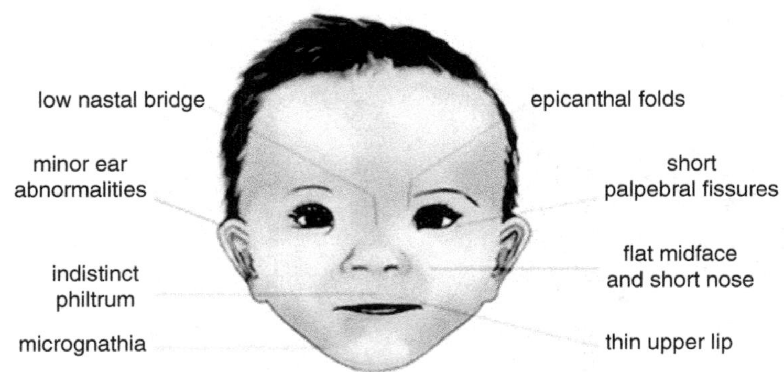

Fig. 2.1 Facial characteristics associated with fetal alcohol exposure

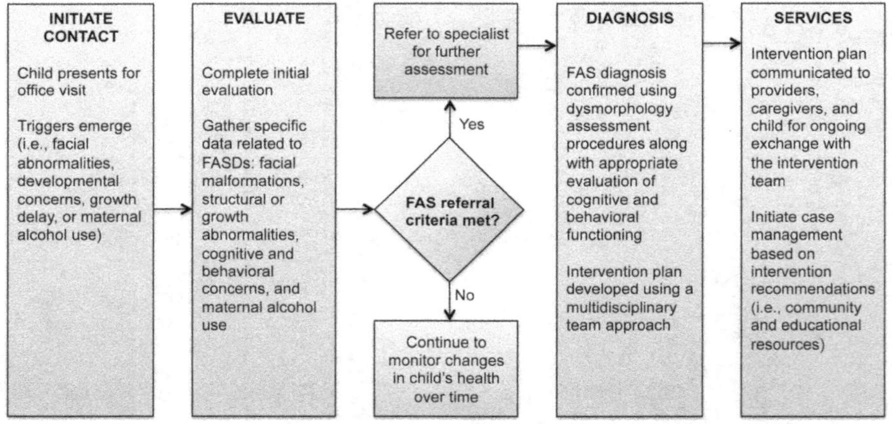

Fig. 2.2 Framework for FAS Diagnosis and Services. Adapted from Fetal Alcohol Syndrome: Guidelines for Referral and Diagnosis. National Center on Birth Defects and Developmental Disabilities, Center for Disease Control and Prevention, Department of Health and Human Services in coordination with the National Task Force on Fetal Alcohol Syndrome and Fetal Alcohol Effect. 2004. http://www.cdc.gov/ncbddd/fasd/documents/FAS_guidelines_accessible.pdf

The majority of children affected by alcohol do not meet all of the physical criteria required for an FAS diagnosis (May et al., 2014). For example, children who present with facial dysmorphology, but do not have growth deficiency or structural brain abnormalities may only meet criteria for partial FAS (pFAS). Most importantly, the majority of children affected by prenatal alcohol exposure do not demonstrate clear facial dysmorphology, which can greatly hinder identification of alcohol-affected individuals. Fetal alcohol spectrum disorders (FASDs) encompass the continuum of effects that result from prenatal alcohol exposure, including FAS (see Table 2.1, Fig. 2.3).

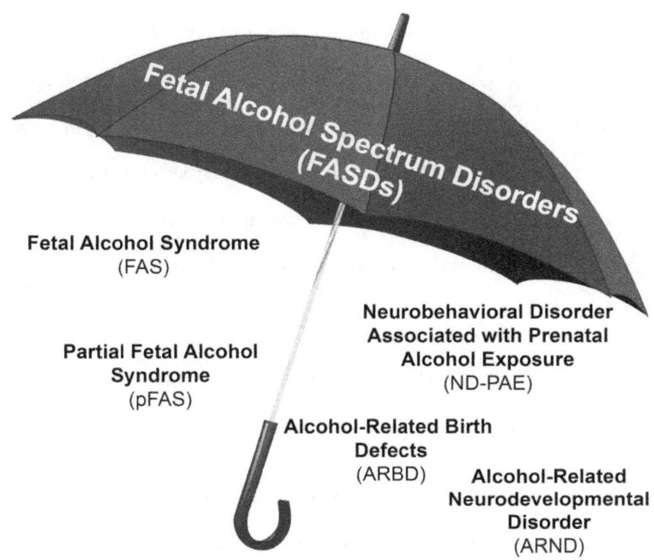

Fig. 2.3 Fetal Alcohol Spectrum Disorders encompass the continuum of potential effects of prenatal alcohol exposure

Recently, the effects of prenatal alcohol exposure have been incorporated into the Diagnostic and Statistical Manual of Mental Disorders (DSM-5) as a condition requiring further study, referred to as Neurobehavioral Disorder Associated with Prenatal Alcohol Exposure (ND-PAE) (American Psychiatric Association, 2013). A similar term, Neurodevelopmental Disorder Associated with Prenatal Alcohol Exposure, is listed as a billable diagnosis as a prototypical example under Other Specified Neurodevelopmental Disorder (American Psychiatric Association, 2013). This difference in terminology (neurobehavioral vs. neurodevelopmental) is likely to cause confusion, especially since the latter diagnosis can be given without attending to the proposed criteria for ND-PAE. The proposed criteria for ND-PAE are listed in Fig. 2.4 and require indication that the individual was exposed to alcohol at some point during gestation (including prior to pregnancy recognition) and that the exposure was more than "minimal." The precise dosage is not specific and relies on clinical judgment, although minimal exposure is defined as 1–13 drinks per month (and never more than two drinks per occasion) prior to pregnancy recognition and/or following pregnancy recognition (American Psychiatric Association, 2013). In addition to exceeding a minimal level of prenatal alcohol exposure, the patient must also have impaired neurocognition, self-regulation, and adaptive functioning. As the location of the disorder in the DSM-5 suggests, there is ongoing research to determine the feasibility, sensitivity, and specificity of the criteria to identify those affected by prenatal alcohol exposure.

Guidelines for alcohol-related diagnoses along the spectrum are developed to ensure valid and reliable identification of those affected by alcohol exposure (Farag, 2014). The greatest consequence of the ongoing debate over the diagnostic criteria

A. More than minimal exposure to alcohol during gestation, including prior to pregnancy recognition. Confirmation of gestational exposure to alcohol may be obtained from maternal self-report of alcohol use during pregnancy, medical or other records, or clinical observation.

B. Impaired neurocognitive functioning as manifested by one or more of the following:

1. Impairment in global intellectual performance (i.e., IQ of 70 or below, or a standard score of 70 or below on a comprehensive developmental assessment).
2. Impairment in executive functioning (e.g., poor planning and organization; inflexibility; difficulty with behavioral inhibition).
3. Impairment in learning (e.g., lower academic achievement than expected for intellectual level; specific learning disability).
4. Memory impairment (e.g., problems remembering information learned recently; repeatedly making the same mistakes; difficulty remembering lengthy verbal instructions).
5. Impairment in visual-spatial reasoning (e.g., disorganized or poorly planned drawings or constructions; problem differentiating left from right).

C. Impaired self-regulation as manifested by one or more of the following:

1. Impairment in mood or behavioral regulation (e.g., mood lability; negative affect or irritability; frequent behavioral outbursts).
2. Attention deficit (e.g., difficulty shifting attention; difficulty sustaining mental effort).
3. Impairment in impulse control (e.g., difficulty waiting turn; difficulty complying with rules).

D. Impairments in adaptive functioning manifested by two or more of the following, one of which must be (1) or (2):

1. Communication deficit (e.g., delayed acquisition of language; difficulty understanding spoken language).
2. Impairment in social communication and interaction (e.g., overly friendly with strangers; difficulty reading social cues; difficulty understanding social consequences).
3. Impairment in daily living skills (e.g., delayed toileting, feeding, or bathing; difficulty managing daily schedule).
4. Impairment in motor skills (e.g., poor fine motor skills development; delayed attainment of gross motor milestones or ongoing deficits in gross motor function; deficits in coordination and balance).

E. The onset of the disorder (symptoms in Criteria B, C, and D) occurs in childhood.

F. The disturbance causes clinically significant distress or impairment in social, academic, occupational, or other important areas of functioning.

G. The disorder is not better explained by the direct physiological effects associated with postnatal use of a substance (e.g., a medication, alcohol or other drugs), a general medical condition (e.g., traumatic brain injury, delirium, dementia), another known teratogen (e.g., fetal hydantoin syndrome), a genetic condition (e.g., Williams syndrome, Down syndrome, Cornelia de Lange syndrome), or environmental neglect.

Fig. 2.4 Criteria for Neurobehavioral Disorder Associated with Prenatal Alcohol Exposure (ND-PAE) listed as a condition for further study in the Diagnostic and Statistical Manual of Mental Disorders—Fifth Edition (DSM-5). Reprinted with permission from the Diagnostic and Statistical Manual of Mental Disorders, Fifth Edition (Copyright ©2013). American Psychiatric Association. All Rights Reserved.

is the risk that affected children and adults may be under-identified or misdiagnosed and therefore underserved. The current diagnostic schemas suffer from various shortcomings, including lack of consensus, lack of validation studies, difficulties in balancing sensitivity and specificity given the variation in clinical presentation, and hardships in educating physicians, dissemination, and implementation (Astley, 2014; Larcher & Brierley, 2014; Salmon & Clarren, 2011).

New objective screening tools, including neonatal testing and the development of potential biomarkers, can assist in the identification of alcohol-exposed children at birth (Koren et al., 2014; Zelner et al., 2010, 2012). Screening techniques are inherently plagued with potential ethical and moral issues. These include the risk of disproportionately targeting specific groups, inaccurate screening, and the concern of stigma and judgment associated with maternal drinking during pregnancy. The controversy regarding the demarcation of viable life and determination of personhood has also led to issues concerning the criminalization of drinking while pregnant (Drabble, Thomas, O'Connor, & Roberts, 2014; Yan, Bell, & Racine, 2014). A recent review of state responses to alcohol use and pregnancy found that there is great variability in the characteristics of policies, ranging from primarily supportive to primarily punitive (Drabble et al., 2014). One issue that arises in testing for alcohol exposure at birth is that even if it is possible to accurately determine prenatal alcohol exposure with adequate sensitivity and specificity, it is not certain that an individual will be negatively affected. Both a false positive and a false negative diagnosis may have detrimental effects throughout a child's development.

While it is difficult to accurately assess drinking, when compared to antenatal or prospective reports, retrospective reports identify 10.8 times as many women as risk drinkers (Hannigan et al., 2010). While retrospective reports were originally considered to be less accurate, changes in motivation and other factors lead them to be a more effective indicator of prenatal exposure that is validated in the prediction of additional behavioral problems compared to antenatal reports (Hannigan et al., 2010). However, despite the validity of retrospective reports, relying on maternal reports alone is not an effective way to identify rates of individuals with prenatal alcohol exposure. A study comparing the prevalence rates of prenatal alcohol exposure based on maternal self-reporting versus objective meconium screening (the earliest stool of the infant) found that the meconium testing yielded over four times as many cases as would have been identified by self-reporting alone (Lange, Shield, Koren, Rehm, & Popova, 2014). Therefore, additional methods of assessing prenatal alcohol exposure may be important to avoid missing affected children.

A pilot study found that ultrasound parameters may allow for early detection of alcohol-mediated negative outcomes resulting from central nervous system dysfunction, which may be more predictive of later dysfunction compared to other screening measures that do not distinguish alcohol-exposed from alcohol-affected outcomes (Kfir et al., 2009). This study found that there were significant differences between alcohol-exposed fetuses and controls in somatic and brain measurements in utero. If these prenatal measurements correlate with subsequent neurodevelopmental outcomes, they may serve as early biomarkers of alcohol exposure as well as early detectors of alcohol-related deficits.

In an effort to increase the identification of children affected by prenatal exposure history, researchers have focused on defining the neurobehavioral patterns associated with FASDs. A variety of screening checklists have been created to facilitate diagnosing FASDs, though with only moderate success (Burd, Klug, Li, Kerbeshian, & Martsolf, 2010; Fitzpatrick et al., 2013). Parent report measures have also been used to help differentiate alcohol-affected individuals from other clinical groups. For example, the Neurobehavioral Screening Test (NST) consists of ten items from a commonly used behavioral scale (the Child Behavior Checklist) (Nash et al., 2006). The NST was tested in a small group of alcohol-exposed children, children with attention-deficit/hyperactivity disorder (ADHD), and controls, with

86 % sensitivity and 82 % specificity for detecting alcohol-exposed children. Certain items from the NST were also able to differentiate children with FASDs from children with oppositional defiant disorder (ODD) and conduct disorder (CD) (Nash, Koren, & Rovet, 2011).

In order to move beyond subjective checklists and parent reporting measures, researchers have attempted to define a sensitive and specific neurobehavioral profile of alcohol-exposed children using objective neuropsychological measures (Jacobson, 1998; Kodituwakku et al., 2006; Mattson et al., 2013; Mattson & Riley, 2011). While classification accuracies have reached adequate levels when comparing alcohol-exposed children to typically developing controls, the classification rates are lower when comparing exposed children to non-exposed children with other diagnoses, such as ADHD (Mattson et al., 2013). Currently, in cases where alcohol exposure is suspected but dysmorphology is not present, the neurobehavioral effects may become the primary tool for identification, acting as a potential diagnostic phenotype.

Individuals with dysmorphology may be identified regardless of the neurobehavioral profile. Therefore, it is important to create a profile that is able to accurately categorize non-dysmorphic children affected by prenatal alcohol exposure. This has been codified in the DSM-5 and is the basis for ND-PAE. A large multi-site study using a standardized neuropsychological battery compared controls, non-exposed children with ADHD, and children who had heavy exposure to alcohol but were not dysmorphic (Mattson et al., 2013). The classification rates were modest when comparing the clinical groups. However, these studies have considerable clinical relevance, as the differential diagnosis between non-dysmorphic alcohol-exposed children and other clinical groups are common within clinical settings.

The combination of a dysmorphology examination and a neurobehavioral assessment may facilitate classification of children where exposure history is unknown. The classification rates for the current brief screeners and the neurobehavioral profile indicate that a more accurate screening tool is needed to help with identification and access to services (Koren et al., 2014; LaFrance et al., 2014). A tiered system of screening tools (dysmorphology, parent report measures, and direct child measures) can assist in identifying children at high risk (Goh et al., 2015). Children who are screened as positive could be referred for a slightly longer testing battery, similar to the FAS referral process (see Fig. 2.2). This type of system would balance the need for feasibility, sensitivity, and specificity. The collaboration of primary care providers, screening tools, and the creation of an effective neurobehavioral profile is imperative, as all are critical steps for getting a child or adult affected by alcohol exposure connected to a system of services.

Prevalence

Although prevalence estimates vary dramatically depending on the sample and diagnostic schema utilized, there is a consensus that heavy prenatal alcohol exposure is a major public health concern and large economic burden (Popova et al., 2013; Stade et al., 2009). Recent estimates using active case ascertainment among first grade children in an American middle class community found the prevalence of FAS was between 6 and 9 children per 1000 (May et al., 2014). The prevalence of FASDs (including FAS) was estimated between 24 and 48 children per 1000. Estimates in other countries and in specific ethnic populations are substantially higher (May et al., 2007a, 2007b, 2009). Further, prevalence rates are extremely high within the foster care system (Burd, Cohen, Shah, & Norris, 2011; Chasnoff, Wells, & King, 2015). Approximately 70 % of children diagnosed with FASDs are currently in or have previously been involved in the foster care system (Burd et al., 2011). As many as 80 % of children within foster or adoptive care who are affected by prenatal alcohol exposure are misdiagnosed or missed completely (Chasnoff et al., 2015).

Impact on the Developing Child

Due to the diffuse teratogenicity of alcohol on the brain, the impact of alcohol exposure on the developing child can occur across physical, cognitive, behavioral, and psychosocial domains (Mattson, Crocker, & Nguyen, 2011). The most severe outcomes of alcohol use during pregnancy are those that result in fetal or newborn death, including miscarriage, stillbirth, and sudden infant death syndrome (Alm et al., 1999; Iyasu et al., 2002). In the surviving child, the possible effects are highly variable, ranging from facial dysmorphology or intellectual disability, to mild behavioral or cognitive deficits. The effects of prenatal alcohol exposure may vary based on timing and amount of exposure in addition to other confounding factors such as individual genetic vulnerability. Based on these facts, the National Institute of Alcohol Abuse and Alcoholism (NIAAA) and the Surgeon General recommend complete abstinence from alcohol during pregnancy (NIAAA, 2013; US Surgeon General, 2005).

Intellectual Functioning

Prenatal exposure to alcohol leads to global cognitive impairment (Mattson et al., 2011; Mattson & Riley, 1998). The heterogeneity of clinical presentation is clear in the range of intelligence scores seen in children on the fetal alcohol spectrum disorder continuum. Full scale intelligence scores are standardized on a scale with a mean of 100 and standard deviation of 15. Scores for children with prenatal alcohol exposure vary widely—from below 50 to over 110, spanning the range from intellectually deficient to above average. Children with FAS have an average IQ of approximately 70, two standard deviations below the mean. However, intellectual deficits can be present with and without dysmorphology (Mattson, Riley, Gramling, Delis, & Jones, 1998) and are apparent across both verbal and nonverbal domains (Mattson & Riley, 1998). The median IQ of over 400 individuals with FASDs (ranging from 6 to 51 years old) was 86 (Streissguth et al., 2004). This finding has been replicated in 8–16 year olds in a recent multisite study (Glass et al., 2013), suggesting the average individual with heavy prenatal alcohol exposure has an intelligence score approximately 1 standard deviation lower than the average non-exposed individual. This suggests that in general, having FAS is related to more severe cognitive deficits overall, however there is a great deal of variability in functioning across the fetal alcohol spectrum.

Importantly, most children with FASDs will not meet the criteria for intellectual disability despite having significant neurobehavioral deficits. Studies found that 24 % of children with FAS and 7–16 % of children with fetal alcohol effects[1] met the basic criteria of having an IQ of below 70 (Streissguth et al., 2004; Streissguth, Barr, Kogan, & Bookstein, 1996). A prospective longitudinal study found that low intellectual functioning coupled with low adaptive functioning leads to a much higher rate of secondary disabilities and adverse life outcomes for people with FASDs (Streissguth, 2007). This may be especially true for individuals who have diminished intellectual capacity but do not meet the diagnosis for intellectual disability and therefore may not qualify for services or interventions.

Even relatively low maternal consumption of alcohol during pregnancy can lead to reductions in global intelligence—consumption of two drinks per day on average was related to a seven point decrement in IQ after accounting for other covariates (Streissguth, Barr, & Sampson, 1990). Mothers with this rate of alcohol consumption during pregnancy are over three times more likely to have a child with subnormal (<85) IQ scores (Streissguth et al., 1990). However, not all studies have found that light alcohol exposure leads to impaired global intellectual functioning (Kelly et al., 2013; Skogerbo et al., 2013). Yet, these results should be reviewed with caution as the methodologies used have been questioned (Powell, 2012) and the results are inconsistent with the majority of the literature, which emphasizes that low-moderate prenatal alcohol exposure should not be considered safe (Jacobson & Jacobson, 2014; O'Leary, Taylor, Zubrick, Kurinczuk, & Bower, 2013).

There are discrepancies on both ends of the spectrum in terms of the relationship between amount of alcohol exposure and outcomes. A recent meta-analysis found a significant, albeit small, association between mild-moderate exposure and behavior and cognition (Flak et al., 2014). On the other hand, children who have histories of heavy prenatal alcohol exposure, even those with facial dysmorphology, may have average IQ scores despite struggling in other domains. This heterogeneity supports the importance of a comprehensive assessment of functioning.

---

[1] Fetal alcohol effects is an outdated term that refers to individuals with prenatal alcohol exposure who have some, but not sufficient features to warrant a diagnosis of FAS.

Academic Functioning

The combination of cognitive and behavioral effects of prenatal alcohol exposure often leads to poor performance in academic achievement (Burd, Cotsonas-Hassler, Martsolf, & Kerbeshian, 2003; Burd, Klug, Martsolf, & Kerbeshian, 2003; Church & Kaltenbach, 1997; Streissguth et al., 1990, 2004). As many as 60 % of clinically referred adolescents over the age of 12 were found to have disrupted school experiences (e.g., suspended, expelled, dropping out from school), and 65 % received some remedial help with reading and math (Streissguth et al., 1996). Impairment in school functioning persists throughout development and occurs in all three major academic domains (math, reading, and writing) to varying degrees (Alati et al., 2013; Goldschmidt, Richardson, Stoffer, Geva, & Day, 1996; Howell, Lynch, Platzman, Smith, & Coles, 2006).

The precise association between amount of alcohol exposure, timing of alcohol exposure, and specific effects on academic functioning has not been fully elucidated. A longitudinal prospective study found a linear dose-response relationship between prenatal alcohol exposure and math (Goldschmidt et al., 1996). This finding remained significant even when controlling for IQ. Interestingly, the relation between alcohol dose, timing of alcohol exposure, and verbal academic domains (reading and spelling) was modeled more accurately using a threshold model of one drink/day during the second trimester.

For children with prenatal exposure to alcohol, deficits in academic achievement exceed what would be expected by intellectual functioning (Kerns, Don, Mateer, & Streissguth, 1997). This exacerbation could be due to the combination of behavioral and cognitive impairments. There are complex interactions between cognitive ability, behavioral functioning, socio-emotional functioning, attention deficits, concomitant psychopathology, environmental supports, school environment, and access to services, all of which can influence academic outcomes (Kable, Taddeo, Strickland, & Coles, 2015).

Mathematics has been the most extensively studied academic area within the realm of prenatal alcohol exposure, as it is thought to be particularly vulnerable to the teratogenic effects of alcohol exposure (Goldschmidt et al., 1996; Howell et al., 2006; Jacobson, Dodge, Burden, Klorman, & Jacobson, 2011; Streissguth et al., 1994a; Streissguth, Barr, Sampson, & Bookstein, 1994b). Children with prenatal exposure to alcohol demonstrate impairments on higher order mathematical reasoning as well as lower order functions such as basic numerical processing, proximity judgment, and cognitive estimation (Coles, Kable, & Taddeo, 2009; Jacobson et al., 2011; Kopera-Frye, Dehaene, & Streissguth, 1996; Meintjes et al., 2010). For example, a longitudinal study compared children with prenatal alcohol exposure (with and without dysmorphology) to other populations that are also at risk for academic and school functioning issues, such as adolescents with low socioeconomic status and students in special education placements (Howell et al., 2006). This study found that children with alcohol exposure and dysmorphology demonstrated lower IQ than all other groups. The non-exposed special education group performed worse on basic reading and spelling, however alcohol-exposed children with dysmorphology performed lowest on mathematics. It appears this effect was the result of difficulties with mathematical reasoning, as there was no difference between groups on a simpler numerical operations task. This supports the suggestion that alcohol-exposed children have greater difficultly on tasks with higher cognitive demands (Kodituwakku et al., 2006).

Recent investigations have begun to identify the underlying cognitive mechanisms of mathematical functioning and the neural correlates of mathematical deficits. One study found that immediate memory and attention contribute to mathematical functioning (Rasmussen & Bisanz, 2009), while another study found that spatial processing had a significant effect on mathematics achievement (Crocker, Riley, & Mattson, 2015). Weak visual-spatial skills have also been related to poor performance on math tests (Kable, Coles, & Taddeo, 2007). In addition to deficits in underlying cognitive mechanisms, structural and functional abnormalities in the brain have been associated with impaired mathematics achievement in alcohol-exposed children (Lebel, Rasmussen, Wyper, Andrew, & Beaulieu, 2010; Santhanam, Li, Hu, Lynch, & Coles, 2009).

While math remains the most studied academic domain in children who have histories of prenatal alcohol exposure, these children are also at risk for impairment in other clinically significant domains. Unlike math, reading abilities have not been the focus of much research, possibly because alcohol-exposed children are not as severely impaired in this domain. As reading is incredibly important for daily functioning, even a lesser impairment may still result in greater functional deficits. Though less work has been done in this area, studies consistently report that children with prenatal alcohol exposure demonstrate deficits in reading and spelling (Adnams et al., 2007; Glass, Graham, Akshoomoff, & Mattson, 2015; Howell et al., 2006; Kodituwakku, 2007; O'Leary et al., 2013; Streissguth, Barr, Carmichael Olson, et al., 1994a). School-age children with FASDs score approximately 1.0–1.5 standard deviations below the mean of typically developing children on basic reading and spelling tasks (Howell et al., 2006). Alcohol-exposed children also demonstrate impairments in the underlying components of literacy skills, including phonological processing and rapid automatized naming (Adnams et al., 2007; Glass et al., 2015; Streissguth, Barr, Carmichael Olson, et al., 1994a). A recent study found that in addition to the expected contributions of phonological processing for spelling, working memory may also be an important consideration in developing interventions for this population (Glass et al., 2015).

Additionally, legible penmanship is a necessary component of academic success, both within the classroom and for standardized testing required in schools. Children with histories of heavy prenatal alcohol exposure have a variety of impairments that might lead to poor handwriting, including motor and visuospatial deficits (Mattson et al., 2011). While there have been anecdotal reports of poor handwriting, only recently has it been addressed in a more systematic manner. In one study, mean handwriting scores for children with FASDs were below average compared to the norms provided by the measure (Duval-White, Jirikowic, Rios, Deitz, & Olson, 2013). However, this study was conducted using a fairly small number of children and no control group.

Neuropsychological Functioning

For children with histories of prenatal alcohol exposure, difficulties with academics may be in part the result of deficits in numerous neuropsychological domains. One of the most prominent areas affected by prenatal alcohol exposure is in the domain of executive functioning. Executive functioning is highly clinically relevant, as it predicts adaptive behavior, social behavior, and theory of mind (Rasmussen, Wyper, & Talwar, 2009; Schonfeld, Paley, Frankel, & O'Connor, 2006; Ware et al., 2012). Children with FASDs struggle with higher order processes in planning, attention, organization, and cognitive flexibility (Green et al., 2009; Rasmussen, Soleimani, & Pei, 2011; Vaurio, Riley, & Mattson, 2008). Alcohol-exposed children demonstrate significant deficits in inhibitory control (Nguyen et al., 2014), which may be related to aberrant neural processes (Fryer et al., 2007b). In addition, alcohol-exposed children often demonstrate deficits in attention, a finding which has been confirmed by both parent reporting and objective measures (Glass et al., 2014). Impaired executive functioning may be substantively related to the high frequency of ADHD in this population (Fryer, McGee, Matt, & Mattson, 2007a). There are some quantitative differences between alcohol-exposed children with and without ADHD, however these distinctions are more apparent in the behavioral domain than in the cognitive domain (Glass et al., 2013; Ware et al., 2014). Deficits have also been reported in working memory, the ability to maintain and manipulate information, which can have a negative impact on both academic and social success (Burden, Jacobson, Sokol, & Jacobson, 2005; Rasmussen et al., 2011; Schonfeld et al., 2006). Poor processing speed and sluggish cognitive tempo (Graham et al., 2013) may present in the classroom as difficulty with interpreting and synthesizing information, inconsistent production of work, difficulty following directions, struggling with classroom routines, and problems keeping up with the class.

In addition to these executive function and processing speed deficits, alcohol-exposed children also demonstrate a delay in verbal skills, both in terms of language and memory. They have delayed language acquisition (Church & Kaltenbach, 1997; O'Leary, Zubrick, Taylor, Dixon, & Bower, 2009) and poor verbal fluency (Schonfeld, Mattson, Lang, Delis, & Riley, 2001). As they get older, these children often demonstrate deficits in both receptive and expressive language (McGee, Bjorkquist, Riley, & Mattson, 2009b). Research on verbal memory in FASDs has found that alcohol-exposed children struggle with encoding information more than retaining information (Kaemingk, Mulvaney, & Halverson, 2003; Mattson, Riley, Delis, Stern, & Jones, 1996; Mattson & Roebuck, 2002), which is different from the pattern seen in children with ADHD (Crocker, Vaurio, Riley, & Mattson, 2011). Alcohol-exposed children, despite poorer learning, demonstrate equivalent relative retention as non-exposed controls, suggesting that once the information is encoded, it can be retained. These deficits persist throughout adolescence; one study found that at the age of 14, initial deficits in encoding and acquisition continue to be responsible for deficits in both immediate and delayed conditions (Willford, Richardson, Leech, & Day, 2004).

Although deficits in verbal learning and memory are well researched and consistently reported, studies on nonverbal learning and memory have yielded less straightforward results (Mattson et al., 1996; Mattson, Autti-Rämö, May, Konovalova, & the CIFASD, 2006; Streissguth et al., 1990; Willoughby, Sheard, Nash, & Rovet, 2008). Children with FASDs have problems in basic visuospatial skills (Mattson & Calarco, 2002; Schonfeld et al., 2001), which can contribute to deficits in more complex tasks required for academic performance (Crocker et al., 2015). Children with heavy prenatal alcohol exposure demonstrate deficits in visual learning and fluency, although these deficits appear to be of the same severity or magnitude as the verbal deficits in these areas (Kaemingk et al., 2003; Schonfeld et al., 2001). There are some differential patterns for visual and verbal information. Once one accounts for initial verbal learning, there are no longer differences in delayed recall of verbal material. For visual information, children with heavy prenatal alcohol exposure recalled less information after a delay even after accounting for initial learning (Mattson & Roebuck, 2002), although these differences are not found universally (Kaemingk et al., 2003).

Emotional and Behavioral Functioning

In many cases, the emotional or behavioral problems associated with prenatal alcohol exposure are the presenting problem that leads a family to seek services. Rates of concomitant psychopathology are high in FASDs, particularly for externalizing disorders such as ADHD (Fryer, McGee, et al., 2007a; Paley, O'Connor, Kogan, & Findlay, 2005; Walthall, O'Connor, & Paley, 2008; Ware et al., 2013). These emotional and behavioral issues may affect academic functioning and psychosocial abilities beyond the effects of lower cognition. High rates of externalizing problems are consistently reported in alcohol-exposed children (Paley et al., 2005; Sood et al., 2001). As children become older, these behaviors can become the basis for psychiatric diagnoses of oppositional defiant disorder, conduct disorder, and delinquent behavior (Fryer, McGee, et al., 2007a; O'Connor & Paley, 2009; Roebuck, Mattson, & Riley, 1999; Schonfeld, Mattson, & Riley, 2005). Alcohol-exposed children also demonstrate higher rates of internalizing behaviors, which in turn can result in other psychiatric diagnoses such as depression and anxiety (Hellemans, Sliwowska, Verma, & Weinberg, 2010; Mattson & Riley, 2000; O'Connor & Paley, 2006). The severity of anxiety, depression, and withdrawal lead to increased rates of self-harm and suicide attempts (Baldwin, 2007). While there are some shared characteristics in social and communication domains with autism spectrum disorders, children with FASDs do not demonstrate the classic repetitive or restrictive behaviors (Stevens, Nash, Koren, & Rovet, 2013).

Other aspects of functioning can also impact a child's academic and social behaviors. For example, children with histories of alcohol exposure also demonstrate impaired sleep habits (Chen, Olson, Picciano, Starr, & Owens, 2012; Jan et al., 2010). Findings indicate that alcohol-exposed children have significantly more sleep disturbances, shortened sleep duration, and an increased rate of night awakenings (Wengel, Hanlon-Dearman, & Fjeldsted, 2011). Sleep is a critical contributor to school performance, with poor sleep quality and sleepiness being related to learning, memory, and academic achievement in a meta-analysis of typically developing children (Dewald, Meijer, Oort, Kerkhof, & Bogels, 2010).

Psychosocial Outcomes

There is strong evidence of impaired social skills in children with prenatal alcohol exposure, which can result in reduced social competence, clinginess, not getting along with others, being teased or bullied, poor social judgment, and issues responding to social cues (Freunscht & Feldmann, 2010; Kully-Martens, Denys, Treit, Tamana, & Rasmussen, 2012; McGee, Bjorkquist, Price, Mattson, & Riley, 2009a; Way & Rojahn, 2012). These social deficits fail to improve with age; as social demands increase, children with FASDs fall even further behind (Crocker, Vaurio, Riley, & Mattson, 2009). Although verbal abilities are sometimes thought to be a relative strength, impairments in these areas can cause difficulties in social communication and conversational exchange (O'Connor et al. 2006, 2012). Alcohol-exposed children have difficulty providing appropriate information in conversations (Coggins, Timler, & Olswang, 2007) and processing social information (McGee, Bjorkquist, Price, et al., 2009a). Further, children with prenatal alcohol exposure struggle to balance linguistic and social-cognitive task demands during conversations (Coggins, Olswang, Carmichael Olson, & Timler, 2003). For example, these children often use ambiguous references and do not appropriately distinguish concepts in their stories (Thorne, Coggins, Carmichael Olson, & Astley, 2007). Inadequate theory of mind is also apparent as alcohol-exposed children fail to consider the perspective of the listener during social interactions (Coggins et al., 2007).

There are many factors that contribute to poor social functioning. Many of these children must contend with the effects of both prenatal alcohol exposure and living in adverse environments (Coggins et al., 2007). The combination of these factors can exacerbate social deficits. In turn, these impairments may affect school performance and academic achievement as well as contribute to the high rates of psychopathology in this population.

As alcohol-exposed children enter their adolescent and teenage years, they are forced to navigate the journey towards independence with additional factors that make the transition even more difficult. Alcohol-exposed adolescents, whether or not they qualify for a diagnosis of intellectual disability, are significantly impaired in their abilities to solve social problems in everyday life (McGee, Fryer, Bjorkquist, Mattson, & Riley, 2008). Even without physical dysmorphology, alcohol-exposed youth demonstrate significant deficits in psychosocial functioning (Roebuck et al., 1999). When matched on IQ, children with FAS still demonstrate social deficits. Therefore, social deficits are beyond what can be expected in low IQ, and findings suggest that these skills may be arrested rather than simply delayed (Thomas, Kelly, Mattson, & Riley 1998).

Impact on Other Areas of Functioning

In addition to the cognitive and behavioral deficits presented above, motor functioning and sensory perception are sensitive to the effects of alcohol. A recent meta-analysis found a significant association between moderate to heavy prenatal alcohol exposure and general motor deficits, particularly in balance and coordination (Lucas et al., 2014). Balance issues in this population are attributed to central core problems and longer latency responses and not entirely the result of vestibular disturbances (Roebuck, Simmons, Richardson, Mattson, & Riley, 1998). A study using a parent reporting measure for children ages 3–6 found that the majority of children with FAS demonstrated clinically relevant delays in general motor development (Kalberg et al., 2006). Fine motor skills were significantly more delayed than gross motor abilities. In a large study, the majority of individuals with FAS or other FASDs demonstrated deficits in motor function (Connor et al., 2006). Children with FASDs demonstrate more variability in performance and more frequently score low average or below on sensory motor measures, particularly in tasks that require visual-motor speed and precision (Jirikowic, Olson, & Kartin, 2008). Unfortunately, these are skills that are required frequently in school settings. These researchers also found that IQ scores may serve as a mediating factor for motor performance or a "surrogate" for neurocognitive deficits. Further, structural and functional differences in neural regions such as the cerebellum (Bookstein, Streissguth, Connor, & Sampson, 2006) and corpus callosum (Wozniak et al., 2009) may contribute to poor motor skills in individuals with FASDs.

Sensory perception deficits are seen at very young ages, with reduced visual acuity noted as early as 6.5 months after birth in a South African cohort even after considering gestational age, birth size, or other neurocognitive deficits (Carter et al., 2005). A diagnosis of FAS is also associated with various measures of hearing, including a developmental delay in auditory maturation, sensorineural hearing loss, and repeated otitis media resulting in conductive hearing loss and central hearing loss (Church, Eldis, Blakley, & Bawle, 1997; Church & Kaltenbach, 1997). One study found very high rates of hearing related issues in children with FAS (Church et al., 1997), however another study looking at children with FASDs found the rates of hearing loss to be no greater than expected (Cohen-Kerem, Bar-Oz, Nulman, Papaioannou, & Koren, 2007). As children with FASDs have visual and auditory sensoriperceptual deficits, which can directly contribute to socio-emotional and school functioning (Jirikowic et al., 2008), they should be screened for early evaluation, detection, and intervention.

Specific Diagnostic Outcomes

In the federal Individuals with Disabilities Education Act (IDEA) of 2007, FAS is listed as a presumptive eligibility diagnosis allowing individuals to obtain services. Unfortunately, the children who are affected by prenatal alcohol exposure but do not meet the criteria for FAS or an intellectual disability (or other eligible diagnosis) may not qualify for these services. For example, children with an alcohol-related neurodevelopmental disorder (the prototypical example of Other Specified Neurodevelopmental Disorder) or the proposed ND-PAE diagnosis may not meet the strict eligibility criteria even though they have similar neurobehavioral impairments as children with FAS (Mattson et al., 1998). The ability to retrospectively and definitively identify alcohol-affected children without the characteristic facial features of FAS remains elusive. Special education and access to services vary by county and state, and therefore the present discussion focuses on nationwide services.

Currently, the most common and feasible method of receiving services for an alcohol-related neurodevelopmental disorder is to qualify for services under a different diagnosis, such as intellectual disability, Other Specified Neurodevelopmental Disorder, or ADHD, or to qualify under a specific catch all category based on functioning and symptomology such as the Other Health Impairment (OHI) category of IDEA. Legal precedents providing services for individuals with intellectual disability, or those requiring similar services, have facilitated access to services in some locations. These services may include a unique type of parenting class, a structure for collaboration between parents, teachers, and counselors, and potentially creating an individualized education plan (IEP). While not all children with FASDs will qualify for an IEP, they may meet criteria under the Section 504 of the Federal Rehabilitation Act of 1973 (*Section 504 of the Federal Rehabilitation Act of 1973*, 29 U.S.C.794, 1973). This can facilitate implementation of individualized classroom accommodations, yet falls short of creating an individualized plan for the student (Senturias, 2014).

While ND-PAE has been added to the DSM-5, it is currently listed as a "condition for further review," making it difficult for children and adolescents to access services as they may not be billable to insurance. In the interim, the DSM includes "Neurodevelopmental Disorder Associated with Prenatal Alcohol Exposure" as an example of Other Specified Neurodevelopmental Disorder (315.8, page 86). Note that the usage of "neurodevelopmental disorder" in the body of the DSM versus "neurobehavioral disorder" in the appendix may cause confusion. Further, the allowed usage of code 315.8 to indicate an alcohol-related disorder can be done without consideration of the criteria of ND-PAE. Individuals with FASDs can require the services of numerous providers, including primary care, specialist centers, occupational therapy, physical therapy, psychosocial skills training, and educational specialists (Rogers-Adkinson & Stuart, 2007). There are several FASD service centers (McFarlane & Rajani, 2007) that provide models for the continued development of resources. However, there is no easy or practical way to standardize the service needs for children with FASDs because each child will have unique patterns of deficits and may require a more individualized approach. Potentially, a modular system of interventions targeted at areas of high risk of deficits may be most effective. Semi-structured interviews revealed that there were no standardized special education classes that were appropriate for all alcohol-affected children (Autti-Rämö, 2000). Instead, each child needed individual supports based on their own patterns of functioning.

Prognosis and Moderating Factors

Until recently, it has not been possible to thoroughly research the developmental trajectory of alcohol exposure. The first cohort of children with FAS were diagnosed in the early 1970s (Jones & Smith, 1973) and are now reaching middle adulthood. There are several large prospective longitudinal studies that are attempting to characterize the effects of alcohol exposure over time, however more research is necessary to fully understand the developmental trajectory (Covington, Nordstrom-Klee, Ager, Sokol, & Delaney-Black, 2002; Elliott, Payne, Morris, Haan, & Bower, 2007; Kuehn et al., 2012; O'Callaghan, O'Callaghan, Najman, Williams, & Bor, 2007; Robinson et al., 2010; Streissguth, 1994c). A recent study of 22-year-olds found that prenatal alcohol exposure was associated with elevated rates of internalizing and externalizing behaviors in adulthood (Day, Helsel, Sonon, & Goldschmidt, 2013).

Adults with FASDs may continue to need support in many areas of their lives due to poor adaptive functioning, even though they may present clinically as cognitively intact. Adults are found to benefit from case management, however many individuals with FAS or another FASD may need continued support in housing, vocational rehabilitation, transportation assistance, and activities of daily living. Adults with prenatal exposure to alcohol have high rates of involvement in the legal system, high rates of substance abuse, and negative long-term outcomes. In one study, over 40 % of adults with FASDs had been incarcerated at some point, 20 % been confined for substance abuse treatment, and 30 % been confined to a mental institution (Streissguth et al., 1996). In spite of these reports, very little is known about the long-term effects of prenatal alcohol exposure as very little research has been conducted to empirically assess adult functioning in this population.

Many factors contribute to poor outcomes in alcohol-exposed children and therefore their deficits may be considered multi-determined (Streissguth et al., 2004). Risk factors commonly associated with alcohol exposure include: poor prenatal care, prenatal exposure to other teratogens (e.g., environmental, other drug exposures), parental psychopathology, neglect, abuse, frequent interactions with the foster care system, and changes in custody (Fagerlund, Autti-Rämö, Hoyme, Mattson, & Korkman, 2011). A longer time spent in residential care is the strongest risk factor associated with behavioral problems for children with prenatal alcohol exposure (Fagerlund et al., 2011). Alcohol-exposed children were also at greater risk of behavioral problems if they were not visibly alcohol affected and thus may not have received the services they needed during critical developmental periods (Fagerlund et al., 2011). Unfortunately, there are multiple systems-level barriers in place that hinder the ability for children and adults with FASDs to receive both diagnostic clarification and adequate services (Petrenko, Tahir, Mahoney, & Chin, 2014a). Children who receive an early diagnosis and are raised in a stable environment are 2–4 times more likely to avoid adverse life outcomes (e.g., disrupted school experiences, trouble with the law, inappropriate sexual behavior, or alcohol and drug problems) (Streissguth et al., 2004). There are also certain protective factors that can help attenuate the secondary disabilities often associated with FASDs, including early identification and diagnostic clarification, early access to effective services, a stable and nurturing home, and not having a history of maltreatment or abuse (Petrenko et al., 2014a; Streissguth et al., 1996, 2004).

Considerations for Prevention/Intervention/School Accommodations and School Reintegration

Prevention

Early identification is a crucial step to improve outcomes for affected individuals and can facilitate the development and implementation of effective treatment (Carmichael et al., 2009). However, identification at any age remains difficult due the heterogeneity in clinical presentation, lack of objective and accurate biomarkers, lack of public awareness, and continued debate regarding the best classification system (Elliot, Payne, Haan, & Bower, 2006; Payne et al., 2011a, 2011b). A survey conducted by the American Academy of Pediatrics and the Centers for Disease Control and Prevention found that "pediatricians are knowledgeable about fetal alcohol syndrome but do not feel adequately trained to integrate the management of this diagnosis or prevention efforts into everyday practice" (Gahagan et al., 2006). Although government services such as the NIAAA warn that there is no safe amount to drink during pregnancy, the effects of light alcohol exposure remain strongly contested in public media (Drabble et al., 2014; NIAAA, 2013). As a result, pregnant women may be receiving mixed messages, which can also hinder prevention efforts.

It is common for women to underreport the amount of alcohol consumed during pregnancy, especially when the amounts are significant (Stockwell et al., 2004). This may be particularly problematic in situations where a woman may feel stigmatized. Women who drink during pregnancy may also not seek proper prenatal care. Even if they attend all prenatal appointments, questions regarding alcohol exposure may not be asked (Morleo et al., 2011). Many practitioners do not feel sufficiently trained in the diagnosis of fetal alcohol spectrum disorders, nor comfortable in talking about alcohol use with pregnant patients (Elliot et al., 2006; Payne et al., 2011b). Thus, it is rarely possible to confirm the accuracy, frequency, and timing of prenatal alcohol exposure.

While it remains difficult to categorize or classify individuals affected by alcohol exposure, there is a consensus regarding the known detrimental effects of alcohol on the developing fetus. Since 1973 when FAS was first identified, the negative effects of heavy prenatal alcohol exposure have been widely studied and accepted by the scientific community, with continued refinement of the neurobehavioral profile (Mattson et al., 2013). This information has resulted in widespread public health campaigns supporting abstinence from alcohol while pregnant. Unfortunately, these methods have not resulted in a significant decrease of drinking during pregnancy over the last decade. In a recent report, between 7.6 and 14.3 % of women who are aware that they are pregnant in the USA report alcohol consumption during their pregnancy, and 1.4 % report binge drinking (Grant et al., 2004; Thomas, Gonneau, Poole, & Cook, 2014).

However, this is likely an underreport of alcohol consumption during pregnancy more generally, as many women may not realize they are pregnant for 5–7 weeks and may continue to drink at high levels prior to pregnancy recognition. Specific maternal risk factors are associated with the development of fetal alcohol spectrum disorders. These include a maternal age of greater than 30 years, specific ethnic and racial backgrounds, lower socioeconomic status, having a previously affected child, undernutrition, and specific genetic backgrounds (Jones, 2011). A greater understanding of risk factors can facilitate more successful and well-informed interventions.

Currently, there are several behavioral interventions aimed at preventing alcohol-exposed pregnancies (Floyd et al., 2007; Hanson & Jensen, 2015; Mengel, Searight, & Cook, 2006). Some programs focus primarily on psychoeducation, as medical professionals at all levels of care have expressed a weakness in knowledge of this area (Payne et al., 2011a, 2011b). Other programs target women through community outreach, counseling sessions, social support, and screening (Floyd et al., 2007; Hanson & Jensen, 2015; Mengel et al., 2006).

As almost half of all pregnancies (49 %) are unplanned, many intervention programs attempt to target women prior to the conception (Finer & Henshaw, 2006). While the rates of unintended pregnancies have declined for college graduates and women of higher socioeconomic status, the rates of unintended pregnancies for unmarried and low-income women between the age of 18–24 remain above the national average (Finer & Henshaw, 2006). CHOICES, an integrated behavioral intervention funded by the CDC, has targeted these high-risk women through randomized controlled trials in a variety of clinical settings including primary care, university hospitals, jails, substance abuse treatment settings, and community settings (Floyd, Ebrahim, Boyle, & Gould, 1999; Hanson & Jensen, 2015; Velasquez, von Sternberg, & Parrish, 2013). Motivational interviewing, personalized feedback, contraceptive counseling, and reducing risky behaviors are the main tenets of the program, which has been demonstrated to be feasible and efficacious.

Another issue complicating the identification of FASDs is the lack of a standardized assessment protocol. One limiting factor of diagnostic clarification in the community setting is access to a trained dysmorphologist or a physician with dysmorphology training needed to make a diagnosis of FAS. Many physicians, including pediatricians, in the USA and abroad lack specific training on identifying FASDs. However, one study found that after a relatively short training session (2 days) many pediatricians were able to accurately diagnose FAS based on physical features—pediatricians' diagnoses were confirmed by the dysmorphologists in 83.5 % of the cases (Jones et al., 2006). Educating our front line medical practitioners is critical to increasing the number of children correctly diagnosed with prenatal alcohol exposure.

Intervention

Key areas of need in the realm of FASDs include a lack of appropriate services, lack of access to existing services, and lack of effective prevention strategies (Carmichael et al., 2009; Ryan, Bonnett, & Gass, 2006). Parents and service providers in focus groups request interventions that are consistent with a positive behavior support network. Specifically, these would include central coordination, early diagnosis, support across the life span, and a strengths-based approach (Petrenko, Tahir, Mahoney, & Chin, 2014b). Caregivers express the need for support from professionals and extended family in the context of a structured environment and greater appreciation and understanding of a specific child's needs (Brown, Sigvaldason, & Bednar, 2005; Grant, Ernst, Streissguth, Phipps, & Gendler, 1996).

There have been several reviews of interventions for children and adolescents with fetal alcohol spectrum disorders within the past decade (Burd, 2006; Kodituwakku, 2010; Paley & O'Connor, 2011; Peadon, Rhys-Jones, Bower, & Elliott, 2009). Interventions must consider the cognitive and behavioral impairments that may affect a child's academic achievement, as both may contribute to deficits in overall functioning (Jirikowic, Gelo, & Astley, 2010). For example, the selective vulnerability of mathematical functioning to prenatal alcohol exposure has led to development of promising math interventions (Coles et al., 2009; Kable et al., 2007). The Math Interactive Learning Experience (MILE) program for children with FASDs focuses on core skill deficits as well as issues that may contribute to poor performance. The program includes lessons on meta-cognitive problem solving skills ("plan-do-review") and learning readiness. In this context, learning readiness involves preparing the child's environment and considering behavioral modifications to ensure that learning can be most successful. The MILE program is individualized to the child's pace, and involves more feedback and active interaction regarding error patterns. In initial studies assessing MILE, the intervention group of 3- to 10-year-olds demonstrated significant improvement in mathematical knowledge, both directly after a 6-week intervention, and 6 months after the intervention was completed (Coles et al., 2009; Kable et al., 2007). A 15-week, randomized clinical trial found that those in the program demonstrated significant gains in math that persisted over six months (Kable et al., 2015). The MILE program was also recently successfully disseminated into community settings, which is an important aspect of all interventions (Kable et al., 2015).

A language and literacy intervention conducted in South Africa has also been successful (Adnams et al., 2007). The program produced significant improvement in certain preliteracy and literacy variables. Despite these gains, alcohol-exposed children were still significantly different from controls, demonstrating improvement but not remediation. For the underlying cognitive mechanisms related to language and literacy, rehearsal training and neurocognitive habilitation training demonstrated improvement, specifically in working memory span and executive functioning (Loomes, Rasmussen, Pei, Manji, & Andrew, 2008). However, it is not clear if these findings generalize beyond the task to school settings (Melby-Lervag & Hulme, 2013).

In addition to the cognitive targets, there have also been interventions focused on the socio-emotional and behavioral concerns in children with heavy prenatal alcohol exposure (Kully-Martens et al., 2012; O'Connor et al., 2012). Some of these interventions are administered to the child directly, such as children's friendship training and adaptive behavior programs. Friendship training demonstrated significant improvement in social skills in children with and without alcohol-exposure

(Keil, Paley, Frankel, & O'Connor, 2010; O'Connor et al., 2012; Paley & O'Connor, 2011). Attempts to improve adaptive behavior and safety behavior have also demonstrated success. A virtual reality intervention for fire and street safety resulted in significantly better knowledge of the intervention, and 72 % of the 32 children were able to generalize their knowledge to behavioral settings (Coles, Strickland, Padgett, & Bellmoff, 2007).

Interventions also include parent-child interaction therapy and family systems models. The Families Moving Forward program has successfully reduced child behavior problems and improved parenting efficacy by combining a developmental systems perspective with a family systems approach (Olson, Oti, Gelo, & Beck, 2009). Likewise, a one-on-one parent mentorship model called Step by Step was also effective in helping caregivers reduce their needs and achieve goals (Denys, Rasmussen, & Henneveld, 2011).

School Accommodations and School Reintegration

A review of FASDs in relation to academic achievement found that successful interventions need to balance the use of environmental modifications and the many additional factors at play with alcohol-affected children (Green, 2007). The heterogeneity of academic, behavioral, and cognitive function in children with FASDs makes it extremely difficult to create a one size fits all academic curriculum. For instance, the range of intellectual function in these children is quite broad, and therefore effective interventions must cater to a wide range of abilities. In addition, programs must understand and address the interplay between cognitive, academic, social, emotional, and behavioral challenges. For example, disruptive behavior may be due to behavioral impulsivity or executive dysfunction, both of which are common in FASDs.

Assessment of school-based services for children with FASDs is a burgeoning area of research. In the classroom, a combination of evidence-based interventions may be the most efficacious, as they can target various areas simultaneously. Since 60–95 % of alcohol-exposed children are diagnosed with ADHD (Fryer, McGee, et al., 2007a; Mattson et al., 2011), it may be worthwhile to investigate the feasibility of repurposing existing, empirically supported ADHD interventions for children with FASDs. Unfortunately, the availability of interventions has fallen far below the needs of alcohol-exposed children, and many of these programs are still being studied to assess generalizability, feasibility, and efficacy. Cognitive deficits such as those well documented in the domains of executive function, learning, and memory must be considered in all aspects of educational intervention, including giving instructions and assignments, arranging the environment, planning transitions, and overall interactions and expectations within the classroom. Other considerations must include the behavioral difficulties as well as auditory and visual perception deficits.

The high variability in IQ scores and differential profiles associated with heavy prenatal alcohol exposure requires a true individualized education plan. Unfortunately, many children with FASDs may not be able to receive services because of strict interpretations of cutoffs, as the majority of affected children have IQ scores in the average or borderline range. In spite of a potentially adequate overall general cognitive ability level, many have a variety of behavioral and cognitive deficits that can dramatically affect performance. Children with average intelligence may benefit from assessment to determine whether specific issues with attention, verbal learning and memory, auditory memory and processing, and executive functioning exist and may be contributing to poor performance. In addition, alcohol-exposed children often present with adaptive functioning deficits and behavioral issues that can interact and limit academic success. Behavioral plans may also be a way to provide support for both the behavioral challenges and the cognitive deficits. Behavioral observations in the classroom are also recommended to understand how the children function when faced with higher cognitive demands and in a more distracting environment.

There continues to be a dearth of research to support the development, implementation, evaluation, and dissemination of interventions despite the known detrimental effects of prenatal alcohol exposure. However, there has been an increase in educational and cognitive interventions that have shown preliminary success. Increased structure, both at home and in the classroom, are useful behavioral tools for children who have low executive functioning.

Most studies of caregivers of children with FASDs focus on understanding caregiver and child interactions at home, but there is little research that has examined how caregivers address issues with schools. One study in a western Canadian province systematically assessed how caregivers behave in response to school difficulties (Swart, Hall, McKee, & Ford, 2014). Caregivers of children with FASDs were found to focus on two themes: orchestrating schooling (e.g., available to be in the classroom, building connections with teachers, anticipating difficulties) and keeping up appearances to avoid being viewed as inadequate parents (e.g., reframing behaviors, controlling access to information, trying to fit in with other parents). These are both areas that should be addressed through intervention.

Conclusion

Since the effects of alcohol exposure are extremely heterogeneous, children who fall under the umbrella of fetal alcohol spectrum disorders often go unrecognized. The lack of early identification can lead to reduced access to services for alcohol-affected individuals. Children with histories of prenatal alcohol exposure must be considered in a holistic manner, as they may present with medical, cognitive, behavioral, and adaptive functioning impairments. An educational plan should be developed with the guidance of a team of specialists that are able to help conceptualize all aspects of the individual's functioning. The interplay between behavior and cognition is incredibly important for both academic and social settings, as they can interact to determine success. Diagnostic clarification and the refinement of a neurobehavioral profile for fetal alcohol spectrum disorders are at the forefront of research focus. While the neurobehavioral profile is not fully elucidated, it is abundantly clear that there are many distinct behavioral and cognitive domains that must be considered while developing and implementing interventions for this population.

References

Adnams, C. M., Sorour, P., Kalberg, W. O., Kodituwakku, P., Perold, M. D., Kotze, A., ... May, P. A. (2007). Language and literacy outcomes from a pilot intervention study for children with fetal alcohol spectrum disorders in South Africa. *Alcohol, 41*(6), 403–414. doi:10.1016/j.alcohol.2007.07.005.

Alati, R., Davey Smith, G., Lewis, S. J., Sayal, K., Draper, E. S., Golding, J., ... Gray, R. (2013). Effect of prenatal alcohol exposure on childhood academic outcomes: Contrasting maternal and paternal associations in the ALSPAC study. *PloS One, 8*(10), e74844. doi:10.1371/journal.pone.0074844.

Alm, B., Wennergren, G., Norvenius, G., Skjaerven, R., Oyen, N., Helweg-Larsen, K., ... Irgens, L. M. (1999). Caffeine and alcohol as risk factors for sudden infant death syndrome. Nordic Epidemiological SIDS Study. *Archives of Disease in Childhood, 81*(2), 107–111.

American Academy of Pediatrics Committee on Substance Abuse and Committee on Children with Disabilities. (2000). Fetal alcohol syndrome and alcohol-related neurodevelopmental disorders. *Pediatrics, 106*(2), 358–361.

American Psychiatric Association. (2013). *Diagnostic and statistical manual of mental disorders* (5th ed.). Arlington, VA: American Psychiatric Association.

Astley, S. J. (2004). *Diagnostic guide for fetal alcohol spectrum* disorders: The 4-digit diagnostic code (3rd ed.). Seattle, WA: University of Washington Publication Services. http://depts.washington.edu/fasdpn/pdfs/guide2004.pdf.

Astley, S. J. (2013). Validation of the fetal alcohol spectrum disorder (FASD) 4-digit diagnostic code. *Journal of Population Therapeutics and Clinical Pharmacology, 20*(3), e416–e467.

Astley, S. J. (2014). The value of a FASD diagnosis (2013). *Journal of Population Therapeutics and Clinical Pharmacology, 21*(1), e81–e105.

Autti-Rämö, I. (2000). Twelve-year follow-up of children exposed to alcohol in utero. *Developmental Medicine and Child Neurology, 42*(6), 406–411.

Baldwin, M. R. (2007). Fetal alcohol spectrum disorders and suicidality in a healthcare setting. *International Journal of Circumpolar Health, 66*(Suppl 1), 54–60.

Bertrand, J., Floyd, R. L., Weber, M. K., O'Connor, M., Riley, E., Johnson, K. A., ... FAS/FAE, N. T. F. O. (2004). Fetal alcohol syndrome: Guidelines for referral and diagnosis. Atlanta, GA: Center for Disease Control and Prevention.

Bookstein, F. L., Streissguth, A. P., Connor, P. D., & Sampson, P. D. (2006). Damage to the human cerebellum from prenatal alcohol exposure: The anatomy of a simple biometrical explanation. *The Anatomical Record, 289*(5), 195–209. doi:10.1002/ar.b.20114.

Brown, J. D., Sigvaldason, N., & Bednar, L. M. (2005). Foster parent perceptions of placement needs for children with a fetal alcohol spectrum disorder. *Children and Youth Services Review, 27*(3), 309–327. doi:10.1016/j.childyouth.2004.10.008.

Burd, L. (2006). Interventions in FASD: We must do better. *Child: Care, Health and Development, 33*, 398–400.

Burd, L., Cohen, C., Shah, R., & Norris, J. (2011). A court team model for young children in foster care: The role of prenatal alcohol and fetal alcohol spectrum disorders. *Journal of Psychiatry & Law, 39*(1), 179–191. doi:10.1177/009318531103900107.

Burd, L., Cotsonas-Hassler, T. M., Martsolf, J. T., & Kerbeshian, J. (2003). Recognition and management of fetal alcohol syndrome. *Neurotoxicology and Teratology, 25*(6), 681–688.

Burd, L., Klug, M. G., Li, Q., Kerbeshian, J., & Martsolf, J. T. (2010). Diagnosis of fetal alcohol spectrum disorders: A validity study of the fetal alcohol syndrome checklist. *Alcohol, 44*(7–8), 605–614.

Burd, L., Klug, M. G., Martsolf, J. T., & Kerbeshian, J. (2003). Fetal alcohol syndrome: Neuropsychiatric phenomics. *Neurotoxicology and Teratology, 25*(6), 697–705. doi:10.1016/j.ntt.2003.07.014.

Burden, M. J., Jacobson, S. W., Sokol, R. J., & Jacobson, J. L. (2005). Effects of prenatal alcohol exposure on attention and working memory at 7.5 years of age. *Alcoholism: Clinical and Experimental Research, 29*(3), 443–452.

Carmichael Olson, H., Ohlemiller, M. M., O'Connor, M. J., Brown, C. W., Morris, C. A., & Damus, K. (2009). A call to action: Advancing essential services and research on fetal alcohol spectrum disorders: A report of the National Task Force on Fetal Alcohol Syndrome and Fetal Alcohol Effect (U. S. D. o. H. a. H. Services., Trans.).

Carter, R. C., Jacobson, S. W., Molteno, C. D., Chiodo, L. M., Viljoen, D., & Jacobson, J. L. (2005). Effects of prenatal alcohol exposure on infant visual acuity. *Journal of Pediatrics, 147*(4), 473–479. doi:10.1016/j.jpeds.2005.04.063.

Chasnoff, I. J., Wells, A. M., & King, L. (2015). Misdiagnosis and missed diagnoses in foster and adopted children with prenatal alcohol exposure. *Pediatrics*. doi:10.1542/peds.2014-2171.

Chen, M. L., Olson, H. C., Picciano, J. F., Starr, J. R., & Owens, J. (2012). Sleep problems in children with fetal alcohol spectrum disorders. *Journal of Clinical Sleep Medicine, 8*(4), 421–429. doi:10.5664/jcsm.2038.

Church, M. W., Eldis, F., Blakley, B. W., & Bawle, E. V. (1997). Hearing, language, speech, vestibular, and dentofacial disorders in fetal alcohol syndrome. *Alcoholism: Clinical and Experimental Research, 21*(2), 227–237.

Church, M. W., & Kaltenbach, J. A. (1997). Hearing, speech, language, and vestibular disorders in the fetal alcohol syndrome: A literature review. *Alcoholism: Clinical and Experimental Research, 21*(3), 495–512.

Clarren, S. K., Chudley, A. E., Wong, L., Friesen, J., & Brant, R. (2010). Normal distribution of palpebral fissure lengths in Canadian school age children. *Canadian Journal of Clinical Pharmacology, 17*, e67–e78.

Coggins, T. E., Olswang, L. B., Carmichael Olson, H., & Timler, G. R. (2003). On becoming socially competent communicators: The challenge for children with fetal alcohol exposure. *International Review of Research in Mental Retardation, 27*, 121–150. doi:10.1016/S0074-7750(03)27004-X.

Coggins, T. E., Timler, G. R., & Olswang, L. B. (2007). A state of double jeopardy: Impact of prenatal alcohol exposure and adverse environments on the social communicative abilities of school-age children with fetal alcohol spectrum disorder. *Language, Speech, and Hearing Services in Schools, 38*(2), 117–127. doi:10.1044/0161-1461(2007/012).

Cohen-Kerem, R., Bar-Oz, B., Nulman, I., Papaioannou, V. A., & Koren, G. (2007). Hearing in children with fetal alcohol spectrum disorder (FASD). *Canadian Journal of Clinical Pharmacology, 14*(3), e307–e312.

Coles, C. D., Kable, J. A., & Taddeo, E. (2009). Math performance and behavior problems in children affected by prenatal alcohol exposure: Intervention and follow-up. *Journal of Developmental and Behavioral Pediatrics, 30*(1), 7–15. doi:10.1097/DBP.0b013e3181966780.

Coles, C. D., Strickland, D. C., Padgett, L., & Bellmoff, L. (2007). Games that "work": Using computer games to teach alcohol-affected children about fire and street safety. *Research in Developmental Disabilities, 28*(5), 518–530. doi:10.1016/j.ridd.2006.07.001.

Connor, P. D., Sampson, P. D., Streissguth, A. P., Bookstein, F. L., & Barr, H. M. (2006). Effects of prenatal alcohol exposure on fine motor coordination and balance: A study of two adult samples. *Neuropsychologia, 44*(5), 744–751.

Covington, C. Y., Nordstrom-Klee, B., Ager, J., Sokol, R., & Delaney-Black, V. (2002). Birth to age 7 growth of children prenatally exposed to drugs. A prospective cohort study. *Neurotoxicology and Teratology, 24*(4), 489–496.

Crocker, N., Riley, E. P., & Mattson, S. N. (2015). Visual-spatial abilities relate to mathematics achievement in children with heavy prenatal alcohol exposure. *Neuropsychology, 29*(1), 108–116. doi:10.1037/neu0000094.

Crocker, N., Vaurio, L., Riley, E. P., & Mattson, S. N. (2009). Comparison of adaptive behavior in children with heavy prenatal alcohol exposure or attention-deficit/hyperactivity disorder. *Alcoholism: Clinical and Experimental Research, 33*(11), 2015–2023. doi:10.1111/j.1530-0277.2009.01040.x.

Crocker, N., Vaurio, L., Riley, E. P., & Mattson, S. N. (2011). Comparison of verbal learning and memory in children with heavy prenatal alcohol exposure or attention-deficit/hyperactivity disorder. *Alcoholism: Clinical and Experimental Research, 35*(6), 1114–1121. doi:10.1111/j.1530-0277.2011.01444.x.

Day, N. L., Helsel, A., Sonon, K., & Goldschmidt, L. (2013). The association between prenatal alcohol exposure and behavior at 22 years of age. *Alcoholism: Clinical and Experimental Research, 37*(7), 1171–1178. doi:10.1111/acer.12073.

Denys, K., Rasmussen, C., & Henneveld, D. (2011). The effectiveness of a community-based intervention for parents with FASD. *Community Mental Health Journal, 47*(2), 209–219. doi:10.1007/s10597-009-9273-9.

Dewald, J. F., Meijer, A. M., Oort, F. J., Kerkhof, G. A., & Bogels, S. M. (2010). The influence of sleep quality, sleep duration and sleepiness on school performance in children and adolescents: A meta-analytic review. *Sleep Medicine Reviews, 14*(3), 179–189. doi:10.1016/j.smrv.2009.10.004.

Drabble, L., Thomas, S., O'Connor, L., & Roberts, S. C. (2014). State responses to alcohol use and pregnancy: Findings from the alcohol policy information system (APIS). *Journal of Social Work Practice in the Addictions, 14*(2), 191–206. doi:10.1080/1533256X.2014.900409.

Duval-White, C. J., Jirikowic, T., Rios, D., Deitz, J., & Olson, H. C. (2013). Functional handwriting performance in school-age children with fetal alcohol spectrum disorders. *American Journal of Occupational Therapy, 67*(5), 534–542. doi:10.5014/ajot.2013.008243.

Elliot, E. J., Payne, J., Haan, E., & Bower, C. (2006). Diagnosis of foetal alcohol syndrome and alcohol use in pregnancy: A survey of paediatricians' knowledge, attitudes and practice. *Journal of Paediatrics and Child Health, 42*(11), 698–703.

Elliott, E. J., Payne, J. M., Morris, A., Haan, E., & Bower, C. A. (2007). Fetal alcohol syndrome: A prospective national surveillance study. *Archives of Disease in Childhood, 93*(9), 732–737.

Fagerlund, Å., Autti-Rämö, I., Hoyme, H. E., Mattson, S. N., & Korkman, M. (2011). Risk factors for behavioural problems in foetal alcohol spectrum disorders. *Acta Paediatrica, 100*(11), 1481–1488. doi:10.1111/j.1651-2227.2011.02354.x.

Farag, M. (2014). Diagnostic issues affecting the epidemiology of fetal alcohol spectrum disorders. *Journal of Population Therapeutics and Clinical Pharmacology, 21*(1), e153–e158.

Finer, L. B., & Henshaw, S. K. (2006). Disparities in rates of unintended pregnancy in the United States, 1994 and 2001. *Perspectives on Sexual and Reproductive Health, 38*(2), 90–96. doi:10.1363/psrh.38.090.06.

Fitzpatrick, J. P., Latimer, J., Ferreira, M., Martiniuk, A. L., Peadon, E., Carter, M., … Elliott, E. J. (2013). Development of a reliable questionnaire to assist in the diagnosis of Fetal Alcohol Spectrum Disorders (FASD). *BMC Pediatrics, 13*, 33. doi:10.1186/1471-2431-13-33.

Flak, A. L., Su, S., Bertrand, J., Denny, C. H., Kesmodel, U. S., & Cogswell, M. E. (2014). The association of mild, moderate, and binge prenatal alcohol exposure and child neuropsychological outcomes: A meta-analysis. *Alcoholism: Clinical and Experimental Research, 38*(1), 214–226. doi:10.1111/acer.12214.

Floyd, R. L., Ebrahim, S. H., Boyle, C. A., & Gould, D. W. (1999). Observations from the CDC. Preventing alcohol-exposed pregnancies among women of childbearing age: The necessity of a preconceptional approach. *Journal of Women's Health & Gender-Based Medicine, 8*(6), 733–736. doi:10.1089/152460999319048.

Floyd, R. L., Sobell, M., Velasquez, M. M., Ingersoll, K., Nettleman, M., Sobell, L., … Project, C. E. S. G. (2007). Preventing alcohol-exposed pregnancies: A randomized controlled trial. *American Journal of Preventive Medicine, 32*(1), 1–10. doi:10.1016/j.amepre.2006.08.028.

Freunscht, I., & Feldmann, R. (2010). Young adults with fetal alcohol syndrome (FAS): Social, emotional and occupational development. *Klinische Padiatrie, 223*(1), 33–37. doi:10.1055/s-0030-1261927.

Fryer, S. L., McGee, C. L., Matt, G. E., & Mattson, S. N. (2007). Evaluation of psychopathological conditions in children with heavy prenatal alcohol exposure. *Pediatrics, 119*(3), E733–E741. doi:10.1542/peds.2006-1606.

Fryer, S. L., Tapert, S. F., Mattson, S. N., Paulus, M. P., Spadoni, A. D., & Riley, E. P. (2007). Prenatal alcohol exposure affects frontal-striatal BOLD response during inhibitory control. *Alcoholism: Clinical and Experimental Research, 31*(8), 1415–1424. doi:10.1111/j.1530-0277.2007.00443.x.

Gahagan, S., Sharpe, T. T., Brimacombe, M., Fry-Johnson, Y., Levine, R., Mengel, M., … Brenneman, G. (2006). Pediatricians' knowledge, training, and experience in the care of children with fetal alcohol syndrome. *Pediatrics, 118*(3), e657–e668. doi:10.1542/peds.2005-0516.

Glass, L., Graham, D. M., Akshoomoff, N., & Mattson, S. N. (2015). Cognitive factors contributing to spelling performance in children with prenatal alcohol exposure. *Neuropsychology.* doi:10.1037/neu0000185.

Glass, L., Graham, D. M., Deweese, B. N., Jones, K. L., Riley, E. P., & Mattson, S. N. (2014). Correspondence of parent report and laboratory measures of inattention and hyperactivity in children with heavy prenatal alcohol exposure. *Neurotoxicology and Teratology, 42*, 43–50. doi:10.1016/j.ntt.2014.01.007.

Glass, L., Ware, A. L., Crocker, N., Deweese, B. N., Coles, C. D., Kable, J. A., … Collaborative Initiative on Fetal Alcohol Spectrum, D. (2013). Neuropsychological deficits associated with heavy prenatal alcohol exposure are not exacerbated by ADHD. *Neuropsychology, 27*(6), 713–724. doi:10.1037/a0033994.

Goh, P. K., Doyle, L. R., Glass, L., Jones, K. L., Riley, E. P., Coles, C. D., Hoyme, H. E., Kable, J. A., May, P. A., Kalberg, W. O., Sowell, E. R., Wozniak, J. R., Mattson, S. N., & the CIFASD. (2016). A clinically useful decision tree to identify children affected by prenatal alcohol exposure. *Manuscript under review.*

Goldschmidt, L., Richardson, G. A., Stoffer, D. S., Geva, D., & Day, N. L. (1996). Prenatal alcohol exposure and academic achievement at age six: A nonlinear fit. *Alcoholism: Clinical and Experimental Research, 20*(4), 763–770.

Graham, D. M., Crocker, N., Deweese, B. N., Roesch, S. C., Coles, C. D., Kable, J. A., … the CIFASD. (2013). Prenatal alcohol exposure, attention-deficit/hyperactivity disorder, and sluggish cognitive tempo. *Alcoholism: Clinical and Experimental Research, 37*(Suppl 1), E338–E346. doi:10.1111/j.1530-0277.2012.01886.x.

Grant, T. M., Ernst, C. C., Streissguth, A. P., Phipps, P., & Gendler, B. (1996). When case management isn't enough: A model of paraprofessional advocacy for drug- and alcohol-abusing mothers. *Journal of Case Management, 5*(1), 3–11.

Grant, T., Huggins, J., Connor, P., Pedersen, J. Y., Whitney, N., & Streissguth, A. (2004). A pilot community intervention for young women with fetal alcohol spectrum disorders. *Community Mental Health Journal, 40*(6), 499–511.

Green, J. H. (2007). Fetal alcohol spectrum disorders: Understanding the effects of prenatal alcohol exposure and supporting students. *Journal of School Health, 77*(3), 103–108. doi:10.1111/j.1746-1561.2007.00178.x.

Green, C. R., Mihic, A. M., Nikkel, S. M., Stade, B. C., Rasmussen, C., Munoz, D. P., & Reynolds, J. N. (2009). Executive function deficits in children with fetal alcohol spectrum disorders (FASD) measured using the Cambridge Neuropsychological Tests Automated Battery (CANTAB). *Journal of Child Psychology and Psychiatry and Allied Disciplines, 50*(6), 688–697. doi:10.1111/j.1469-7610.2008.01990.x.

Hall, J. G., Froster-Iskenius, U. G., & Allanson, J. E. (1989). Handbook of normal physical measurements. New York: Oxford University Press.

Hall, J. G. (2010). New palpebral fissure measurements. *American Journal of Medical Genetics Part A, 152A*, 1870.

Hannigan, J. H., Chiodo, L. M., Sokol, R. J., Janisse, J., Ager, J. W., Greenwald, M. K., & Delaney-Black, V. (2010). A 14-year retrospective maternal report of alcohol consumption in pregnancy predicts pregnancy and teen outcomes. *Alcohol, 44*(7–8), 583–594. doi:10.1016/j.alcohol.2009.03.003.

Hanson, J. D., & Jensen, J. (2015). Importance of social support in preventing alcohol-exposed pregnancies with American Indian communities. *Journal of Community Health, 40*(1), 138–146. doi:10.1007/s10900-014-9911-1.

Hellemans, K. G., Sliwowska, J. H., Verma, P., & Weinberg, J. (2010). Prenatal alcohol exposure: Fetal programming and later life vulnerability to stress, depression and anxiety disorders. *Neuroscience and Biobehavioral Reviews, 34*(6), 791–807. doi:10.1016/j.neubiorev.2009.06.004.

Howell, K. K., Lynch, M. E., Platzman, K. A., Smith, G. H., & Coles, C. D. (2006). Prenatal alcohol exposure and ability, academic achievement, and school functioning in adolescence: A longitudinal follow-up. *Journal of Pediatric Psychology, 31*(1), 116–126. doi:10.1093/jpepsy/jsj029.

Hoyme, H. E., May, P. A., Kalberg, W. O., Kodituwakku, P., Gossage, J. P., Trujillo, P. M., … Robinson, L. K. (2005). A practical clinical approach to diagnosis of fetal alcohol spectrum disorders: Clarification of the 1996 institute of medicine criteria. *Pediatrics, 115*(1), 39–47. doi:10.1542/peds.2004-0259.

Iyasu, S., Randall, L. L., Welty, T. K., Hsia, J., Kinney, H. C., Mandell, F., … Willinger, M. (2002). Risk factors for sudden infant death syndrome among northern plains Indians. *Journal of the American Medical Association, 288*(21), 2717–2723.

Jacobson, S. W. (1998). Specificity of neurobehavioral outcomes associated with prenatal alcohol exposure. *Alcoholism: Clinical and Experimental Research, 22*(2), 313–320.

Jacobson, J. L., Dodge, N. C., Burden, M. J., Klorman, R., & Jacobson, S. W. (2011). Number processing in adolescents with prenatal alcohol exposure and ADHD: Differences in the neurobehavioral phenotype. *Alcoholism: Clinical and Experimental Research, 35*(3), 431–442. doi:10.1111/j.1530-0277.2010.01360.x.

Jacobson, S. W., & Jacobson, J. L. (2014). The risk of low-to-moderate prenatal alcohol exposure on child academic underachievement and behaviour may be difficult to measure and should not be underestimated. *Evidence-Based Medicine, 19*(2), e7. doi:10.1136/eb-2013-101535.

Jan, J. E., Asante, K. O., Conry, J. L., Fast, D. K., Bax, M. C., Ipsiroglu, O. S., … Wasdell, M. B. (2010). Sleep health issues for children with FASD: Clinical considerations. *International Journal of Pediatrics, 2010*, Article ID 639048. doi:10.1155/2010/639048.

Jirikowic, T., Gelo, J., & Astley, S. (2010). Children and youth with fetal alcohol spectrum disorders: Summary of intervention recommendations after clinical diagnosis. *Intellectual and Developmental Disabilities, 48*(5), 330–344. doi:10.1352/1934-9556-48.5.330.

Jirikowic, T., Olson, H. C., & Kartin, D. (2008). Sensory processing, school performance, and adaptive behavior of young school-age children with fetal alcohol spectrum disorders. *Physical & Occupational Therapy in Pediatrics, 28*(2), 117–136.

Jones, K. L. (2011). The effects of alcohol on fetal development. *Birth Defects Research Part C: Embryo Today: Reviews, 93*(1), 3–11. doi:10.1002/bdrc.20200.

Jones, K. L., & Smith, D. W. (1973). Recognition of the fetal alcohol syndrome in early infancy. *Lancet, 302*(7836), 999–1001.

Jones, K. L., Robinson, L. K., Bakhireva, L. N., Marintcheva, G., Storojev, V., Strahova, A., … Chambers, C. D. (2006). Accuracy of the diagnosis of physical features of fetal alcohol syndrome by pediatricians after specialized training. *Pediatrics, 118*(6), e1734–e1738. doi:10.1542/peds.2006-1037.

Kable, J. A., Coles, C. D., & Taddeo, E. (2007). Socio-cognitive habilitation using the math interactive learning experience program for alcohol-affected children. *Alcoholism: Clinical and Experimental Research, 31*(8), 1425–1434. doi:10.1111/j.1530-0277.2007.00431.x.

Kable, J. A., Taddeo, E., Strickland, D., & Coles, C. D. (2015). Community translation of the Math Interactive Learning Experience Program for children with FASD. *Research in Developmental Disabilities, 39*, 1–11. doi:10.1016/j.ridd.2014.12.031.

Kaemingk, K. L., Mulvaney, S., & Halverson, P. T. (2003). Learning following prenatal alcohol exposure: Performance on verbal and visual multitrial tasks. *Archives of Clinical Neuropsychology, 18*(1), 33–47.

Kalberg, W. O., Provost, B., Tollison, S. J., Tabachnick, B. G., Robinson, L. K., Hoyme, H. E., … May, P. A. (2006). Comparison of motor delays in young children with fetal alcohol syndrome to those with prenatal alcohol exposure and with no prenatal alcohol exposure. *Alcoholism: Clinical and Experimental Research, 30*(12), 2037–2045.

Keil, V., Paley, B., Frankel, F., & O'Connor, M. J. (2010). Impact of a social skills intervention on the hostile attributions of children with prenatal alcohol exposure. *Alcoholism: Clinical and Experimental Research, 34*(2), 231–241. doi:10.1111/j.1530-0277.2009.01086.x.

Kelly, Y., Iacovou, M., Quigley, M. A., Gray, R., Wolke, D., Kelly, J., & Sacker, A. (2013). Light drinking versus abstinence in pregnancy – Behavioural and cognitive outcomes in 7-year-old children: A longitudinal cohort study. *BJOG: An International Journal of Obstetrics and Gynaecology, 120*(11), 1340–1347. doi:10.1111/1471-0528.12246.

Kerns, K. A., Don, A., Mateer, C. A., & Streissguth, A. P. (1997). Cognitive deficits in nonretarded adults with fetal alcohol syndrome. *Journal of Learning Disabilities, 30*(6), 685–693.

Kfir, M., Yevtushok, L., Onishchenko, S., Wertelecki, W., Bakhireva, L., Chambers, C. D., … Hull, A. D. (2009). Can prenatal ultrasound detect the effects of in-utero alcohol exposure? A pilot study. *Ultrasound in Obstetrics and Gynecology, 33*(6), 683–689. doi:10.1002/uog.6379.

Kodituwakku, P. W. (2007). Defining the behavioral phenotype in children with fetal alcohol spectrum disorders: A review. *Neuroscience and Biobehavioral Reviews, 31*(2), 192–201. doi:10.1016/j.neubiorev.2006.06.020.

Kodituwakku, P. W. (2010). A neurodevelopmental framework for the development of interventions for children with fetal alcohol spectrum disorders. *Alcohol, 44*(7–8), 717–728.

Kodituwakku, P., Coriale, G., Fiorentino, D., Aragon, A. S., Kalberg, W. O., Buckley, D., … May, P. A. (2006). Neurobehavioral characteristics of children with fetal alcohol spectrum disorders in communities from Italy: Preliminary results. *Alcoholism: Clinical and Experimental Research, 30*(9), 1551–1561. doi:10.1111/j.1530-0277.2006.00187.x.

Kopera-Frye, K., Dehaene, S., & Streissguth, A. P. (1996). Impairments of number processing induced by prenatal alcohol exposure. *Neuropsychologia, 34*(12), 1187–1196.

Koren, G., Chudley, A., Loock, C., MacLeod, S. M., Orrbine, E., Rosales, T., … Sarkar, M. (2014). Screening and referral to identify children at risk for FASD: Search for new methods 2006–2013. *Journal of Population Therapeutics and Clinical Pharmacology, 21*(2), e260–e265.

Kuehn, D., Aros, S., Cassorla, F., Avaria, M., Unanue, N., Henriquez, C., … Mills, J. L. (2012). A prospective cohort study of the prevalence of growth, facial, and central nervous system abnormalities in children with heavy prenatal alcohol exposure. *Alcoholism: Clinical and Experimental Research, 36*(10), 1811–1819. doi:10.1111/j.1530-0277.2012.01794.x.

Kully-Martens, K., Denys, K., Treit, S., Tamana, S., & Rasmussen, C. (2012). A review of social skills deficits in individuals with fetal alcohol spectrum disorders and prenatal alcohol exposure: Profiles, mechanisms, and interventions. *Alcoholism: Clinical and Experimental Research, 36*(4), 568–576. doi:10.1111/j.1530-0277.2011.01661.x.

LaFrance, M. A., McLachlan, K., Nash, K., Andrew, G., Loock, C., Oberlander, T. F., … Rasmussen, C. (2014). Evaluation of the neurobehavioral screening tool in children with fetal alcohol spectrum disorders (FASD). *Journal of Population Therapeutics and Clinical Pharmacology, 21*(2), e197–e210.

Lange, S., Shield, K., Koren, G., Rehm, J., & Popova, S. (2014). A comparison of the prevalence of prenatal alcohol exposure obtained via maternal self-reports versus meconium testing: A systematic literature review and meta-analysis. *BMC Pregnancy and Childbirth, 14*, 127. doi:10.1186/1471-2393-14-127.

Larcher, V., & Brierley, J. (2014). Fetal alcohol syndrome (FAS) and fetal alcohol spectrum disorder (FASD)-diagnosis and moral policing; an ethical dilemma for paediatricians. *Archives of Disease in Childhood, 99*(11), 969–970. doi:10.1136/archdischild-2014-306774.

Lebel, C., Rasmussen, C., Wyper, K., Andrew, G., & Beaulieu, C. (2010). Brain microstructure is related to math ability in children with fetal alcohol spectrum disorder. *Alcoholism: Clinical and Experimental Research, 34*(2), 354–363. doi:10.1111/j.1530-0277.2009.01097.x.

Loomes, C., Rasmussen, C., Pei, J., Manji, S., & Andrew, G. (2008). The effect of rehearsal training on working memory span of children with fetal alcohol spectrum disorder. *Research in Developmental Disabilities, 29*(2), 113–124. doi:10.1016/j.ridd.2007.01.001.

Lucas, B. R., Latimer, J., Pinto, R. Z., Ferreira, M. L., Doney, R., Lau, M., … Elliott, E. J. (2014). Gross motor deficits in children prenatally exposed to alcohol: A meta-analysis. *Pediatrics, 134*(1), e192–e209. doi:10.1542/peds.2013-3733.

Mattson, S. N., Autti-Rämö, I., May, P. A., Konovalova, V., & the CIFASD. (2006). Spatial learning and navigation deficits in an international sample of children with heavy prenatal alcohol exposure. Presented at the Thirteenth Congress of the International Society for Biomedical Research on Alcoholism, Sydney, Australia, September 2006. *Alcoholism: Clinical and Experimental Research, 30*(9), 176A.

Mattson, S. N., & Calarco, K. E. (2002). "What" and "where" visuospatial processing in children with heavy prenatal alcohol exposure. *Journal of the International Neuropsychological Society, 8*(4), 513.

Mattson, S. N., Crocker, N., & Nguyen, T. T. (2011). Fetal alcohol spectrum disorders: Neuropsychological and behavioral features. *Neuropsychology Review, 21*(2), 81–101. doi:10.1007/s11065-011-9167-9.

Mattson, S. N., & Riley, E. P. (1998). A review of the neurobehavioral deficits in children with fetal alcohol syndrome or prenatal exposure to alcohol. *Alcoholism: Clinical and Experimental Research, 22*(2), 279–294.

Mattson, S. N., & Riley, E. P. (2000). Parent ratings of behavior in children with heavy prenatal alcohol exposure and IQ-matched controls. *Alcoholism: Clinical and Experimental Research, 24*(2), 226–231. doi:10.1111/j.1530-0277.2000.tb04595.x.

Mattson, S. N., & Riley, E. P. (2011). The quest for a neurobehavioral profile of heavy prenatal alcohol exposure. *Alcohol Research and Health, 34*(1), 51–55.

Mattson, S. N., Riley, E. P., Delis, D. C., Stern, C., & Jones, K. L. (1996). Verbal learning and memory in children with fetal alcohol syndrome. *Alcoholism: Clinical and Experimental Research, 20*(5), 810–816. doi:10.1111/j.1530-0277.1996.tb05256.x.

Mattson, S. N., Riley, E. P., Gramling, L., Delis, D. C., & Jones, K. L. (1998). Neuropsychological comparison of alcohol-exposed children with or without physical features of fetal alcohol syndrome. *Neuropsychology, 12*(1), 146–153.

Mattson, S. N., & Roebuck, T. M. (2002). Acquisition and retention of verbal and nonverbal information in children with heavy prenatal alcohol exposure. *Alcoholism: Clinical and Experimental Research, 26*(6), 875–882. doi:10.1111/j.1530-0277.2002.tb02617.x.

Mattson, S. N., Roesch, S. C., Glass, L., Deweese, B. N., Coles, C. D., Kable, J. A., … the CIFASD. (2013). Further development of a neurobehavioral profile of fetal alcohol spectrum disorders. *Alcoholism: Clinical and Experimental Research, 37*(3), 517–528. doi:10.1111/j.1530-0277.2012.01952.x.

May, P. A., Gossage, J. P., Marais, A. S., Adnams, C. M., Hoyme, H. E., Jones, K. L., … Viljoen, D. L. (2007a). The epidemiology of fetal alcohol syndrome and partial FAS in a South African community. *Drug and Alcohol Dependence, 88*(2–3), 259–271.

May, P. A., Miller, J. H., Goodhart, K. A., Maestas, O. R., Buckley, D., Trujillo, P. M., & Gossage, J. P. (2007b). Enhanced case management to prevent fetal alcohol spectrum disorders in Northern Plains communities. *Maternal Child Health Journal, 12*(6), 747–759.

May, P. A., Gossage, J. P., Kalberg, W. O., Robinson, L. K., Buckley, D., Manning, M., & Hoyme, H. E. (2009). Prevalence and epidemiologic characteristics of FASD from various research methods with an emphasis on recent in-school studies. *Developmental Disabilities Research Reviews, 15*(3), 176–192. doi:10.1002/ddrr.68.

May, P. A., Baete, A., Russo, J., Elliott, A. J., Blankenship, J., Kalberg, W. O., … Hoyme, H. E. (2014). Prevalence and characteristics of fetal alcohol spectrum disorders. *Pediatrics, 134*(5), 855–866. doi:10.1542/peds.2013-3319.

McFarlane, A., & Rajani, H. (2007). Rural FASD diagnostic services model: Lakeland Centre for fetal alcohol spectrum disorder. *Canadian Journal of Clinical Pharmacology, 14*(3), e301–e306.

McGee, C. L., Bjorkquist, O. A., Price, J. M., Mattson, S. N., & Riley, E. P. (2009). Social information processing skills in children with histories of heavy prenatal alcohol exposure. *Journal of Abnormal Child Psychology, 37*(6), 817–830. doi:10.1007/s10802-009-9313-5.

McGee, C. L., Bjorkquist, O. A., Riley, E. P., & Mattson, S. N. (2009). Impaired language performance in young children with heavy prenatal alcohol exposure. *Neurotoxicology and Teratology, 31*(2), 71–75. doi:10.1016/j.ntt.2008.09.004.

McGee, C. L., Fryer, S. L., Bjorkquist, O. A., Mattson, S. N., & Riley, E. P. (2008). Deficits in social problem solving in adolescents with prenatal exposure to alcohol. *American Journal of Drug and Alcohol Abuse, 34*(4), 423–431. doi:10.1080/00952990802122630.

Meintjes, E. M., Jacobson, J. L., Molteno, C. D., Gatenby, J. C., Warton, C., Cannistraci, C. J., … Jacobson, S. W. (2010). An FMRI study of number processing in children with fetal alcohol syndrome. *Alcoholism: Clinical and Experimental Research, 34*(8), 1450–1464. doi:10.1111/j.1530-0277.2010.01230.x.

Melby-Lervag, M., & Hulme, C. (2013). Is working memory training effective? A meta-analytic review. *Developmental Psychology, 49*(2), 270–291. doi:10.1037/A0028228.

Mengel, M. B., Searight, H. R., & Cook, K. (2006). Preventing alcohol-exposed pregnancies. *Journal of the American Board of Family Medicine, 19*(5), 494–505.

Morleo, M., Woolfall, K., Dedman, D., Mukherjee, R., Bellis, M. A., & Cook, P. A. (2011). Underreporting of foetal alcohol spectrum disorders: An analysis of hospital episode statistics. *BMC Pediatrics, 11*, 14. doi:10.1186/1471-2431-11-14.

Nash, K., Koren, G., & Rovet, J. (2011). A differential approach for examining the behavioural phenotype of fetal alcohol spectrum disorders. *Journal of Population Therapeutics and Clinical Pharmacology, 18*(3), 440–453.

Nash, K., Rovet, J., Greenbaum, R., Fantus, E., Nulman, I., & Koren, G. (2006). Identifying the behavioural phenotype in fetal alcohol spectrum disorder: Sensitivity, specificity and screening potential. *Archives of Women's Mental Health, 9*(4), 181–186. doi:10.1007/s00737-006-0130-3.

Nguyen, T. T., Glass, L., Coles, C. D., Kable, J. A., May, P. A., Kalberg, W. O., … the CIFASD. (2014). The clinical utility and specificity of parent report of executive function among children with prenatal alcohol exposure. *Journal of the International Neuropsychological Society, 20*(7), 704–716. doi:10.1017/S1355617714000599.

NIAAA. (2013). *NIAAA Director's Report on Institute Activities to the 134th Meeting of the National Advisory Council on Alcohol Abuse and Alcoholism.*

O'Callaghan, F. V., O'Callaghan, M., Najman, J. M., Williams, G. M., & Bor, W. (2007). Prenatal alcohol exposure and attention, learning and intellectual ability at 14 years: A prospective longitudinal study. *Early Human Development, 83*(2), 115–123.

O'Connor, M. J., & Paley, B. (2006). The relationship of prenatal alcohol exposure and the postnatal environment to child depressive symptoms. *Journal of Pediatric Psychology, 31*(1), 50–64. doi:10.1093/jpepsy/jsj021.

O'Connor, M. J., & Paley, B. (2009). Psychiatric conditions associated with prenatal alcohol exposure. *Dev Disabil Res Rev, 15*(3), 225–234. doi:10.1002/ddrr.74.

O'Connor, M. J., Frankel, F., Paley, B., Schonfeld, A. M., Carpenter, E., Laugeson, E. A., & Marquardt, R. (2006). A controlled social skills training for children with fetal alcohol spectrum disorders. *Journal of Consulting and Clinical Psychology, 74*(4), 639–648.

O'Connor, M. J., Laugeson, E. A., Mogil, C., Lowe, E., Welch-Torres, K., Keil, V., & Paley, B. (2012). Translation of an evidence-based social skills intervention for children with prenatal alcohol exposure in a community mental health setting. *Alcoholism: Clinical and Experimental Research, 36*(1), 141–152. doi:10.1111/j.1530-0277.2011.01591.x.

O'Leary, C. M., Taylor, C., Zubrick, S. R., Kurinczuk, J. J., & Bower, C. (2013). Prenatal alcohol exposure and educational achievement in children aged 8–9 years. *Pediatrics, 132*(2), e468–e475. doi:10.1542/peds.2012-3002.

O'Leary, C., Zubrick, S. R., Taylor, C. L., Dixon, G., & Bower, C. (2009). Prenatal alcohol exposure and language delay in 2-year-old children: The importance of dose and timing on risk. *Pediatrics, 123*(2), 547–554. doi:10.1542/peds.2008-0459.

Olson, H. C., Oti, R., Gelo, J., & Beck, S. (2009). "Family matters:" Fetal alcohol spectrum disorders and the family. *Dev Disabil Res Rev, 15*(3), 235–249. doi:10.1002/ddrr.65.

Paley, B., & O'Connor, M. J. (2011). Behavioral interventions for children and adolescents with fetal alcohol spectrum disorders. *Alcohol Research & Health, 34*(1), 64–75.

Paley, B., O'Connor, M. J., Kogan, N., & Findlay, R. (2005). Prenatal alcohol exposure, child externalizing behavior, and maternal stress. *Parenting: Science and Practice, 5*(1), 29–56.

Payne, J., France, K., Henley, N., D'Antoine, H., Bartu, A., O'Leary, C., … Bower, C. (2011a). Changes in health professionals' knowledge, attitudes and practice following provision of educational resources about prevention of prenatal alcohol exposure and fetal alcohol spectrum disorder. *Paediatric and Perinatal Epidemiology, 25*(4), 316–327. doi:10.1111/j.1365-3016.2011.01197.x.

Payne, J. M., France, K. E., Henley, N., D'Antoine, H. A., Bartu, A. E., Mutch, R. C., … Bower, C. (2011b). Paediatricians' knowledge, attitudes and practice following provision of educational resources about prevention of prenatal alcohol exposure and fetal alcohol spectrum disorder. *Journal of Paediatrics and Child Health, 47*(10), 704–710. doi:10.1111/j.1440-1754.2011.02037.x.

Peadon, E., Rhys-Jones, B., Bower, C., & Elliott, E. J. (2009). Systematic review of interventions for children with fetal alcohol spectrum disorders. *BMC Pediatrics, 9*, 35. doi:10.1186/1471-2431-9-35.

Petrenko, C. L., Tahir, N., Mahoney, E. C., & Chin, N. P. (2014a). Prevention of secondary conditions in fetal alcohol spectrum disorders: Identification of systems-level barriers. *Maternal and Child Health Journal, 18*(6), 1496–1505. doi:10.1007/s10995-013-1390-y.

Petrenko, C. L., Tahir, N., Mahoney, E. C., & Chin, N. P. (2014b). A qualitative assessment of program characteristics for preventing secondary conditions in individuals with fetal alcohol spectrum disorders. *Journal of Population Therapeutics and Clinical Pharmacology, 21*(2), e246–e259.

Popova, S., Lange, S., Burd, L., Chudley, A. E., Clarren, S. K., & Rehm, J. (2013). Cost of fetal alcohol spectrum disorder diagnosis in Canada. *PLoS One, 8*(4), 6. doi:10.1371/journal.pone.0060434.

Powell, G. (2012). Danish studies suggesting low and moderate prenatal alcohol exposure has no adverse effects on children aged 5 years did not use appropriate or effective measures of executive functioning. *BJOG: An International Journal of Obstetrics and Gynaecology, 119*(13), 1669–1670. doi:10.1111/1471-0528.12005. author reply 1673-1665.

Rasmussen, C., & Bisanz, J. (2009). Executive functioning in children with fetal alcohol spectrum disorders: Profiles and age-related differences. *Child Neuropsychology, 15*(3), 201–215. doi:10.1080/09297040802385400.

Rasmussen, C., Soleimani, M., & Pei, J. (2011). Executive functioning and working memory deficits on the CANTAB among children with prenatal alcohol exposure. *Journal of Population Therapeutics and Clinical Pharmacology, 18*(1), e44–e53.

Rasmussen, C., Wyper, K., & Talwar, V. (2009). The relation between theory of mind and executive functions in children with fetal alcohol spectrum disorders. *The Canadian Journal of Clinical Pharmacology, 16*(2), e370–e380.

Robinson, M., Oddy, W. H., McLean, N. J., Jacoby, P., Pennell, C. E., de Klerk, N. H., … Newnham, J. P. (2010). Low-moderate prenatal alcohol exposure and risk to child behavioural development: A prospective cohort study. *BJOG: An International Journal of Obstetrics and Gynaecology, 117*(9), 1139–1150. doi:10.1111/j.1471-0528.2010.02596.x.

Roebuck, T. M., Mattson, S. N., & Riley, E. P. (1999). Behavioral and psychosocial profiles of alcohol-exposed children. *Alcoholism: Clinical and Experimental Research, 23*(6), 1070–1076.

Roebuck, T. M., Simmons, R. W., Richardson, C., Mattson, S. N., & Riley, E. P. (1998). Neuromuscular responses to disturbance of balance in children with prenatal exposure to alcohol. *Alcoholism: Clinical and Experimental Research, 22*(9), 1992–1997.

Rogers-Adkinson, D. L., & Stuart, S. K. (2007). Collaborative services: Children experiencing neglect and the side effects of prenatal alcohol exposure. *Language, Speech, and Hearing Services in Schools, 38*(2), 149–156. doi:10.1044/0161-1461(2007/015).

Ryan, D. M., Bonnett, D. M., & Gass, C. B. (2006). Sobering thoughts: Town hall meetings on fetal alcohol spectrum disorders. *American Journal of Public Health, 96*(12), 2098–2101. doi:10.2105/AJPH.2005.062729.

Salmon, A., & Clarren, S. K. (2011). Developing effective, culturally appropriate avenues to FASD diagnosis and prevention in northern Canada. *International Journal of Circumpolar Health, 70*(4), 428–433.

Santhanam, P., Li, Z., Hu, X., Lynch, M. E., & Coles, C. D. (2009). Effects of prenatal alcohol exposure on brain activation during an arithmetic task: An fMRI study. *Alcoholism: Clinical and Experimental Research, 33*(11), 1901–1908. doi:10.1111/j.1530-0277.2009.01028.x.

Schonfeld, A. M., Mattson, S. N., Lang, A. R., Delis, D. C., & Riley, E. P. (2001). Verbal and nonverbal fluency in children with heavy prenatal alcohol exposure. *Journal of Studies on Alcohol and Drugs, 62*(2), 239–246.

Schonfeld, A. M., Mattson, S. N., & Riley, E. P. (2005). Moral maturity and delinquency after prenatal alcohol exposure. *Journal of Studies on Alcohol, 66*(4), 545–554.

Schonfeld, A. M., Paley, B., Frankel, F., & O'Connor, M. J. (2006). Executive functioning predicts social skills following prenatal alcohol exposure. *Child Neuropsychology, 12*(6), 439–452. doi:10.1080/09297040600611338.

Senturias, Y. S. (2014). Fetal alcohol spectrum disorders: An overview for pediatric and adolescent care providers. *Current Problems in Pediatric and Adolescent Health Care, 44*(4), 74–81. doi:10.1016/j.cppeds.2013.12.012.

Skogerbo, A., Kesmodel, U. S., Denny, C. H., Kjaersgaard, M. I., Wimberley, T., Landro, N. I., & Mortensen, E. L. (2013). The effects of low to moderate alcohol consumption and binge drinking in early pregnancy on behaviour in 5-year-old children: A prospective cohort study on 1628 children. *BJOG: An International Journal of Obstetrics and Gynaecology, 120*(9), 1042–1050. doi:10.1111/1471-0528.12208.

Sood, B., Delaney-Black, V., Covington, C., Nordstrom-Klee, B., Ager, J., Templin, T., … Sokol, R. J. (2001). Prenatal alcohol exposure and childhood behavior at age 6 to 7 years: I. dose-response effect. *Pediatrics, 108*(2), E34.

Stade, B., Ali, A., Bennett, D., Campbell, D., Johnston, M., Lens, C., … Koren, G. (2009). The burden of prenatal exposure to alcohol: Revised measurement of cost. *Canadian Journal of Clinical Pharmacology, 16*(1), e91–e102.

Stevens, S. A., Nash, K., Koren, G., & Rovet, J. (2013). Autism characteristics in children with fetal alcohol spectrum disorders. *Child Neuropsychology, 19*(6), 579–587. doi:10.1080/09297049.2012.727791.

Stockwell, T., Donath, S., Cooper-Stanbury, M., Chikritzhs, T., Catalano, P., & Mateo, C. (2004). Under-reporting of alcohol consumption in household surveys: A comparison of quantity-frequency, graduated-frequency and recent recall. *Addiction, 99*(8), 1024–1033. doi:10.1111/j.1360-0443.2004.00815.x.

Streissguth, A. P., Sampson, P. D., Olson, H. C., Bookstein, F. L., Barr, H. M., Scott, M., … Mirsky, A. F. (1994c). Maternal drinking during pregnancy: Attention and short-term memory in 14-year-old offspring – A longitudinal prospective study. *Alcoholism: Clinical and Experimental Research, 18*(1), 202–218. doi:10.1111/j.1530-0277.1994.tb00904.x.

Streissguth, A. P. (2007). Offspring effects of prenatal alcohol exposure from birth to 25 years: The Seattle prospective longitudinal study. *Journal of Clinical Psychology in Medical Settings, 14*, 81–101.

Streissguth, A. P., Barr, H. M., Carmichael Olson, H., Sampson, P. D., Bookstein, F. L., & Burgess, D. M. (1994). Drinking during pregnancy decreases word attack and arithmetic scores on standardized tests: Adolescent data from a population-based prospective study. *Alcoholism: Clinical and Experimental Research, 18*(2), 248–254.

Streissguth, A. P., Barr, H. M., Kogan, J., & Bookstein, F. L. (1996). *Final report: Understanding the occurrence of secondary disabilities in clients with fetal alcohol syndrome (FAS) and fetal alcohol effects (FAE)*. Seattle, WA: University of Washington Publication Services.

Streissguth, A. P., Barr, H. M., Sampson, P. D., & Bookstein, F. L. (1994). Prenatal alcohol and offspring development: The first fourteen years. *Drug and Alcohol Dependence, 36*, 89–99.

Streissguth, A. P., Barr, H. M., & Sampson, P. D. (1990). Moderate prenatal alcohol exposure: Effects on child IQ and learning problems at age 7 1/2 years. *Alcoholism: Clinical and Experimental Research, 14*(5), 662–669.

Streissguth, A. P., Bookstein, F. L., Barr, H. M., Sampson, P. D., O'Malley, K., & Young, J. K. (2004). Risk factors for adverse life outcomes in fetal alcohol syndrome and fetal alcohol effects. *Journal of Developmental and Behavioral Pediatrics, 25*(4), 228–238.

Surgeon General, U. S. (2005). *Advisory on alcohol use in pregnancy*. Washington, DC: US Department of Health and Human Services.

Swart, S., Hall, W. A., McKee, W. T., & Ford, L. (2014). Caregivers' management of schooling for their children with fetal alcohol spectrum disorder. *Qualitative Health Research, 24*(11), 1540–1552. doi:10.1177/1049732314545497.

Thomas, L. T., Gaitantzis, Y. A., & Frias, J. L. (1987). Palpebral fissure length from 29 weeks to 14 years. *Journal of Pediatrics, 111*(2), 267–268.

Thomas, G., Gonneau, G., Poole, N., & Cook, J. (2014). The effectiveness of alcohol warning labels in the prevention of fetal alcohol spectrum disorder: A brief review. *International Journal of Alcohol and Drug Research, 3*(1), 91–103. doi:10.7895/ijadr.vXiY.126.

Thomas, S. E., Kelly, S. J., Mattson, S. N., & Riley, E. P. (1998). Comparison of social abilities of children with fetal alcohol syndrome to those of children with similar IQ scores and normal controls. *Alcoholism: Clinical and Experimental Research, 22*(2), 528–533.

Thorne, J. C., Coggins, T. E., Carmichael Olson, H., & Astley, S. J. (2007). Exploring the utility of narrative analysis in diagnostic decision making: Picture-bound reference, elaboration, and fetal alcohol spectrum disorders. *Journal of Speech, Language, and Hearing Research, 50*(2), 459–474.

Vaurio, L., Riley, E. P., & Mattson, S. N. (2008). Differences in executive functioning in children with heavy prenatal alcohol exposure or attention-deficit/hyperactivity disorder. *Journal of the International Neuropsychological Society, 14*(1), 119–129. doi:10.1017/S1355617708080144.

Velasquez, M. M., von Sternberg, K., & Parrish, D. E. (2013). CHOICES: An integrated behavioral intervention to prevent alcohol-exposed pregnancies among high-risk women in community settings. *Social Work in Public Health, 28*(3-4), 224–233. doi:10.1080/19371918.2013.759011.

Walthall, J. C., O'Connor, M. J., & Paley, B. (2008). A comparison of psychopathology in children with and without prenatal alcohol exposure. *Mental Health Aspects of Developmental Disabilities, 11*(3), 69–78.

Ware, A. L., Crocker, N., O'Brien, J. W., Deweese, B. N., Roesch, S. C., Coles, C. D., ... the CIFASD. (2012). Executive function predicts adaptive behavior in children with histories of heavy prenatal alcohol exposure and attention-deficit/hyperactivity disorder. *Alcoholism: Clinical and Experimental Research, 36*(8), 1431–1341. doi:10.1111/j.1530-0277.2011.01718.x.

Ware, A. L., O'Brien, J. W., Crocker, N., Deweese, B. N., Roesch, S. C., Coles, C. D., ... the CIFASD. (2013). The effects of prenatal alcohol exposure and attention-deficit/hyperactivity disorder on psychopathology and behavior. *Alcoholism: Clinical and Experimental Research, 37*(3), 507–516. doi:10.1111/j.1530-0277.2012.01953.x.

Ware, A. L., Glass, L., Crocker, N., Deweese, B. N., Coles, C. D., Kable, J. A., ...the CIFASD. (2014). Effects of prenatal alcohol exposure and attention-deficit/hyperactivity disorder on adaptive functioning. *Alcoholism: Clinical and Experimental Research, 38*(5), 1439–1447. doi:10.1111/acer.12376.

Way, E. L., & Rojahn, J. (2012). Psycho-social characteristics of children with prenatal alcohol exposure, compared to children with down syndrome and typical children. *Journal of Developmental and Physical Disabilities, 24*(3), 247–268. doi:10.1007/S10882-012-9269-1.

Wengel, T., Hanlon-Dearman, A. C., & Fjeldsted, B. (2011). Sleep and sensory characteristics in young children with fetal alcohol spectrum disorder. *Journal of Developmental and Behavioral Pediatrics, 32*(5), 384–392. doi:10.1097/DBP.0b013e3182199694.

Willford, J. A., Richardson, G. A., Leech, S. L., & Day, N. L. (2004). Verbal and visuospatial learning and memory function in children with moderate prenatal alcohol exposure. *Alcoholism: Clinical and Experimental Research, 28*(3), 497–507.

Willoughby, K. A., Sheard, E. D., Nash, K., & Rovet, J. (2008). Effects of prenatal alcohol exposure on hippocampal volume, verbal learning, and verbal and spatial recall in late childhood. *Journal of the International Neuropsychological Society, 14*(6), 1022–1033. doi:10.1017/S1355617708081368.

Wozniak, J. R., Muetzel, R. L., Mueller, B. A., McGee, C. L., Freerks, M. A., Ward, E. E., … Lim, K. O. (2009). Microstructural corpus callosum anomalies in children with prenatal alcohol exposure: An extension of previous diffusion tensor imaging findings. *Alcoholism: Clinical and Experimental Research, 33*(10), 1825–1835. doi:10.1111/j.1530-0277.2009.01021.x.

Yan, A., Bell, E., & Racine, E. (2014). Ethical and social challenges in newborn screening for prenatal alcohol exposure. *The Canadian Journal of Neurological Sciences, 41*(1), 115–118.

Zelner, I., Shor, S., Gareri, J., Lynn, H., Roukema, H., Lum, L., … Koren, G. (2010). Universal screening for prenatal alcohol exposure: A progress report of a pilot study in the region of Grey Bruce, Ontario. *Therapeutic Drug Monitoring, 32*(3), 305–310. doi:10.1097/FTD.0b013e3181dca381.

Zelner, I., Shor, S., Lynn, H., Roukema, H., Lum, L., Eisinga, K., & Koren, G. (2012). Neonatal screening for prenatal alcohol exposure: Assessment of voluntary maternal participation in an open meconium screening program. *Alcohol, 46*(3), 269–276. doi:10.1016/j.alcohol.2011.09.029.

Chapter 3
In Utero Exposure to Nicotine, Cocaine, and Amphetamines

Lynn T. Singer, Meeyoung O. Min, Adelaide Lang, and Sonia Minnes

Introduction

Nicotine, cocaine, and amphetamines (methamphetamine, amphetamine, and 3,4, methylenedioxymethamphetamine, "MDMA or Ecstasy") are psychomotor stimulants, a class of drugs in which significant sensorimotor activation occurs with drug administration (Meyer & Quenzer, 2005). Stimulants are drugs that enhance alertness and attention, increase arousal and behavioral excitement, and have a high potential for producing mental and physiological dependence. They vary in their legality, therapeutic use, mode and pattern of intake, pharmacologic actions, and prevalence of use, as well as in the sociodemographic and personality characteristics of women who choose to continue to use them during pregnancy despite strong medical contraindications. Importantly, our understanding of the effects of these stimulants on fetal and child developmental outcomes varies considerably across specific substances. Some stimulants, such

L.T. Singer, Ph.D. (✉)
Case Western Reserve University, 2040 Adelbert Road, Cleveland, OH 44106, USA
e-mail: Lynn.Singer@case.edu

M.O. Min, Ph.D. • S. Minnes, Ph.D.
Case Western Reserve University, 10900 Euclid Avenue, Cleveland, OH 44106, USA
e-mail: Meeyoung.Min@case.edu; Sonia.Minnes@case.edu

A. Lang, Ph.D.
Case Western Reserve University, 11635 Euclid Avenue, Cleveland, OH 44106, USA
e-mail: Adelaide.Lang@case.edu

C. Riccio, J. Sullivan (eds.), *Pediatric Neurotoxicology*, Specialty Topics in Pediatric Neuropsychology, DOI 10.1007/978-3-319-32358-9_3

as cocaine and nicotine, are subjects of a large body of research, while there is virtually no information on the effects of prescribed amphetamines or MDMA on long-term child development.

A significant issue in current research on the behavioral teratology of stimulants is that women who use stimulants during pregnancy, particularly those that are illegal, are virtually all polydrug users. They also tend to be heavier users of other drugs, such as marijuana, opiates, and alcohol that serve to mitigate the excitatory "highs" of stimulants. Thus, untangling the prenatal effects of any one drug on child development becomes difficult because stimulant drugs are likely to cause dependence and are rarely used alone. In studies of cocaine-exposed infants, their mothers self-reported using higher amounts of alcohol, marijuana, and nicotine during pregnancy in addition to cocaine than did control groups in which women reported alcohol, marijuana, and nicotine, but not cocaine use (Coles, Bard, Platzman, & Lynch, 1999; Eyler, Behnke, Conlon, Woods, & Wobie, 1998; Singer, Arendt et al., 2002). Similarly, in a study in the UK, the majority of women who used MDMA recreationally during pregnancy also used alcohol, tobacco, and marijuana, as well as psychedelic drugs like LSD and ketamine (Singer et al., 2012a).

Other factors affecting understanding of the outcomes of children exposed to stimulants in utero are the legality of the drug as well as the psychological and sociodemographic characteristics of the users. Exposure levels to illegal stimulants, such as cocaine, MDMA, and methamphetamines, are difficult to quantify accurately, while nicotine and prescription stimulant amphetamines, such as Ritalin, Concerta, Adderall, and Vyvanse, are federally regulated and provide more precise measures of the dose of drug exposure to the fetus if maternal reports are accurate. With illegal stimulants, data may be unreliable as fear of incarceration or loss of child custody may lead pregnant women to deny or minimize the amount of the drug used. However, even when legal, when harmful effects to the fetus are widely publicized, such as with alcohol or tobacco, pregnant women are reluctant to admit use to avoid social disapproval, so that denial or minimization of use occurs.

Finally, assessing the relative risks of various stimulants is difficult because the type of stimulant used by women during pregnancy is frequently confounded with the social and psychological characteristics of the users. The extensive data base now available on the sequelae of prenatal cocaine exposure is derived primarily from studies of offspring of poor, urban, largely minority women recruited during the "crack-cocaine" epidemic of the late 1980s and 1990s in the USA. There are no comparable studies available for children of women of middle socioeconomic status, so it is difficult to separate the biological effects of cocaine exposure from the effects of violence exposure, poor education, and poverty of the cohorts studied. The few studies available of prescription amphetamines, alternatively, are derived from studies of middle socioeconomic status volunteers with preexisting attentional deficits, so that effects on offspring may not be generalizable to other populations that do not share genetic factors or caregiving characteristics associated with a parent with ADHD. Despite these caveats, a substantial body of research that can begin to inform public health efforts for prevention and intervention has begun to emerge documenting the outcomes of various cohorts of children exposed prenatally to stimulants. In light of the different research findings associated with different types of stimulants, in this chapter we discuss the developmental outcomes of in utero exposure to nicotine, cocaine, and amphetamines in separate sections.

Nicotine

Definitional Issues and Prevalence

Nicotine, an alkaloid found in tobacco leaves, is the primary psychoactive component of tobacco. While there are over 4000 chemicals in tobacco smoke that may be toxic, substantial evidence exists that nicotine is a key ingredient with adverse effects on brain development (Dwyer, McQuown, & Leslie, 2009). Despite widespread public health warnings, about 15.4 % of pregnant women aged 15–44 in the USA smoke tobacco during their pregnancies (Substance Abuse and Mental Health Services Administration, 2014). While some women quit smoking prior to or during pregnancy, about 10.7 % of pregnant women continue to smoke through their third trimester. Smoking during pregnancy occurs in all socioeconomic and ethnic groups, but rates are higher in low socioeconomic populations, those under age 25, and those with less education. Of those who quit smoking during pregnancy, up to 40 % relapse within 6 months after delivery (Centers for Disease Control and Prevention, 2013). Thus, adverse effects of smoking can continue after birth by transmission through breast milk (Primo, Ruela, Brotto, Garcia, & Ede Lima, 2013) and exposure to second hand smoke (US Department of Health and Human Services, 2006).

Impact on the Developing Child

Nicotine crosses the placenta readily and may reach fetal concentrations much higher than maternal levels, contributing to reduced oxygen supply, undernourishment of the fetus, and vasoconstrictor effects on the placenta and umbilical cord (Behnke, Smith, Committee on Substance Abuse, & Committee on Fetus and Newborn, 2013). The adverse physical effects of smoking during pregnancy include increased risk for miscarriage, stillbirth, infant mortality, Sudden Infant Death Syndrome (SIDS), preterm birth, fetal growth retardation, and low birthweight (National Institute on Drug Abuse—US Department of Health and Human Services, National Institutes of Health, 2012). Relationships between maternal smoking in pregnancy and childhood obesity, elevated blood pressure, and Type II diabetes have also been found (Rogers, 2009). Exposure to secondhand smoke can cause additional health problems such as asthma attacks, bronchitis, respiratory infections, ear infections, and SIDS (Centers for Disease Control and Prevention, 2014, March 5).

Animal studies indicate that prenatal exposure to nicotine disrupts the timing of trophic events linked to nicotinic cholinergic receptors, leading to premature onset of cell differentiation at the expense of replication, alteration of cell signaling, brain cell death or structural alterations in regional brain areas, and effects on the neurotransmitter systems involving dopamine, serotonin, and norepinephrine (Slikker, Xu, Levin, & Slotkin, 2005). In rats, these brain changes are associated with locomotor hyperactivity and reduced cognitive function. A review of the literature on brain structure and function in humans (Bublitz & Stroud, 2012) indicates that prenatal nicotine exposure is associated with decreased volume/thickness of the cerebellum and corpus callosum, increased auditory brainstem responses in infants, and lack of coordination across brain regions in response inhibition, memory, and attention tasks in adolescents. Alterations in these brain regions have also been linked to deficits in cognitive abilities, auditory processing, social development, and ADHD.

Numerous studies have identified neurobehavioral abnormalities in nicotine-exposed infants including greater excitability, arousal, muscle tension, more signs of stress/abstinence, greater need for touch to be calmed, poorer self-regulation, and greater negative affect (Barros, Mitsuhiro, Chalem, Laranjeira, & Guinsburg, 2011; Law et al., 2003; Schuetze & Eiden, 2007; Stroud et al., 2009) compared to unexposed infants. This early compromised neurobehavior may predict persistent adverse outcomes in childhood, particularly behavioral difficulties (Hernandez-Martinez, Arija Val, Escribano Subias, & Canals Sans, 2012; Stroud et al., 2009).

Intellectual Functioning

Many studies have found a relationship between prenatal nicotine exposure and lower IQ scores on intelligence measures across childhood and adolescence. A systematic review of the literature (Clifford, Lang, & Chen, 2012) indicated that the reductions in IQ tend to be small and effects sometimes attenuated or eliminated after adjustment for maternal intelligence, maternal education, SES, sibling relationships, and infant birth weight. Heavier exposure to nicotine is associated with lower overall intelligence scores (Batty, Der, & Deary, 2006; Fried, Watkinson, & Gray, 2003; Mortensen, Michaelsen, Sanders, & Reinisch, 2005).

Academic Functioning

A limited number of studies investigated the link between prenatal tobacco exposure and academic achievement. In one prospective birth cohort study, school age children of mothers who smoked during pregnancy performed more poorly on tests of arithmetic and spelling, after adjustment for risk factors (Batstra, Hadders-Algra, & Neeleman, 2003). Other studies found dose–response associations between exposure and school age children's reading skills after adjusting for socioeconomic status, type of school attended, and prenatal and postnatal characteristics (Cho, Frijters, Zhang, Miller, & Gruen, 2013; Fried, Watkinson, & Siegel, 1997). In studies that measured academic achievement using school grades or grade point average

(D'Onofrio et al., 2010; Lambe, Hultman, Torrang, Maccabe, & Cnattingius, 2006; Martin, Dombrowski, Mullis, Wisenbaker, & Huttunen, 2006) exposed children (age 12) and adolescents (age 15) had a higher risk of lower grade performance compared to non-exposed peers. However, when compared to siblings differentially exposed to maternal smoking during pregnancy, there were no differences in academic achievement in two large epidemiological studies (D'Onofrio et al., 2010; Lambe et al., 2006), suggesting the confounding role of genetic and familial factors.

Neuropsychological Functioning

Studies investigating the effect of prenatal nicotine exposure on executive functions such as memory, attention, self-regulation, and response inhibition have produced mixed findings. At preschool age, nicotine-exposed 4-year-old children demonstrated poorer selective attention than unexposed children (Noland et al., 2005). Maternal smoking during pregnancy was also associated with a decrease of 4-year-old children's global cognitive scores, and poorer executive function and working memory (Julvez et al., 2007). In 3-year-old children, prenatal tobacco exposure was related to lower motivational, but not cognitive self-regulation (Wiebe et al., 2015).

At school age, prenatal cigarette exposure has been associated with impaired speed of executive attention in 5–7-year-old children (Mezzacappa, Buckner, & Earls, 2011). Seven- to nine-year-olds exposed to prenatal smoking had poor emotional inhibitory control in a dose response manner but no relationship was found on a measure of cognitive inhibitory control (Huijbregts, Warren, de Sonneville, & Swaab-Barneveld, 2008). Significant associations between prenatal tobacco exposure and 10-year-olds' lower performance on tasks measuring verbal learning, design memory, problem solving, mental flexibility, and eye-hand coordination were reported (Cornelius, Ryan, Day, Goldschmidt, & Willford, 2001) but no differences were found in attention deficits or increased activity on a continuous performance task.

In adolescence, a relationship between prenatal cigarette smoking and auditory memory has been noted (Fried et al., 2003). However, an extensive neuropsychological battery of cognitive tests given to a large sample of 12–18-year-olds with and without prenatal nicotine exposure found no effects on any cognitive ability (IQ, academic achievement, executive functions) with cases matched by maternal education (Kafouri et al., 2009). The wide variety of neuropsychological measures used across different methodological approaches makes it difficult to draw definitive conclusions about prenatal nicotine exposure and its impact on specific executive function abilities (Clifford et al., 2012).

Language Functioning

Prenatal tobacco exposure has been linked to reduced language skills in childhood. In a polydrug exposed sample of children followed prospectively from birth to age 6, cigarette exposure was associated with lower receptive language scores (Lewis, Kirchner, et al. 2007). Lower auditory processing and receptive language skills have also been reported through age 12 (Fried et al., 1997). One large prospective birth cohort related higher prenatal nicotine exposure to poorer performance on language tasks and increased risk of language impairment at age 8 after adjusting for socioeconomic status, type of school attended, and parental interaction (Eicher et al., 2013).

Emotional and Behavioral Functioning

There are mixed findings on the association between prenatal nicotine exposure and child internalizing symptoms such as depression or anxiety, with some studies finding an association (Ashford, van Lier, Timmermans, Cuijpers, & Koot, 2008; Menezes et al., 2013; Moylan et al., 2015), while others did not (Brion et al., 2010; Lavigne et al., 2011). Prenatal nicotine exposure has been linked to a range of externalizing behavior problems consistently including inattention, hyperactivity, impulsivity, oppositional behavior, aggression, rule-breaking, delinquency, and peer problems, across childhood and adolescence (Cornelius et al., 2011; Cornelius, Goldschmidt, DeGenna, Day, & Goldschmidt, 2007; Day, Richardson, Goldschmidt, & Cornelius, 2000; Gatzke-Kopp & Beauchaine, 2007). Whether these effects are causal or due to genetic and other family environment factors remains a question (D'Onofrio et al., 2008, 2012; D'Onofrio, Van Hulle, Goodnight, Rathouz, & Lahey, 2012). A recent genetically sensitive study that examined the relationship between maternal smoking during pregnancy and conduct problems in children reared by biological and adoptive mothers across three pooled study samples found smoking during pregnancy to be a risk factor for offspring externalizing behavior problems even after control for child-rearing practices and the home environment (Gaysina et al., 2013). A comprehensive overview of prenatal nicotine exposure and behavioral findings of attentional, externalizing and internalizing problems concluded there is evidence of increased risk of conduct or externalizing problems in children (Tiesler & Heinrich, 2014).

Prenatal nicotine exposure increases the risk of early tobacco use as well as multiple substance use in adolescents (Goldschmidt, Cornelius, & Day, 2012; Lotfipour et al., 2009). Family background factors (D'Onofrio, Rickert, et al., 2012; D'Onofrio, Ricker, et al., 2012) and current maternal smoking and peer smoking (Cornelius, Leech, Goldschmidt, & Day, 2005) likely play confounding roles. Maternal smoking during pregnancy has been associated with increased risk of nicotine dependence in offspring (Buka, Shenassa, & Niaura, 2003), nearly doubling the risk that the child will meet diagnostic criteria for lifetime tobacco dependence in adulthood, if that child starts smoking.

Specific Diagnostic Outcomes

Maternal smoking during pregnancy is one of the most commonly cited prenatal risks associated with ADHD, with dose–response relationships evident (Thapar, Cooper, Eyre, & Langley, 2013). The risk of developing ADHD in children exposed in utero to nicotine ranges from 2.4 to 3.4 times higher than among unexposed children (Zhou et al., 2014). It is unclear whether the association is causal or due to confounding genetic or other household-level factors, in light of studies finding no association with increased ADHD risk that controlled for these factors (D'Onofrio et al., 2008; Thapar et al., 2009).

Support for the association of smoking during pregnancy and the diagnosis of conduct disorder (CD), a severe and persistent pattern of antisocial behavior, has also been found (Wakschlag, Pickett, Cook, Benowitz, & Leventhal, 2002). In particular, children born to mothers who smoke more than a half pack of cigarettes per day during pregnancy are up to four times more likely to have CD, and to have increased rates of oppositional defiant disorder (ODD) (Zhou et al., 2014). While some argue that these findings cannot be interpreted as causal (D'Onofrio, Van Hulle, et al., 2012), others (Slotkin, 2013; Tiesler & Heinrich, 2014) believe that the bulk of the evidence supports prenatal tobacco exposure as contributing to subsequent conduct problems in offspring.

Prognosis and Moderating Factors

The adverse effects of prenatal nicotine exposure on cognitive and behavioral outcomes have been shown to persist well into young adulthood (Cornelius, Goldschmidt, & Day, 2012; Mortensen et al., 2005). Low birth weight, maternal intelligence and education, SES, and other family environment factors (e.g., learning stimulation in the home) all play a role in the relationship between exposure and cognitive functioning (Clifford et al., 2012). A number of moderating factors have been demonstrated in the pathway from prenatal tobacco exposure to disruptive behaviors as well, including gender (early studies indicated the link was stronger in boys but recent findings are more contradictory), SES, parental psychopathology (e.g., ADHD or antisocial/criminal behavior), and caregiving environment (e.g., parental responsiveness) (Agrawal et al., 2010; Wakschlag et al., 2011).

Considerations for Prevention/Intervention

To prevent the negative effects of prenatal nicotine exposure on child development, women are advised to quit smoking before becoming pregnant. Once pregnant, smoking cessation should be done as early as possible to reduce impact on the developing fetus. Psychosocial support is an effective, evidence-based smoking cessation treatment for pregnant women, particularly if incentives are included. However, the safety and efficacy of pharmacotherapy during pregnancy (e.g., nicotine replacement therapy) remain unclear (Meernik & Goldstein, 2015).

For women who smoked during pregnancy, periodic developmental and behavioral assessment of their young children may identify early learning or behavioral problems requiring intervention. Parent training, behavior modification and wraparound services that target multiple family risk factors may reduce externalizing behaviors, while medication management may be warranted if a child is formally diagnosed with an attention deficit disorder. Specific interventions that target self-regulatory skills may alter trajectories toward severe behavior problems in children with prenatal tobacco exposure (Wiebe et al., 2015). School accommodations for learning, attention and/or disruptive behaviors may also become necessary if problems persist in childhood and adolescence.

Prenatal Cocaine Exposure

Definitional Issues and Prevalence

Cocaine is one of the most commonly abused illicit drugs in the USA and Europe. During the "cocaine epidemic" in the USA of the late 1980s and early 1990s it was estimated that 50,000–100,000 children were born prenatally with cocaine exposure each year, with higher rates reported in urban areas (National Institute on Drug Abuse, 1996; Ostrea, Brady, Gause, Raymundo, & Stevens, 1992). Although the annual rate of affected births has dropped since then, it is currently estimated that nearly 7.5 million children have been affected by prenatal cocaine exposure (PCE) in the USA (Chae & Covington, 2009). Worldwide, 0.5–3 % of pregnant women are estimated to use cocaine (Lamy & Thibaut, 2010).

Cocaine use in expensive powder form became prevalent in the 1980s when portrayed as a "safe" drug by President Carter's drug "czar". By the 1990s, a cheap smokable "crack" form had been manufactured and epidemic use occurred in major urban areas, primarily by poor, minority men and women. Information on developmental outcomes comes primarily from a number of large prospective birth cohort studies initiated by the NIH in the early 1990s, and drug effects are confounded with the environmental risks associated with "crack" cocaine use in poor urban areas.

Impact on the Developing Child

Maternal cocaine use exposes the fetal brain to a powerful stimulant that readily crosses the fetal blood–brain barrier and can act directly to disrupt monoamine neurotransmitter systems important for directing fetal brain development (Kosofsky, Wilkins, Gressens, & Evrard, 1994; McCarthy, Kabir, Bhide, & Kosofsky, 2014) particularly in brain areas known to impact reward systems and executive function (McCarthy et al., 2014). Prenatal cocaine exposure can also act indirectly via its vasoconstrictive properties that limit oxygen and nutrition to the developing fetal brain (Smeriglio & Wilcox, 1999). A number of well-controlled prospective studies indicate that PCE affects fetal physical growth, resulting in an increased likelihood of preterm birth, low birth weight, shorter birth length, smaller head circumference, and growth retardation, an indication of potential developmental delay (Gouin,

Murphy, Shah, & Knowledge Synthesis Group on Determinants of Low Birth Weight and Preterm Births, 2011). Recent data suggest PCE is associated with persistent disruption in dopamine signaling, changes in pyramidal neuron dendritic structure, and fewer GABA neurons, all of which can compromise the dopamine-rich prefrontal cortex (McCarthy et al., 2014; Thompson, Levitt, & Stanwood, 2009). These structural brain differences may underlie cognitive deficits, including executive function, attention, and inhibitory control, in prenatally cocaine exposed children.

Brain imaging studies of cocaine-exposed children have consistently noted morphologic differences from non-exposed samples. These include less gray matter in the parietal and occipital lobes and lower volume of the corpus callosum in 7–8-year-olds (Singer et al., 2006), lower volume of the right anterior cerebellum at 11 years of age, and smaller caudate at adolescence (Avants et al., 2007).

Intellectual Functioning

Although global cognitive deficits have been noted in cohorts of children 1–3 years of age with PCE (Behnke, Smith, & Committee on Substance Abuse, & Committee on Fetus and Newborn, 2013; Richardson, Goldschmidt, & Willford, 2008; Singer et al., 2002), specific, rather than overall cognitive differences have been found in older children with PCE. School age PCE cohorts and comparison substance-exposed children had mean IQ scores between 0.5 and 1.0 SD below the mean, reflective of their poor urban environments, low SES, and elevated lead levels (Ackerman, Riggins, & Black, 2010).

Academic Functioning

PCE has not been directly associated with child academic achievement (Frank et al., 2005; Singer et al., 2008). However, PCE children were 2.8 times more likely to demonstrate learning disabilities than non-exposed peers at age 7 (Morrow et al., 2006) and to need individualized education plans and special support services (Levine et al., 2008) than non-exposed children. At 4 years, cocaine-exposed boys had deficits in arithmetic skills compared to non-exposed peers (Singer et al., 2004).

Neuropsychological Functioning

PCE appears to disrupt specific neuropsychological functions, including attention, executive function, and visual perceptual organization, especially difficulties with sustained (Bandstra, Morrow, Anthony, Accornero, & Fried, 2001) and selective (Savage, Brodsky, Malmud, Giannetta, & Hurt, 2005) attention. PCE children were more likely to demonstrate commission errors (Noland et al., 2005) at age 4, and omission errors and slower reaction times at ages 5–7 (Accornero, Anthony, Morrow, Xue, & Bandstra, 2006; Roth, Isquith, & Gioia, 2005).

Negative effects of PCE on EF have been found via experimental neuropsychological tasks during infancy (Noland et al., 2003) and on standard neuropsychological assessments at elementary school age (Eyler et al., 2009; Mayes, Molfese, Key, & Hunter, 2005) and at adolescence (Richardson, Goldschmidt, Larkby, & Day, 2015). In a study of inhibitory control using the Stroop interference task (Bridgett & Mayes, 2011), children with PCE made more errors than non-cocaine exposed (NCE) children at 7 years, but had more age related improvements between 7 and 12 years. While girls in both groups improved faster than boys, PCE girls did not catch up to their NCE peers.

Gender specific effects were also found in a study using parental ratings of EF that assessed functional aspects of school and home life. At 12 years, girls with PCE were rated by caregivers to have more problems in metacognition (planning/organizing and self-monitoring) but not behavioral regulation (Min et al., 2014a, Min, Minnes, Yoon, Short, & Singer, 2014b). In contrast, PCE effects were found in boys only using a computerized go/no-go task (Carmody, Bennett, & Lewis, 2011). Boys with heavier PCE showed deficits in attention and inhibitory behaviors at ages 6, 9, and 11. Negative effects of heavier PCE on inhibitory control at 8.5–11 years of age were found compared to lighter PCE and NCE (Rose-Jacobs et al., 2009), but no effects were noted at 12–14 years of age (Rose-Jacobs et al., 2011).

The Cleveland Prenatal Cocaine Study found that children with PCE had deficits on Perceptual Reasoning tasks from the Wechsler IQ tests at ages 4, 9, and 15 (Singer et al., 2004, 2008; Singer, Minnes, Min, Lewis, & Short, 2015). These IQ tasks of Block Design, Picture Arrangement, and Object Assembly measure nonverbal reasoning, visual-spatial processing, visual-perceptual organization, and the ability to learn new information.

Emotional and Behavioral Functioning

In the preschool years, studies provide conflicting evidence of PCE effects on behavior (Dixon, Kurtz, & Chin, 2008). However, findings on behavioral regulation converge at school age with few exceptions (Ackerman et al., 2010). PCE effects have been found on child-reported symptoms of Oppositional Defiant Disorder (ODD) and ADHD at 6 years (Linares et al., 2006), on caregiver-reported aggressive and delinquent behavior at 9 years (McLaughlin et al., 2011), on child-reported depressive symptoms and teacher-rated anxious/depressed behavior at 10 years (Richardson, Larkby, Goldschmidt, & Day, 2013), on teacher- and caregiver-rated externalizing behavior problems at 7, 9, and 11 years (Bada et al., 2011), and on child-reported externalizing behavior at 12 (Min, Minnes, Lang, et al., 2014a) and 15 years (Min, Minnes, Lang, et al., 2014a; Min, Minnes, Yoon, et al., 2014b; Richardson et al., 2013). Mixed findings of PCE by gender on behavioral adjustment have been noted, with PCE boys showing more clinically significant externalizing and delinquent behaviors using teacher ratings (Delaney-Black et al., 2000) and self-report (Bennett, Marini, Berzenski, Carmody, & Lewis, 2013) while other studies report effects of PCE in girls only (McLaughlin et al., 2011; Minnes et al.,

2010; Sood et al., 2005). The negative effects of PCE on externalizing behaviors have been consistent across ages with small effect sizes at 0.20 SD on average (Ackerman et al., 2010; Singer et al., 2015).

PCE effects have been noted in adolescence on substance use (Delaney-Black et al., 2011; Frank et al., 2011; Minnes et al., 2014; Richardson et al., 2013) and early sexual behavior (De Genna, Goldschmidt, & Richardson, 2014; Min, Minnes, Lang, Yoon, & Singer, 2015). PCE adolescents self-reported more substance use related problems at age 15, and were more likely to experience accidents, forgetfulness, and mood swings when using alcohol or drugs (Min, Minnes, Lang, et al., 2014a).

Language Functioning

Studies of language development in PCE children have also been consistent even after controlling for multiple prenatal and environmental confounders (Ackerman et al., 2010; Lambert & Bauer, 2012). The Miami Prenatal Cocaine study (Bandstra et al., 2011) reported a gradient (dose-dependent) relationship between PCE and lower receptive, expressive, and total language scores at 3, 5, and 12 years of age, with expressive language being most affected. Deficits in expressive language observed at age 3 years persisted to age 12 years. The Cleveland study (Lewis, Kirchner, et al., 2007; Singer et al., 2001) found stable negative effects of cocaine on expressive language skills across 1, 2, 4, and 6 years of age (Lewis, Fulton, et al., 2007; Lewis, Kirchner, et al., 2007). This cohort continued to show PCE-associated language deficits related to syntax and phonological awareness at age 10 (Lewis et al., 2011) and 12 years (Lewis et al., 2013). Gender differences were noted with PCE girls differentially affected at age 10, consistent with other research.

Specific Diagnostic Outcomes

Studies from two birth cohorts (Linares et al., 2006; Morrow et al., 2009) reported that ADHD and ODD were associated with prenatal cocaine exposure although these findings should be considered preliminary until replicated.

Prognosis and Moderating Factors

The net effect of PCE is in the range of small to medium effect sizes. Children prenatally exposed to cocaine are likely to continue to have functional deficits due to the teratogenic effects of PCE and from associated risk factors (low SES, caregivers' ongoing substance use, poor parenting, and violence exposure). Compromised development in language skills, neuropsychological functioning, and externalizing behavior problems may lead to cascading effects in other developmental domains. As noted previously, gender may moderate PCE effects on behavior, but findings to date have been inconsistent.

Considerations for Prevention/Intervention

Interventions that provide stimulating, responsive caregiving may mitigate PCE effects in some aspects of development. In addition, drug treatment of maternal depressive symptoms during pregnancy may also mitigate harmful effects on the fetus (Singer et al., 2002; Singer, Salvator, et al., 2002). Preschool enrichment positively affected 4 year IQ in PCE children (Frank et al., 2005). A substantial (20–25 %) portion of PCE children from the Cleveland cohort placed in nonrelative foster-adoptive care had better quality home environments with lower lead levels, and caregivers with higher verbal skills and less depression than children with their biologic families. They also had better cognitive (Singer et al., 2004, 2008) and language (Lewis et al., 2011) outcomes compared to those in biological relative care through school age, that were positively correlated with the length of time in better caregiving environments (Singer et al., 2004). However, these protective effects were not found for behavioral outcomes (Linares et al., 2006; McLaughlin et al., 2011; Min, Minnes, Lang, et al., 2014a; Min, Minnes, Yoon, et al., 2014b; Minnes et al., 2010).

Amphetamines, Methamphetamine, and MDMA (3,4-Methylenedioxymethamphetamine)

Definitional Issues and Prevalence

Amphetamine and its related compounds are synthetic psychostimulants that resemble the neurotransmitter dopamine in chemical structure, accounting for their effects on the dopaminergic system. Amphetamine, methamphetamine, and 3,4, methylenedioxymethamphetamine (MDMA, "Ecstasy") are highly similar, but not identical, psychostimulants. They cross the placenta to increase the levels of norepinephrine, dopamine, and serotonin in the synaptic cleft via transporter reuptake inhibition (Ross, Graham, Money, & Stanwood, 2015). Amphetamine is composed of two distinct compounds, dextroamphetamine and levoamphetamine, and medications containing amphetamine are prescribed for narcolepsy, obesity, ADHD, and Parkinson's Disease. Prescription drugs containing amphetamine, such as Ritalin, Vyvanse, Adderall, and Concerta are frequently used by women of child bearing age with obesity and ADHD, but the prevalence of women using amphetamines for nonmedical reasons is currently unknown.

Methamphetamine and MDMA are illicit drugs that are part of the collective group of amphetamines. Substance Abuse and Mental Health Services Administration (2014) estimates that .3 % of adults age 18–25 reported using methamphetamine in the past month. The only study to assess methamphetamine prevalence in pregnant women found that 5 % of women in selected hospitals self-reported use in the US areas with significant overall use (Arria et al., 2006). Methamphetamine is more rapidly transported across the blood–brain barrier than amphetamine (Barr et al., 2006), with a higher potential for addiction.

MDMA, while similar to amphetamine, has additional hallucinogenic properties (Parrott, 2014) and a particular affinity for the serotonin transporter (Green, Mechan, Elliott, O'Shea, & Colado, 2003) in that 80 % of serotonin stores can be depleted in one episode. Usually taken in pill form, more recently MDMA has been popularized as "Molly", a powder form wrongly perceived as a safe form of the drug. MDMA has been called an "enactogen" referring to users' subjective experience of empathy, euphoria, and emotional warmth while using and has been used therapeutically to treat posttraumatic stress disorder.

MDMA is widely used recreationally throughout Europe, Australia, and the USA. Johnston et al. (2014) found 5.6 % of 12th graders in the USA reporting lifetime use of Ecstasy and Substance Abuse and Mental Health Services Administration (2014) reported 12.8 % of 18–25-year-olds with lifetime use. Amphetamine type stimulants have highest prevalence rates in New Zealand, Australia, and the western USA (Mohan, 2014). Their use has been increasing, moving eastward from epidemics first noted in the western and southwestern parts of the USA (Nordahl, Salo, & Leamon, 2003). Although effects of amphetamine type stimulants have been extensively studied in adults (Berman, Kuczenski, McCracken, & London, 2009; Nordahl et al., 2003; Parrott, 2014), the impact of prenatal exposure to these stimulants on child development has not been well documented.

Impact on the Developing Child

Given their similarities of action at the cellular level, the four major follow-up studies of prenatal amphetamine exposure will be summarized together. These studies include an early uncontrolled study from Sweden of growth and development of 65 children exposed to amphetamines through early adolescence (Billing, Eriksson, Larsson, & Zetterstrom, 1980). The New Zealand IDEAL study, a prospective, longitudinal, well-controlled study, has been following 100 methamphetamine-exposed children in comparison to similar non-exposed children since 2006 (Wouldes et al., 2014). The US IDEAL study recruited 204 methamphetamine-exposed and 208 non-exposed matched comparison children from four US sites (Los Angeles, CA; Des Moines, IA; Tulsa, OK; Honolulu, HI) and has followed them until 7.5 years old. The Drugs and Infancy Study (DAISY), a prospective longitudinal cohort design, followed 28 MDMA-exposed and 68 non-exposed infants from birth to 2 years of age using a volunteer sample of middle class recreational drug users from London, England. Infants were evaluated at 1, 4, 12, 18, and 24 months of age. The DAISY Study is the only available study worldwide to investigate prenatal MDMA exposure effects in humans (Moore et al., 2010).

Amphetamine exposure in pregnancy was associated with low birthweight and prematurity in one meta-analysis of ten small studies (Ladhani, Shah, Murphy, & Knowledge Synthesis Group on Determinants of Preterm/LBW Births, 2011). Several studies, including IDEAL, found that prenatal methamphetamine exposure was also related to prematurity, fetal growth retardation, and decreased birthweight, length, and head circumference (Smith et al., 2003). Methamphetamine-exposed infants appear to largely catch up in growth by 3 years of age. However, imaging studies indicated lower volume of the caudate nucleus and decreased cortical thickness at age 3 years in the same study (Zabaneh et al., 2012). In contrast, no differences were found in the DAISY study in birth complications or growth parameters, but MDMA exposure was associated with more male births, similar to findings of alterations in sex ratios seen with other toxins (Mocarelli et al., 2000; Singer, Moore, Fulton, et al., 2012a). One infant in the MDMA-exposed group in this study was diagnosed with Townes-Brocks Syndrome, a rare congenital anomaly that could not be attributed to MDMA exposure (Singer et al., 2012b). However, the finding is consistent with a study that found a 4–7 times higher risk of congenital malformations in a series of 136 MDMA-exposed pregnancies (McElhatton, Bateman, Evans, Pughe, & Thomas, 1999).

Structural brain abnormalities have been identified in children with prenatal methamphetamine exposure, i.e., regional brain volume reductions in the putamen, globus pallidus, hippocampus, and caudate and decreased cortical thickness (Chang et al., 2004), and lower apparent diffusion coefficient (ADC) in frontal and parietal white matter (Cloak, Ernst, Fujii, Hedemark, & Chang, 2009; Zabaneh et al., 2012). There are no similar studies of amphetamine or MDMA exposed infants.

Intellectual Functioning

Amphetamine-exposed children at age 4 had lower IQ scores, although in the average range of functioning, compared to a community sample in Sweden (Billing, Eriksson, Steneroth, & Zetterström, 1985). However, no differences in cognitive development related to methamphetamine exposure were found from 1–3 years of age on the Bayley Scales of Infant Development—Second Edition (BSID-II) relative to non-exposed children in the IDEAL Study through 7.5 years (Smith et al., 2011) nor in a small experimental study (Piper et al., 2011).

Similarly, no global differences on the MDI of the BSID-II between MDMA-exposed and non-exposed infants were found in the DAISY study. More heavily exposed infants achieved an MDI of 98.5 ± 11 vs. 103.4 ± 6 and 103.4 ± 9 for lighter exposed and non-exposed. However, heavier MDMA exposure prenatally was predictive of a lower Mental Development Index score at 12 months only (Singer, Moore, Min, et al., 2012b) at an age when the MDI items are heavily dependent on motor skills.

Academic Functioning

Fifteen percent of 14–15-year-old amphetamine-exposed children were 1 year behind their school-age peers in the Swedish study, with problems in language and mathematics (Cernerud, Eriksson, Jonsson, Steneroth, & Zetterstrom, 1996) but there are no other reports on school achievement related to methamphetamine, MDMA, or amphetamine-exposed children.

Neuropsychological Functioning

The US IDEAL study identified lower grasping scores on the Peabody Developmental Motor Scales (PDMS-2) associated with heavier methamphetamine exposure from 1 to 3 years, but did not find a relationship with fine or gross motor skills on the Bayley Scales of Psychomotor Development Index (PDI) (Smith et al., 2011). Similar, but even more consistent motor deficits were found in MDMA-exposed infants in the DAISY study. At 4 months, MDMA-exposed infants were slower moving and more delayed as assessed by the motor subscale of the Behavioral Rating Scale (BRS) of the BSID-II, and more heavily exposed infants performed more poorly than comparison infants on the Alberta Infant Motor Scale (AIMS) (Singer, Moore, Fulton, et al., 2012a). By 12 months, significant delays in motor skills were identified for more heavily exposed MDMA infants on the BSID-II PDI and the BRS motor quality scale (Singer, Moore, Min, et al., 2012b). By 2 years, heavily MDMA-exposed infants still lagged behind the lighter and non-exposed comparison groups (Singer et al., 2015; Singer, Minnes, Min, Lewis, Lang, et al., 2015; Singer, Minnes, Min, Lewis, & Short, 2015).

Other specific deficits have been found related to methamphetamine exposure in preschool and early school age children. A subsample from the US IDEAL study was administered the Conner's Kiddie Continuous Performance Test (K-CPT) at age 5.5 years. While no differences were found in omission or commission errors or reaction time for correct trials, prenatal exposure was associated with outcomes predictive of ADHD. In a sample of 31, 7–9-year-old methamphetamine-exposed children compared to 35 non-exposed on the Conner's Parent Rating Scale at 7.5 years, exposed children were 2.8 times more likely to be rated to have cognitive problem scores above average. Parents rated their children to have more problems in executive function and the children were more likely to show poorer performance in spatial memory compared to non-exposed children (Roussotte et al., 2011).

Emotional and Behavioral Functioning

Aggressive behavior and poorer social functioning were related to the amount and duration of prenatal amphetamine exposure in the Swedish cohort at 8 years (Billing, Eriksson, Jonsson, Steneroth, & Zetterström, 1994). Likewise, in the US IDEAL study, higher emotional reactivity and more anxiety, depressive, and ADHD symptoms were found at preschool age, but not at 7 1/2 years when using parent report (Smith et al., 2015). In the DAISY study, no effects of MDMA exposure were found on emotional regulation up to 2 years of age (Singer, Moore, Min, Goodwin, Turner, et al., 2015).

Impact on Other Areas of Functioning

The amphetamine exposed children in the Swedish cohort displayed deficits in math, language, and physical fitness activities at 14 years compared to normative groups (Cernerud et al., 1996), but no specific functional deficits have been noted in either the US or New Zealand IDEAL studies or the MDMA DAISY Study, although follow-up extends only from 2 to 7.5 years of age.

Specific Diagnostic Outcomes

Preschool outcomes in the US IDEAL Study suggested that ADHD was potentially related to methamphetamine exposure, a finding not replicated at early school age (Diaz et al., 2014).

Prognosis and Moderating Factors

The early identification of motor, executive function, and behavior regulation problems across these four cohorts raises concern about long-term school achievement and conduct problems in stimulant exposed children, although definitive outcomes await larger and longer term studies. As with cocaine and nicotine, environmental factors can either increase or decrease developmental risk. The IDEAL studies identified methamphetamine use to be associated with maternal psychiatric symptoms of paranoia, depression, suicidal ideation, and psychosis (Smith et al., 2015), problems that could be expected to affect child behavior. The Swedish cohort mothers had significant problems with alcoholism, also related to child outcomes (Billing, Eriksson, Steneroth, & Zetterstrom, 1988). In the DAISY study, no clinically significant differences in psychological distress symptoms in MDMA using women were noted although depressive symptoms were higher. These symptoms abated over the first year after infant birth coincident with decreased use of MDMA (Turner et al., 2014).

Considerations for Prevention/Intervention

Pregnant women should be apprised of the addictive potential of amphetamine type stimulants. Non-pharmacologic treatments for ADHD and weight control should be considered as first line interventions to prevent addiction. Treatment of depression, alcohol and substance use prenatally may mitigate physiologic effects on the fetus and improve maternal–child interactions after birth. As motor delays can be identified early in development, and have been noted in the longitudinal studies, early screening and intervention for amphetamine-exposed infants is warranted.

Conclusion

Prenatal nicotine exposure is robustly associated with externalizing behavior problems and, to a lesser extent, compromised cognitive functioning and academic achievement and an increased risk of teen tobacco and other substance use. While the exact causal mechanisms of these associations are not yet determined in humans, the adverse effects of prenatal nicotine exposure persist on a long-term basis. Public health education efforts about the dangers of smoking during pregnancy are warranted. The increasing use among young people of alternative tobacco products perceived to be less harmful, such as e-cigarettes, smokeless tobacco, and hookahs, is an area of needed future research.

Prenatal cocaine exposure is associated with compromised language development, suboptimal executive functions, and greater externalizing behavior problems, as well as an increased risk of teen substance use and early sexual behavior, reflecting long-lasting teratogenic effects of PCE. Amphetamines are among the most poorly researched stimulants regarding use during pregnancy and impact on the developing child, despite their widespread legal and illegal use, with no controlled longitudinal studies beyond the preschool years. Limited data available suggest significant effects on brain development, behavioral adjustment, and motor skills, although the research literature is too small to allow firm conclusions to be drawn.

Acknowledgement This study was supported by grant RO1-DA07957 NIH—National Institute on Drug Abuse.

References

Accornero, V. H., Anthony, J. C., Morrow, C. E., Xue, L., & Bandstra, E. S. (2006). Prenatal cocaine exposure: An examination of childhood externalizing and internalizing behavior problems at age 7 years. *Epidemiologia E Psichiatria Sociale, 15*(1), 20–29.

Ackerman, J. P., Riggins, T., & Black, M. M. (2010). A review of the effects of prenatal cocaine exposure among school-aged children. *Pediatrics, 125*(3), 554–565. doi:10.1542/peds.2009-0637.

Agrawal, A., Scherrer, J. F., Grant, J. D., Sartor, C. E., Pergadia, M. L., Duncan, A. E., et al. (2010). The effects of maternal smoking during pregnancy on offspring outcomes. *YPMED Preventive Medicine, 50*(1), 13–18.

Arria, A. M., Derauf, C., Lagasse, L. L., Grant, P., Shah, R., Smith, L., et al. (2006). Methamphetamine and other substance use during pregnancy: Preliminary estimates from the infant development, environment, and lifestyle (IDEAL) study. *Maternal and Child Health Journal, 10*(3), 293–302. doi:10.1007/s10995-005-0052-0.

Ashford, J., van Lier, P. A., Timmermans, M., Cuijpers, P., & Koot, H. M. (2008). Prenatal smoking and internalizing and externalizing problems in children studied from childhood to late adolescence. *Journal of the American Academy of Child and Adolescent Psychiatry, 47*(7), 779–787. doi:10.1097/CHI.0b013e318172eefb.

Avants, B. B., Hurt, H., Giannetta, J. M., Epstein, C. L., Shera, D. M., Rao, H., et al. (2007). Effects of heavy in utero cocaine exposure on adolescent caudate morphology. *Pediatric Neurology, 37*(4), 275–279. doi:S0887-8994(07)00328-1 [pii].

Bada, H. S., Bann, C. M., Bauer, C. R., Shankaran, S., Lester, B., LaGasse, L., et al. (2011). Preadolescent behavior problems after prenatal cocaine exposure: Relationship between teacher and caretaker ratings (maternal lifestyle study). *Neurotoxicology and Teratology, 33*(1), 78–87. doi:10.1016/j.ntt.2010.06.005.

Bandstra, E. S., Morrow, C. E., Accornero, V. H., Mansoor, E., Xue, L., & Anthony, J. C. (2011). Estimated effects of in utero cocaine exposure on language development through early adolescence. *Neurotoxicology and Teratology, 33*(1), 25–35. doi:10.1016/j.ntt.2010.07.001.

Bandstra, E. S., Morrow, C. E., Anthony, J. C., Accornero, V. H., & Fried, P. A. (2001). Longitudinal investigation of task persistence and sustained attention in children with prenatal cocaine exposure. *Neurotoxicology and Teratology, 23*(6), 545–559.

Barr, A. M., Panenka, W. J., MacEwan, G. W., Thornton, A. E., Lang, D. J., Honer, W. G., et al. (2006). The need for speed: An update on methamphetamine addiction. *Journal of Psychiatry & Neuroscience, 31*(5), 301–313.

Barros, A. M., Mitsuhiro, S. S., Chalem, E., Laranjeira, R. R., & Guinsburg, R. (2011). Prenatal tobacco exposure is related to neurobehavioral modifications in infants of adolescent mothers. *Clinics (Sao Paulo, Brazil), 66*(9), 1597–1603.

Batstra, L., Hadders-Algra, M., & Neeleman, J. (2003). Effect of antenatal exposure to maternal smoking on behavioural problems and academic achievement in childhood: Prospective evidence from a Dutch birth cohort. *Early Human Development, 75*(1-2), 21–33.

Batty, G. D., Der, G., & Deary, I. J. (2006). Effect of maternal smoking during pregnancy on offspring's cognitive ability: Empirical evidence for complete confounding in the US national longitudinal survey of youth. *Pediatrics, 118*(3), 943–950.

Behnke, M., Smith, V. C., & Committee on Substance Abuse, & Committee on Fetus and Newborn. (2013). Prenatal substance abuse: Short- and long-term effects on the exposed fetus. *Pediatrics, 131*(3), 1009–1024. doi:10.1542/peds.2012-3931.

Bennett, D. S., Marini, V. A., Berzenski, S. R., Carmody, D. P., & Lewis, M. (2013). Externalizing problems in late childhood as a function of prenatal cocaine exposure and environmental risk. *Journal of Pediatric Psychology, 38*(3), 296–308. doi:10.1093/jpepsy/jss117.

Berman, S. M., Kuczenski, R., McCracken, J. T., & London, E. D. (2009). Potential adverse effects of amphetamine treatment on brain and behavior: A review. *Molecular Psychiatry, 14*(2), 123–142.

Billing, L., Eriksson, M., Jonsson, B., Steneroth, G., & Zetterström, R. (1994). The influence of environmental factors on behavioural problems in 8-year-old children exposed to amphetamine during fetal life. *Child Abuse & Neglect, 18*(1), 3–9.

Billing, L., Eriksson, M., Larsson, G., & Zetterstrom, R. (1980). Amphetamine addiction and pregnancy. III. One year follow-up of the children. Psychosocial and pediatric aspects. *Acta Paediatrica Scandinavica, 69*(5), 675–680.

Billing, L., Eriksson, M., Steneroth, G., & Zetterström, R. (1985). Pre-school children of amphetamine-addicted mothers. I. Somatic and psychomotor development. *Acta Paediatrica Scandinavica, 74*(2), 179–184.

Billing, L., Eriksson, M., Steneroth, G., & Zetterstrom, R. (1988). Predictive indicators for adjustment in 4-year-old children whose mothers used amphetamine during pregnancy. *Child Abuse & Neglect, 12*(4), 503–507. doi: 0145-2134(88)90067-1 [pii].

Bridgett, D. J., & Mayes, L. C. (2011). Development of inhibitory control among prenatally cocaine exposed and non-cocaine exposed youths from late childhood to early adolescence: The effects of gender and risk and subsequent aggressive behavior. *Neurotoxicology and Teratology, 33*(1), 47–60. doi:10.1016/j.ntt.2010.08.002.

Brion, M. J., Victora, C., Matijasevich, A., Horta, B., Anselmi, L., Steer, C., et al. (2010). Maternal smoking and child psychological problems: Disentangling causal and noncausal effects. *Pediatrics, 126*(1), e57–e65. doi:10.1542/peds.2009-2754.

Bublitz, M. H., & Stroud, L. R. (2012). Maternal smoking during pregnancy and offspring brain structure and function: Review and agenda for future research. *Nicotine & Tobacco Research, 14*(4), 388–397. doi:10.1093/ntr/ntr191.

Buka, S. L., Shenassa, E. D., & Niaura, R. (2003). Elevated risk of tobacco dependence among offspring of mothers who smoked during pregnancy: A 30-year prospective study. *The American Journal of Psychiatry, 160*(11), 1978–1984.

Carmody, D. P., Bennett, D. S., & Lewis, M. (2011). The effects of prenatal cocaine exposure and gender on inhibitory control and attention. *Neurotoxicology and Teratology, 33*(1), 61–68. doi:10.1016/j.ntt.2010.07.004.

Centers for Disease Control and Prevention. (2013). Trends in smoking before, during, and after pregnancy: Pregnancy risk assessment monitoring system (PRAMS), United States, 40 sites, 2000–2010. *Morbidity and Mortality Weekly Report, 62*(6), 1–19.

Centers for Disease Control and Prevention. (2014). *Fact sheet: Health effects of secondhand smoke, March 5*. Atlanta, GA: Centers for Disease Control and Prevention. Retrieved from http://Www.cdc.gov/tobacco/data_statistics/fact_sheets/secondhand_smoke/health_effects.

Cernerud, L., Eriksson, M., Jonsson, B., Steneroth, G., & Zetterstrom, R. (1996). Amphetamine addiction during pregnancy: 14-year follow-up of growth and school performance. *Acta Paediatrica, 85*, 204–208.

Chae, S. M., & Covington, C. Y. (2009). Biobehaivoral outcomes in adolescents and young adults prenatally exposed to cocaine: Evidence from animal models. *Biological Research for Nursing, 10*, 318–330.

Chang, L., Smith, L. M., LoPresti, C., Yonekura, M. L., Kuo, J., Walot, I., & Ernst, T. (2004). Smaller subcortical volumes and cognitive deficits in children with prenatal methamphetamine exposure. *Psychiatry Research, 132*(2), 95–106. doi:S0925-4927(04)00073-3 [pii].

Cho, K., Frijters, J. C., Zhang, H., Miller, L. L., & Gruen, J. R. (2013). Prenatal exposure to nicotine and impaired reading performance. *The Journal of Pediatrics, 162*(4), 713–718.e2. doi:10.1016/j.jpeds.2012.09.041.

Clifford, A., Lang, L., & Chen, R. (2012). Effects of maternal cigarette smoking during pregnancy on cognitive parameters of children and young adults: A literature review. *NTT Neurotoxicology and Teratology, 34*(6), 560–570.

Cloak, C. C., Ernst, T., Fujii, L., Hedemark, B., & Chang, L. (2009). Lower diffusion in white matter of children with prenatal methamphetamine exposure. *Neurology, 72*(24), 2068–2075. doi:10.1212/01.wnl.0000346516.49126.20.

Coles, C. D., Bard, K. A., Platzman, K. A., & Lynch, M. E. (1999). Attentional response at eight weeks in prenatally drug-exposed and preterm infants. *Neurotoxicology and Teratology, 21*(5), 527–537. doi:S0892-0362(99)00023-9 [pii].

Cornelius, M. D., De Genna, N. M., Leech, S. L., Willford, J. A., Goldschmidt, L., & Day, N. L. (2011). Effects of prenatal cigarette smoke exposure on neurobehavioral outcomes in 10-year-old children of adolescent mothers. *Neurotoxicology and Teratology, 33*(1), 137–144. doi:10.1016/j.ntt.2010.08.006.

Cornelius, M. D., Goldschmidt, L., DeGenna, N., Day, N. L., & Goldschmidt, L. (2007). Smoking during teenage pregnancies: Effects on behavioral problems in offspring. *Nicotine & Tobacco Research, 9*(7), 739–750.

Cornelius, M. D., Goldschmidt, L., & Day, N. L. (2012). Prenatal cigarette smoking: Long-term effects on young adult behavior problems and smoking behavior. *NTT Neurotoxicology and Teratology, 34*(6), 554–559.

Cornelius, M. D., Leech, S. L., Goldschmidt, L., & Day, N. L. (2005). Is prenatal tobacco exposure a risk factor for early adolescent smoking? A follow-up study. *NTT Neurotoxicology and Teratology, 27*(4), 667–676.

Cornelius, M. D., Ryan, C. M., Day, N. L., Goldschmidt, L., & Willford, J. A. (2001). Prenatal tobacco effects on neuropsychological outcomes among preadolescents. *Journal of Developmental and Behavioral Pediatrics, 22*(4), 217–225.

Day, N. L., Richardson, G. A., Goldschmidt, L., & Cornelius, M. D. (2000). Effects of prenatal tobacco exposure on preschoolers' behavior. *Journal of Developmental and Behavioral Pediatrics, 21*(3), 180–188.

De Genna, N., Goldschmidt, L., & Richardson, G. A. (2014). Prenatal cocaine exposure and age of sexual initiation: Direct and indirect effects. *Drug and Alcohol Dependence, 145*, 194–200. doi:10.1016/j.drugalcdep.2014.10.011.

Delaney-Black, V., Chiodo, L. M., Hannigan, J. H., Greenwald, M. K., Janisse, J., Patterson, G., et al. (2011). Prenatal and postnatal cocaine exposure predict teen cocaine use. *Neurotoxicology and Teratology, 33*(1), 110–119. doi:10.1016/j.ntt.2010.06.011.

Delaney-Black, V., Covington, C., Templin, T., Ager, J., Nordstrom-Klee, B., Martier, S., et al. (2000). Teacher-assessed behavior of children prenatally exposed to cocaine. *Pediatrics, 106*(4), 782–791.

Diaz, S. D., Smith, L. M., LaGasse, L. L., Derauf, C., Newman, E., Shah, R., et al. (2014). Effects of prenatal methamphetamine exposure on behavioral and cognitive findings at 7.5 years of age. *The Journal of Pediatrics, 164*(6), 1333–1338. doi:10.1016/j.jpeds.2014.01.053.

Dixon, D. R., Kurtz, P. F., & Chin, M. D. (2008). A systematic review of challenging behaviors in children exposed prenatally to substances of abuse. *Research in Developmental Disabilities, 29*(6), 483–502. doi:S0891-4222(07)00051-0 [pii].

D'Onofrio, B, M., Van Hulle, C. A., Waldman, I. D., Rodgers, J. L., Harden, K. P., Rathouz, P. J., & Lahey, B. B. (2008). Smoking during pregnancy and offspring externalizing problems: An exploration of genetic and environmental confounds. *Development and Psychopathology, 20*(1), 139–164. doi:10.1017/S0954579408000072.

D'Onofrio, B. M., Rickert, M. E., Langstrom, N., Donahue, K. L., Coyne, C. A., Larsson, H., et al. (2012). Familial confounding of the association between maternal smoking during pregnancy and offspring substance use and problems. *Archives of General Psychiatry, 69*(11), 1140–1150. doi:10.1001/archgenpsychiatry.2011.2107.

D'Onofrio, B. M., Singh, A. L., Iliadou, A., Lambe, M., Hultman, C. M., Neiderhiser, J. M., et al. (2010). A quasi-experimental study of maternal smoking during pregnancy and offspring academic achievement. *Child Development, 81*(1), 80–100.

D'Onofrio, B. M., Van Hulle, C. A., Goodnight, J. A., Rathouz, P. J., & Lahey, B. B. (2012). Is maternal smoking during pregnancy a causal environmental risk factor for adolescent antisocial behavior? Testing etiological theories and assumptions. *Psychological Medicine, 42*(7), 1535–1545.

Dwyer, J. B., McQuown, S. C., & Leslie, F. M. (2009). The dynamic effects of nicotine on the developing brain. *Pharmacology & Therapeutics, 122*(2), 125–139. doi:10.1016/j.pharmthera.2009.02.003.

Eicher, J. D., Powers, N. R., Cho, K., Miller, L. L., Mueller, K. L., Ring, S. M., et al. (2013). Associations of prenatal nicotine exposure and the dopamine related genes ANKK1 and DRD2 to verbal language. *PloS One, 8*(5), e63762. doi:10.1371/journal.pone.0063762.

Eyler, F. D., Behnke, M., Conlon, M., Woods, N. S., & Wobie, K. (1998). Birth outcome from a prospective, matched study of prenatal crack/cocaine use: II. Interactive and dose effects on neurobehavioral assessment. *Pediatrics, 101*(2), 237–241.

Eyler, F. D., Warner, T. D., Behnke, M., Hou, W., Wobie, K., & Garvan, C. W. (2009). Executive functioning at ages 5 and 7 years in children with prenatal cocaine exposure. *Developmental Neuroscience, 31*(1-2), 121–136. doi:10.1159/000207500.

Frank, D. A., Rose-Jacobs, R., Beeghly, M., Wilbur, M., Bellinger, D., & Cabral, H. (2005). Level of prenatal cocaine exposure and 48-month IQ: Importance of preschool enrichment. *Neurotoxicology and Teratology, 27*(1), 15–28.

Frank, D. A., Rose-Jacobs, R., Crooks, D., Cabral, H. J., Gerteis, J., Hacker, K. A., et al. (2011). Adolescent initiation of licit and illicit substance use: Impact of intrauterine exposures and post-natal exposure to violence. *Neurotoxicology and Teratology, 33*(1), 100–109. doi:10.1016/j.ntt.2010.06.002.

Fried, P. A., Watkinson, B., & Gray, R. (2003). Differential effects on cognitive functioning in 13- to 16-year-olds prenatally exposed to cigarettes and marihuana. *Neurotoxicology and Teratology, 25*(4), 427–436.

Fried, P. A., Watkinson, B., & Siegel, L. S. (1997). Reading and language in 9- to 12-year olds prenatally exposed to cigarettes and marijuana. *Neurotoxicology and Teratology, 19*(3), 171–183. doi:S0892036297000159 [pii].

Gatzke-Kopp, L. M., & Beauchaine, T. P. (2007). Direct and passive prenatal nicotine exposure and the development of externalizing psychopathology. *Child Psychiatry and Human Development, 38*(4), 255–269. doi:10.1007/s10578-007-0059-4.

Gaysina, D., Fergusson, D. M., Leve, L. D., Horwood, J., Reiss, D., Shaw, D. S., et al. (2013). Maternal smoking during pregnancy and offspring conduct problems: Evidence from 3 independent genetically sensitive research designs. *JAMA Psychiatry, 70*(9), 956–963.

Goldschmidt, L., Cornelius, M. D., & Day, N. L. (2012). Prenatal cigarette smoke exposure and early initiation of multiple substance use. *Nicotine & Tobacco Research, 14*(6), 694–702. doi:10.1093/ntr/ntr280.

Gouin, K., Murphy, K., Shah, P. S., & Knowledge Synthesis Group on Determinants of Low Birth Weight and Preterm Births. (2011). Effects of cocaine use during pregnancy on low birthweight and preterm birth: Systematic review and metaanalyses. *American Journal of Obstetrics and Gynecology, 204*(4), 340.e1-340.1. doi:10.1016/j.ajog.2010.11.013.

Green, A. R., Mechan, A. O., Elliott, J. M., O'Shea, E., & Colado, M. I. (2003). The pharmacology and clinical pharmacology of 3,4-methylenedioxymethamphetamine (MDMA, "ecstasy"). *Pharmacology Review, 55*(3), 463–508.

Hernandez-Martinez, C., Arija Val, V., Escribano Subias, J., & Canals Sans, J. (2012). A longitudinal study on the effects of maternal smoking and secondhand smoke exposure during pregnancy on neonatal neurobehavior. *Early Human Development, 88*(6), 403–408. doi:10.1016/j.earlhumdev.2011.10.004.

Huijbregts, S. C., Warren, A. J., de Sonneville, L. M., & Swaab-Barneveld, H. (2008). Hot and cool forms of inhibitory control and externalizing behavior in children of mothers who smoked during pregnancy: An exploratory study. *Journal of Abnormal Child Psychology, 36*(3), 323–333. doi:10.1007/s10802-007-9180-x.

Johnston, L. D., O'Malley, P. M., Miech, R. A., Bachman, J. G., & Schulenberg, J. E. (2014). *Monitoring the future, national survey results on drug use 2014 overview key findings on adolescent drug use*. Ann Arbor, MI: Institute for Social Research, the University of Michigan.

Julvez, J., Ribas-Fitó, N., Torrent, M., Forns, M., Garcia-Esteban, R., & Sunyer, J. (2007). Maternal smoking habits and cognitive development of children at age 4 years in a population-based birth cohort. *International Journal of Epidemiology, 36*(4), 825–832.

Kafouri, S., Leonard, G., Perron, M., Richer, L., Seguin, J. R., Veillette, S., et al. (2009). Maternal cigarette smoking during pregnancy and cognitive performance in adolescence. *International Journal of Epidemiology, 38*(1), 158–172. doi:10.1093/ije/dyn250.

Kosofsky, B. E., Wilkins, A. S., Gressens, P., & Evrard, P. (1994). Transplacental cocaine exposure: A mouse model demonstrating neuroanatomic and behavioral abnormalities. *Journal of Child Neurology, 9*(3), 234–241.

Ladhani, N. N., Shah, P. S., Murphy, K. E., & Knowledge Synthesis Group on Determinants of Preterm/LBW Births. (2011). Prenatal amphetamine exposure and birth outcomes: A systematic review and metaanalysis. *American Journal of Obstetrics and Gynecology, 205*(3), 219e1–219.e7. doi:10.1016/j.ajog.2011.04.016.

Lambe, M., Hultman, C., Torrang, A., Maccabe, J., & Cnattingius, S. (2006). Maternal smoking during pregnancy and school performance at age 15. *Epidemiology (Cambridge, MA), 17*(5), 524–530. doi:10.1097/01.ede.0000231561.49208.be.

Lambert, B. L., & Bauer, C. R. (2012). Developmental and behavioral consequences of prenatal cocaine exposure: A review. *Journal of Perinatology, 32*(11), 819–828. doi:10.1038/jp.2012.90.

Lamy, S., & Thibaut, F. (2010). Psychoactive substance use during pregnancy: A review. [Etat des lieux de la consommation de substances psychoactives par les femmes enceintes]. *L'Encephale, 36*(1), 33–38. doi:10.1016/j.encep.2008.12.009.

Lavigne, J. V., Hopkins, J., Gouze, K. R., Bryant, F. B., LeBailly, S. A., Binns, H. J., & Lavigne, P. M. (2011). Is smoking during pregnancy a risk factor for psychopathology in young children? A methodological caveat and report on preschoolers. *Journal of Pediatric Psychology, 36*(1), 10–24. doi:10.1093/jpepsy/jsq044.

Law, K. L., Stroud, L. R., LaGasse, L. L., Niaura, R., Liu, J., & Lester, B. M. (2003). Smoking during pregnancy and newborn neurobehavior. *Pediatrics, 111*(6 Pt 1), 1318–1323.

Levine, T. P., Liu, J., Das, A., Lester, B., Lagasse, L., Shankaran, S., et al. (2008). Effects of prenatal cocaine exposure on special education in school-aged children. *Pediatrics, 122*(1), e83–e91. doi:10.1542/peds.2007-2826.

Lewis, B. A., Kirchner, H. L., Short, E. J., Minnes, S., Weishampel, P., Satayathum, S., et al. (2007). Prenatal cocaine and tobacco effects on children's language trajectories. *Pediatrics, 120*(1), 78–85.

Lewis, B. A., Minnes, S., Short, E. J., Min, M. O., Wu, M., Lang, A., et al. (2013). Language outcomes at 12 years for children exposed prenatally to cocaine. *Journal of Speech Language and Hearing Research, 56*(5), 1662–1676. doi:10.1044/1092-4388(2013/12-0119).

Lewis, B. A., Minnes, S., Short, E. J., Weishampel, P., Satayathum, S., Min, M. O., et al. (2011). The effects of prenatal cocaine on language development at 10 years of age. *Neurotoxicology and Teratology, 33*(1), 17–24. doi:10.1016/j.ntt.2010.06.006.

Linares, T. J., Singer, L. T., Kirchner, H. L., Short, E. J., Min, M. O., Hussey, P., et al. (2006). Mental health outcomes of cocaine-exposed children at 6 years of age. *Journal of Pediatric Psychology, 31*(1), 85–97. doi:10.1093/jpepsy/jsj020.

Lotfipour, S., Ferguson, E., Leonard, G., Perron, M., Pike, B., Richer, L., et al. (2009). Orbitofrontal cortex and drug use during adolescence: Role of prenatal exposure to maternal smoking and BDNF genotype. *Archives of General Psychiatry, 66*(11), 1244–1252. doi:10.1001/archgenpsychiatry.2009.124.

Martin, R. P., Dombrowski, S. C., Mullis, C., Wisenbaker, J., & Huttunen, M. O. (2006). Smoking during pregnancy: Association with childhood temperament, behavior, and academic performance. *Journal of Pediatric Psychology, 31*(5), 490–500.

Mayes, L. C., Molfese, D. L., Key, A. P., & Hunter, N. C. (2005). Event-related potentials in cocaine-exposed children during a Stroop task. *Neurotoxicology and Teratology, 27*(6), 797–813.

McCarthy, D. M., Kabir, Z. D., Bhide, P. G., & Kosofsky, B. E. (2014). Effects of prenatal exposure to cocaine on brain structure and function. *Progress in Brain Research, 211*, 277–289. doi:10.1016/B978-0-444-63425-2.00012-X.

McElhatton, P. R., Bateman, D. N., Evans, C., Pughe, K. R., & Thomas, S. H. (1999). Congenital anomalies after prenatal ecstasy exposure. *Lancet, 354*(9188), 1441–1442.

McLaughlin, A. A., Minnes, S., Singer, L. T., Min, M., Short, E. J., Scott, T. L., et al. (2011). Caregiver and self-report of mental health symptoms in 9-year old children with prenatal cocaine exposure. *Neurotoxicology and Teratology, 33*(5), 582–591. doi:10.1016/j.ntt.2011.03.002.

Meernik, C., & Goldstein, A. O. (2015). A critical review of smoking, cessation, relapse and emerging research in pregnancy and post-partum. *British Medical Bulletin, 114*(1), 135–146. doi:10.1093/bmb/ldv016.

Menezes, A. M., Murray, J., Laszlo, M., Wehrmeister, F. C., Hallal, P. C., Goncalves, H., et al. (2013). Happiness and depression in adolescence after maternal smoking during pregnancy: Birth cohort study. *PLoS One, 8*(11), e80370. doi:10.1371/journal.pone.0080370.

Meyer, J. S., & Quenzer, L. F. (2005). *Psychopharmacology: Drugs, the brain, and behavior*. Sunderland, MA: Sinauer Associates, Publishers.

Mezzacappa, E., Buckner, J. C., & Earls, F. (2011). Prenatal cigarette exposure and infant learning stimulation as predictors of cognitive control in childhood. *Developmental Science, 14*(4), 881–891. doi:10.1111/j.1467-7687.2011.01038.x.

Min, M. O., Minnes, S., Lang, A., Weishampel, P., Short, E. J., Yoon, S., et al. (2014a). Externalizing behavior and substance use related problems at 15 years in prenatally cocaine exposed adolescents. *Journal of Adolescence, 37*(3), 269–279. doi:10.1016/j.adolescence.2014.01.004.

Min, M. O., Minnes, S., Lang, A., Yoon, S., & Singer, L. T. (2015). Effects of prenatal cocaine exposure on early sexual behavior: Gender difference in externalizing behavior as a mediator. *Drug and Alcohol Dependence, 153*, 59–65. doi:10.1016/j.drugalcdep.2015.06.009.

Min, M. O., Minnes, S., Yoon, S., Short, E. J., & Singer, L. T. (2014b). Self-reported adolescent behavioral adjustment: Effects of prenatal cocaine exposure. *Journal of Adolescence Health, 55*(2), 167–174. doi:10.1016/j.jadohealth.2013.12.032.

Minnes, S., Singer, L. T., Kirchner, H. L., Short, E., Lewis, B., Satayathum, S., et al. (2010). The effects of prenatal cocaine exposure on problem behavior in children 4-10 years. *Neurotoxicology and Teratology, 32*(4), 443–451. doi:10.1016/j.ntt.2010.03.005.

Minnes, S., Singer, L., Min, M. O., Wu, M., Lang, A., & Yoon, S. (2014). Effects of prenatal cocaine/polydrug exposure on substance use by age 15. *Drug and Alcohol Dependence, 134*, 201–210. doi:10.1016/j.drugalcdep.2013.09.031.

Mocarelli, P., Gerthoux, P. M., Ferrari, E., Patterson, D. G., Kieszak, J. S. M., Brambilla, P., et al. (2000). Paternal concentrations of dioxin and sex ratio of offspring. *Lancet, 355*(9218), 1858–1863.

Mohan, J. (Ed.). (2014). *World drug report 2014*. Vienna: United Nations Office on Drugs and Crime. No. ISBN 978-92-1-056752-7; pp 2, 3, 123–152.

Moore, D. G., Turner, J. D., Parrott, A. C., Goodwin, J. E., Fulton, S. E., Min, M. O., et al. (2010). During pregnancy, recreational drug-using women stop taking ecstasy (3,4-methylenedioxy-N-methylamphetamine) and reduce alcohol consumption, but continue to smoke tobacco and cannabis: Initial findings from the development and infancy study. *Journal of Psychopharmacology, 24*(9), 1403–1410. doi:10.1177/0269881109348165.

Morrow, C. E., Accornero, V. H., Xue, L., Manjunath, S., Culbertson, J. L., Anthony, J. C., et al. (2009). Estimated risk of developing selected DSM-IV disorders among 5-year-old children with prenatal cocaine exposure. *Journal of Child and Family Studies, 18*(3), 356–364.

Morrow, C. E., Culbertson, J. L., Accornero, V. H., Xue, L., Anthony, J. C., & Bandstra, E. S. (2006). Learning disabilities and intellectual functioning in school-aged children with prenatal cocaine exposure. *Developmental Neuropsychology, 30*(3), 905–931. doi:10.1207/s15326942dn3003_8.

Mortensen, E. L., Michaelsen, K. F., Sanders, S. A., & Reinisch, J. M. (2005). A dose-response relationship between maternal smoking during late pregnancy and adult intelligence in male offspring. *Paediatric and Perinatal Epidemiology, 19*(1), 4–11.

Moylan, S., Gustavson, K., Overland, S., Karevold, E. B., Jacka, F. N., Pasco, J. A., & Berk, M. (2015). The impact of maternal smoking during pregnancy on depressive and anxiety behaviors in children: The Norwegian mother and child cohort study. *BMC Medicine, 13*(1), 24-014-0257-4. doi:10.1186/s12916-014-0257-4.

National Institute on Drug Abuse. (1996). *National pregnancy and health survey: Drug use among women delivering live births, 1992*. (No. NIH publication no. 96-3819). doi:10.3886/ICPSR02835.v2.

National Institute on Drug Abuse – US Department of Health and Human Services, National Institutes of Health. (2012). *Smoking and pregnancy – what are the risks*. (No. NIH Publication Number 12-4342).

Noland, J. S., Singer, L. T., Arendt, R. E., Minnes, S., Short, E. J., & Bearer, C. F. (2003). Executive functioning in preschool-age children prenatally exposed to alcohol, cocaine, and marijuana. *Alcoholism, Clinical and Experimental Research, 27*(4), 647–656. doi:10.1097/01.ALC.0000060525.10536.F6.

Noland, J. S., Singer, L. T., Short, E. J., Minnes, S., Arendt, R. E., Kirchner, H. L., et al. (2005). Prenatal drug exposure and selective attention in preschoolers. *Neurotoxicology and Teratology, 27*(3), 429–438. doi:10.1016/j.ntt.2005.02.001.

Nordahl, T. E., Salo, R., & Leamon, M. (2003). Neuropsychological effects of chronic methamphetamine use on neurotransmitters and cognition: A review. *The Journal of Neuropsychiatry and Clinical Neurosciences, 15*(3), 317–325.

Ostrea, E. M., Brady, M., Gause, S., Raymundo, A. L., & Stevens, M. (1992). Drug screening of newborns by meconium analysis: A large-scale, prospective, epidemiologic study. *Pediatrics, 89*(1), 107–113.

Parrott, A. C. (2014). Why all stimulant drugs are damaging to recreational users: An empirical overview and psychobiological explanation. *Human Psychopharmacology: Clinical and Experimental, 30*(4), 213–224. doi:10.1002/hup.2468.

Piper, B. J., Acevedo, S. F., Kolchugina, G. K., Butler, R. W., Corbett, S. M., Honeycutt, E. B., et al. (2011). Abnormalities in parentally rated executive function in methamphetamine/polysubstance exposed children. *Pharmacology, Biochemistry, and Behavior, 98*(3), 432–439. doi:10.1016/j.pbb.2011.02.013.

Primo, C. C., Ruela, P. B., Brotto, L. D., Garcia, T. R., & Ede Lima, F. (2013). Effects of maternal nicotine on breastfeeding infants. *Revista Paulista De Pediatria, 31*(3), 392–397. doi:10.1590/S0103-05822013000300018.

Richardson, G. A., Goldschmidt, L., Larkby, C., & Day, N. L. (2015). Effects of prenatal cocaine exposure on adolescent development. *Neurotoxicology and Teratology, 49*, 41–48. doi:S0892-0362(15)00035-5 [pii].

Richardson, G. A., Goldschmidt, L., & Willford, J. (2008). The effects of prenatal cocaine use on infant development. *Neurotoxicology and Teratology, 30*(2), 96–106.

Richardson, G. A., Larkby, C., Goldschmidt, L., & Day, N. L. (2013). Adolescent initiation of drug use: Effects of prenatal cocaine exposure. *Journal of the American Academy of Child & Adolescent Psychiatry, 52*(1), 37–46. doi:10.1016/j.jaac.2012.10.011.

Rogers, J. M. (2009). Tobacco and pregnancy. *Reproductive Toxicology (Elmsford, NY), 28*(2), 152–160. doi:10.1016/j.reprotox.2009.03.012.

Rose-Jacobs, R., Soenksen, S., Appugliese, D. P., Cabral, H. J., Richardson, M. A., Beeghly, M., et al. (2011). Early adolescent executive functioning, intrauterine exposures and own drug use. *Neurotoxicology and Teratology, 33*(3), 379–392. doi:10.1016/j.ntt.2011.02.013.

Rose-Jacobs, R., Waber, D., Beeghly, M., Cabral, H., Appugleise, D., Heeren, T., et al. (2009). Intrauterine cocaine exposure and executive functioning in middle childhood. *Neurotoxicology and Teratology, 31*(3), 159–168. doi:10.1016/j.ntt.2008.12.002.

Ross, E. J., Graham, D. L., Money, K. M., & Stanwood, G. D. (2015). Developmental consequences of fetal exposure to drugs: What we know and what we still must learn. *Neuropsychopharmacology, 40*(1), 61–87. doi:10.1038/npp.2014.147.

Roth, R. M., Isquith, P. K., & Gioia, G. A. (2005). Executive function: Concepts, assessment and intervention. In G. P. Koocher, J. C. Norcross, & S. S. Hill (Eds.), *Psychologists' desk reference* (2nd ed., pp. 38–41). New York, NY: Oxford University Press.

Roussotte, F. F., Bramen, J. E., Nunez, S. C., Quandt, L. C., Smith, L., O'Connor, M. J., et al. (2011). Abnormal brain activation during working memory in children with prenatal exposure to drugs of abuse: The effects of methamphetamine, alcohol, and polydrug exposure. *NeuroImage, 54*(4), 3067–3075. doi:10.1016/j.neuroimage.2010.10.072.

Savage, J., Brodsky, N. L., Malmud, E., Giannetta, J. M., & Hurt, H. (2005). Attentional functioning and impulse control in cocaine-exposed and control children at age ten years. *Journal of Developmental and Behavioral Pediatrics, 26*(1), 42–47. doi:00004703-200502000-00010 [pii].

Schuetze, P., & Eiden, R. D. (2007). The association between prenatal exposure to cigarettes and infant and maternal negative affect. *Infant Behavior & Development, 30*(3), 387–398. doi:S0163-6383(06)00073-7.

Singer, L. T., Arendt, R., Minnes, S., Salvator, A., Siegel, A. C., & Lewis, B. A. (2001). Developing language skills of cocaine-exposed infants. *Pediatrics, 107*, 1057–1064.

Singer, L. T., Arendt, R., Minnes, S., Farkas, K., Salvator, A., Kirchner, H. L., et al. (2002). Cognitive and motor outcomes of cocaine-exposed infants. *JAMA, 287*(15), 1952–1960.

Singer, L. T., Lewin, J., Minnes, S., Weishampel, P., Drake, K., Satayathum, S., et al. (2006). Neuroimaging of 7 to 8 year-old children exposed prenatally to cocaine. *Neurotoxicology and Teratology, 28*, 393–396.

Singer, L. T., Minnes, S., Min, M. O., Lewis, B. A., Lang, A., & Wu, M. (2015). Prenatal cocaine, alcohol, and tobacco effects on adolescent attention/inhibition [Abstract]. *Neurotoxicology and Teratology*, Presented at the 2015 NBTS Annual Meeting, Montreal, Canada, June 27–July 1, 2015.

Singer, L. T., Minnes, S., Min, M. O., Lewis, B. A., & Short, E. J. (2015). Prenatal cocaine exposure and child outcomes: A conference report based on a prospective study from cleveland. *Human Psychopharmacology: Clinical and Experimental, Special Edition, 30*, 285–289. doi:10.1002/hup.2454.

Singer, L. T., Minnes, S., Short, E., Arendt, R., Farkas, K., Lewis, B., et al. (2004). Cognitive outcomes of preschool children with prenatal cocaine exposure. *JAMA, 291*(20), 2448–2456. doi:10.1001/jama.291.20.2448.

Singer, L. T., Moore, D. G., Fulton, S., Goodwin, J., Turner, J. J. D., Min, M. O., et al. (2012). Neurobehavioral outcomes of infants exposed to MDMA (ecstasy) and other recreational drugs during pregnancy. *Neurotoxicology and Teratology, 34*(3), 303–310. doi:10.1016/j.ntt.2012.02.001.

Singer, L. T., Moore, D. G., Min, M. O., Goodwin, J., Turner, J. J. D., Fulton, S., et al. (2012). One-year outcomes of prenatal exposure to MDMA and other recreational drugs. *Pediatrics, 130*(3), 407–413. doi:10.1542/peds.2012-0666.

Singer, L. T., Moore, D. G., Min, M. O., Goodwin, J., Turner, J.J., Fulton, S., & Parrott, A. C. (2015). Developmental outcomes of 3,4-methylenedioxymethamphetamine (ecstasy)-exposed infants in the UK. *Human Psychopharmacology: Clinical and Experimental, Special Edition, 30*(4), 290–294. doi:10.1002/hup.2459.

Singer, L. T., Nelson, S., Short, E., Min, M. O., Lewis, B., Russ, S., & Minnes, S. (2008). Prenatal cocaine exposure: Drug and environmental effects at 9 years. *The Journal of Pediatrics, 153*(1), 105–111. doi:10.1016/j.jpeds.2008.01.001.

Singer, L. T., Salvator, A., Arendt, R., Minnes, S., Farkas, K., & Kliegman, R. (2002). Effects of cocaine/polydrug exposure and maternal psychological distress on infant birth outcomes. *Neurotoxicology and Teratology, 24*(2), 127–135.

Slikker, W. J., Xu, Z. A., Levin, E. D., & Slotkin, T. A. (2005). Mode of action: Disruption of brain cell replication, second messenger, and neurotransmitter systems during development leading to cognitive dysfunction—developmental neurotoxicity of nicotine. *Critical Reviews in Toxicology, 35*(8-9), 703–711.

Slotkin, T. A. (2013). Maternal smoking and conduct disorder in the offspring. *JAMA Psychiatry, 70*(9), 901–902.

Smeriglio, V. L., & Wilcox, H. C. (1999). Prenatal drug exposure and child outcome. past, present, future. *Clinics in Perinatology, 26*(1), 1–16.

Smith, L. M., Diaz, S., LaGasse, L. L., Wouldes, T., Derauf, C., Newman, E., et al. (2015). Developmental and behavioral consequences of prenatal methamphetamine exposure: A review of the infant development, environment, and lifestyle (IDEAL) study. *Neurotoxicology and Teratology, 51*, 35–44. doi:10.1016/j.ntt.2015.07.006.

Smith, L. M., LaGasse, L. L., Derauf, C., Newman, E., Shah, R., Haning, W., et al. (2011). Motor and cognitive outcomes through three years of age in children exposed to prenatal methamphetamine. *Neurotoxicology and Teratology, 33*(1), 176–184. doi:10.1016/j.ntt.2010.10.004.

Smith, L., Yonekura, M. L., Wallace, T., Berman, N., Kuo, J., & Berkowitz, C. (2003). Effects of prenatal methamphetamine exposure on fetal growth and drug withdrawal symptoms in infants born at term. *Journal of Developmental and Behavioral Pediatrics, 24*(1), 17–23.

Sood, B. G., Nordstrom, B. B., Covington, C., Sokol, R. J., Ager, J., Janisse, J., et al. (2005). Gender and alcohol moderate caregiver reported child behavior after prenatal cocaine. *Neurotoxicology and Teratology, 27*(2), 191–201. doi:S0892-0362(04)00146-1 [pii].

Stroud, L. R., Paster, R. L., Papandonatos, G. D., Niaura, R., Salisbury, A. L., Battle, C., et al. (2009). Maternal smoking during pregnancy and newborn neurobehavior: Effects at 10 to 27 days. *The Journal of Pediatrics, 154*(1), 10–16. doi:10.1016/j.jpeds.2008.07.048.

Substance Abuse and Mental Health Services Administration. (2014). *Results from the 2013 National survey on drug use and health: Summary of national findings, NSDUH series H-48, HHS publication no. (SMA) 14–4863 Center for behavioral health statistics and quality*. Rockville, MD: Substance Abuse and Mental Health Services Administration.

Thapar, A., Cooper, M., Eyre, O., & Langley, K. (2013). Practitioner review: What have we learnt about the causes of ADHD? *Journal of Child Psychology and Psychiatry, 54*(1), 3–16.

Thapar, A., Rice, F., Hay, D., Boivin, J., Langley, K., van den Bree, M., et al. (2009). Prenatal smoking might not cause attention-deficit/hyperactivity disorder: Evidence from a novel design. *BPS Biological Psychiatry, 66*(8), 722–727.

Thompson, B. L., Levitt, P., & Stanwood, G. D. (2009). Prenatal exposure to drugs: Effects on brain development and implications for policy and education. *Nature Reviews Neuroscience, 10*(4), 303–312. doi:10.1038/nrn2598.

Tiesler, C. M., & Heinrich, J. (2014). Prenatal nicotine exposure and child behavioural problems. *European Child & Adolescent Psychiatry, 23*(10), 913–929. doi:10.1007/s00787-014-0615-y.

Turner, J. J., Parrott, A. C., Goodwin, J., Moore, D. G., Fulton, S., Min, M. O., et al. (2014). Psychiatric profiles of mothers who take ecstasy/MDMA during pregnancy: Reduced depression 1 year after giving birth and quitting ecstasy. *Journal of Psychopharmacology, 28*(1), 55–61. doi:10.1177/0269881113515061.

US Department of Health and Human Services. (2006). *The health consequences of involuntary exposure to tobacco smoke: A report of the surgeon general* (p. 790). Atlanta, GA: US Department of Health and Human Services. Centers for Disease Control and Prevention, Coordinating Center for Health Promotion, National Center for Chronic Disease Prevention and Health Promotion, Office on Smoking and Health.

Wakschlag, L. S., Henry, D. B., Blair, R. J., Dukic, V., Burns, J., & Pickett, K. E. (2011). Unpacking the association: Individual differences in the relation of prenatal exposure to cigarettes and disruptive behavior phenotypes. *Neurotoxicology and Teratology, 33*(1), 145–154. doi:10.1016/j.ntt.2010.07.002.

Wakschlag, L. S., Pickett, K. E., Cook, E. J., Benowitz, N. L., & Leventhal, B. L. (2002). Maternal smoking during pregnancy and severe antisocial behavior in offspring: A review. *American Journal of Public Health, 92*(6), 966–974.

Wiebe, S. A., Clark, C. A., De Jong, D. M., Chevalier, N., Espy, K. A., & Wakschlag, L. (2015). Prenatal tobacco exposure and self-regulation in early childhood: Implications for developmental psychopathology. *Development and Psychopathology, 27*(2), 397–409. doi:10.1017/S095457941500005X.

Wouldes, T. A., LaGasse, L. L., Huestis, M. A., DellaGrotta, S., Dansereau, L. M., & Lester, B. M. (2014). Prenatal methamphetamine exposure and neurodevelopmental outcomes in children from 1 to 3 years. *Neurotoxicology and Teratology, 42*(2), 77–84.

Zabaneh, R., Smith, L. M., LaGasse, L. L., Derauf, C., Newman, E., Shah, R., et al. (2012). The effects of prenatal methamphetamine exposure on childhood growth patterns from birth to 3 years of age. *American Journal of Perinatology, 29*(3), 203–210. doi:10.1055/s-0031-1285094.

Zhou, S., Rosenthal, D. G., Sherman, S., Zelikoff, J., Gordon, T., & Weitzman, M. (2014). Physical, behavioral, and cognitive effects of prenatal tobacco and postnatal secondhand smoke exposure. *Current Problems in Pediatric and Adolescent Health Care, 44*(8), 219–241. doi:10.1016/j.cppeds.2014.03.007.

Chapter 4
Opiates and Marijuana Use During Pregnancy: Neurodevelopmental Outcomes

Leandra Parris

Definitional Issues and Prevalence

Opioids are a class of narcotics that are derived, either naturally or synthetically, from the opium chemical found in the poppy plant (Hart & Ksir, 2015). Opioids bind the opioid receptors in the nervous system and can act as an analgesic to reduce pain. Additional effects include euphoria, decreased respiration, sedation, a scratching reflect known as pruritus, and nausea/vomiting. Over time, those who use opioids can develop a tolerance to their effects and thus require higher and higher doses to achieve the same effect.

The classification of opioids by the US Drug Enforcement Administration (DEA) and the US Food and Drug Administration (FDA) varies based on the potential for dependence and clinical use. For example, the DEA classifies opioids such as methadone and oxycodone as a schedule II drug as these forms of opium have been shown to have some medical benefits but also have a high risk for abuse and dependence. Doctors, to alleviate pain following surgery or injury, may prescribe many of the opioids in this class of narcotics as part of patient care. However, some forms of opioids that are a combination of synthetic and naturally occurring derivatives, such as buprenorphine, have the same medicinal application with lower risks of abuse and dependence and are thus considered a schedule III drug. Heroin, considered one of the most dangerous forms, is labeled as a schedule I drug due to its very high risk for abuse and dependence with no current medical uses.

L. Parris, Ph.D. (✉)
Department of Psychology, Illinois State University,
Campus Box 4620, Normal, IL 61790, USA
e-mail: lnparris@ilstu.edu

C. Riccio, J. Sullivan (eds.), *Pediatric Neurotoxicology*, Specialty Topics in Pediatric Neuropsychology, DOI 10.1007/978-3-319-32358-9_4

When evaluating the use of opioids during pregnancy, the FDA considers most forms of opioids to be class C, which is given to drugs in which both animal and human studies have shown to have a negative impact on fetal development but the benefits of use may outweigh these risks for some patients. However, it should be noted that this classification applies to drugs for which there have not been sufficient control studies in humans. The exception is heroin, for which the FDA provides no classification information.

In determining the prevalence of opioid use during pregnancy, studies have indicated that approximately 21 % of women used a prescribed opioid, most commonly codeine or hydrocodone, at some point during their pregnancy (Desai, Hernandez-Diaz, Bateman, & Huybrechts, 2014). These rates appear to be increasing in the past decade (Desai et al., 2014). According to Azadi and Dildy (2008), approximately 2.6 % of participants in a 2005 investigation tested positive for opioids. The 2013 administration of the National Survey on Drug Use and Health (NSDUH) indicated that approximately 2.5 % of people 12 or older reported using prescription drugs, including opioids, in a nonmedical capacity (Substance Abuse and Mental Health Services Administration, 2009). It was reported that about 289,000 respondents (0.1 %) indicated they were currently using heroin, with 681,000 reporting they had used heroin in the past year. While the report did not provide information regarding how often pregnant women reported using opioids, overall use of illicit drugs while pregnant was around 5.4 % for the 2012 and 2013 years.

Like opioids, the use of marijuana has a long history with records indicating its use by ancient civilizations, including those in Egypt and China (Hart & Ksir, 2015). Marijuana, which is derived from the cannabis plant, has multiple psychoactive, as well as physical, effects. These include euphoria, increased relaxation, and increased appetite. However, additional effects can include paranoia, decreased short-term memory capacity, and decreased functioning of cognitive and motor skills. To date, the long-term effects of marijuana use have not been systematically identified. Initial findings regarding the impact of long-term use of marijuana suggest that chronic use of the drug may not have a lasting impact on cognition (Cohen et al., 2015) or memory (Jager, Kahn, Van Den Brink, Van Ree, & Ramsey, 2006). Further, previously held beliefs regarding the development of amotivational syndrome as a result of chronic use of marijuana have been called into question by some researchers (Hart & Ksir, 2015). However, as research in the area becomes more sophisticated and begins to look at additional, potentially confounding factors, it is possible that such effects may be more clearly delineated in the future (Hart & Ksir, 2015; Schoeler & Bhattacharyya, 2013). Currently, the DEA considers marijuana as a schedule I drug, with high risk for abuse/dependence and no current medical applications. The FDA also does not approve the use of marijuana for medical purposes, with no classification with regard to use during pregnancy. However, there has been growing evidence marijuana may have some medical benefits for patients with glaucoma, currently undergoing radiation therapy, and those who suffer from seizures (Stanhope, Gill, & Rose, 2013). Both the DEA and FDA have indicated support for reevaluating the classification of marijuana given these findings.

According to the NSDUH report, marijuana was the most commonly used drug in 2013. Around 19.8 million (7.5 %) people 12 or older reported using marijuana in the past month, representing approximately 80.6 % of illicit drug users. Research conducted between 2002 and 2007 indicated that approximately 9 % of pregnant women smoked marijuana during the past month, representing the most commonly used illicit drug (Substance Abuse and Mental Health Services Administration, 2009).

Impact on the Developing Child

Opioid and marijuana use during pregnancy has received limited attention in research in comparison to other substances such as cocaine and alcohol. Specific to the study of opioid effects, most studies focused on women participating in methadone treatment for opioid dependence as opposed to the effects of other forms of opioids such as heroin or morphine. Further, many studies investigated these substances in conjunction with other drug forms (e.g., polydrug use), making it hard to determine differences that may be attributed specifically to opioids or marijuana use. While short-term, neonatal effects have been investigated to some degree, less has been done to determine long-term effects of prenatal exposure to opioids and marijuana. Such a dearth of research related to this area has resulted in calls for attention to the topic (e.g., Walhovd et al., 2009). The following sections outline what research has found with regard to various areas of functioning. When possible, both short-term and long-term effects are discussed.

Intellectual Functioning

Prenatal opioid exposure has been shown to have deleterious effects on early cognitive abilities. When examining neural development, researchers have found that in utero exposure to opioids results in decreases in neural plasticity and increased apoptosis, or cell death, in developing brains of rats and humans (Hu, Sheng, Lokensgard, & Peterson, 2002; Schrott, Franklin, & Serrano, 2008). Such changes have been shown to impact the ability to learn. For example, rats with weakened neural plasticity demonstrated a decreased ability to learn and complete maze tasks (Schrott et al., 2008; Steingart et al., 2000). The effects of opioids on learning have been attributed to direct effects of prenatal heroin exposure (Steingart et al., 2000) on the developing brain or possibly a result of withdrawal symptoms (Schrott et al., 2008). These initial findings are important in demonstrating that opioid exposure in utero has the potential to hinder the learning capacity of the child.

Additional studies that examined neonatal exposure to opioids in children have also demonstrated reduced cognitive functioning. For example, Beckwith and Burke (2015) examined children ages 1 month to 42 months of age using the Bayley-III, which assesses cognitive skills such as exploration of objects, understanding how objects relate to one another, the formation of concepts, and memory abilities. The researchers found that participants that had been prenatally exposed to opioids performed lower on these tests when compared to non-exposed children of the same age. Similar research has found that at 1 month, infants exposed to opioids demonstrated more problems with regulating their autonomic responses which may impact learning, though this effect was stronger when the mother reported using both cocaine and opioids during pregnancy (Conradt et al., 2013).

As children age, those exposed to opioids prenatally continue to demonstrate reduced cognitive functioning and developmental delays based on intelligence testing. Research examining 2- and 3-year-old children found that approximately 29 % of children exposed to opioids during pregnancy exhibited significant delays in cognition, such as practical reasoning (Palchik, Einspieler, Evstafeyeva, Talisa, & Marschik, 2013). However, additional research has shown that by the age of 3, children with opiate exposure did not significantly differ in cognitive performance from their same-aged peers, suggesting that these effects may be most noticeable prior to the age of 2 (Messinger et al., 2004).

In contrast, some research findings have suggested that cognitive delays associated with opiate exposure were noted in preschool children and even adolescents. Preschool aged children, ages 5 and 6, exposed to buprenorphine (an opiate used as treatment for opioid-dependency during pregnancy) have demonstrated below average scores on general IQ assessments when compared to non-exposed peers (Wahlsten & Sarman, 2013). Children and adolescents from 5 to 14 years old have also been shown to exhibit greater intellectual difficulties and alterations in neural structure, such as a reduction in size and less white matter, which can have an impact on cognitive abilities (Ornoy, Segal, Bar-Hamburger, & Greenbaum, 2001; Walhovd et al., 2007, 2010). Reduced cognitive functioning was found to be greater in children who were raised in lower socioeconomic status (SES) environments and experienced neglect, with exposed children who were raised in comfortable and supportive home environments demonstrating very little differences in intellectual functioning as compared to non-exposed children (Ornoy et al., 2001). This finding suggests that the effects prenatal opioid exposure on intellectual functioning may depend on the environment and risk factors that the child is exposed to after birth.

There has been limited research regarding the impact of prenatal exposure to marijuana on children's intellectual development and functioning. Initial investigations have demonstrated that mothers who smoked marijuana during pregnancy were more likely to give birth to children who demonstrated challenges in verbal reasoning, quantitative reasoning, and short-term memory abilities (Goldschmidt, Richardson, Willford, & Day, 2008; Richardson, Ryan, Willford, Day, & Goldschmidt, 2002). Even when controlling for other factors that may impede learning, these effects were demonstrated for children ages 6 and 10, indicating prenatal exposure to marijuana can have long-term consequences (Goldschmidt et al., 2008; Richardson et al., 2002). Further, 10-year-old children who were exposed to marijuana in utero were found to be more impulsive than their counterparts, which can also impact learning and performance on cognitive tasks (Richardson et al., 2002). While deficits were noted in these specific areas of intelligence, an effect of marijuana in utero exposure was not found on scores representing global intellectual functioning (Fried & Smith, 2001).

Academic Functioning

Based on research suggesting that children who are exposed to opioids or marijuana in utero experience deficits in learning and cognitive functioning, it could be reasoned that these children would also demonstrate challenges in academic performance. However, there is a paucity of research investigating this hypothesis. Initial investigations regarding prenatal exposure of marijuana found that exposed children, when compared to unexposed children, demonstrated poorer performance on reading, spelling, and language achievement scores and receive lower ratings of achievement by teachers (Fried, Watkinson, & Siegel, 1997; Goldschmidt, Richardson, Cornelius, & Day, 2004). Specifically, exposure during the third trimester of pregnancy was found to be associated with below average achievement in reading comprehension (Goldschmidt et al., 2004). To date, there have been no studies which specifically examine the effects of prenatal opioid exposure on later academic achievement in children. This represents an area of research which is lacking and requires empirical investigations to help determine the academic prognosis for students who were exposed to opioids and marijuana in utero.

Neuropsychological Functioning

In utero exposure to opioids and marijuana have been shown to have a variety of effects on the neuropsychological functioning of children, including reduced abilities in motor, memory, and executive functioning skills such as attention and impulsivity. In regard to prenatal exposure to opioids, research has shown that these children exhibited deficits in motor skills, such as reflexes, eye-hand coordination, and intentional movement (Wahlsten & Sarman, 2013). However, these effects may be short-term in nature (Jansson, DePietro, & Elko, 2005). Further, when assessed as infants and toddlers, children exposed to opioids did not demonstrate significant difficulties with motor tasks (Beckwith & Burke, 2015). This suggests that while differences in motor movements may be noted early in life (Palchik et al., 2013), these effects appear to lessen over time as the child develops. It is possible that immediate postnatal treatment may decrease the amount of time it takes for these challenges to decline; however, research is required to examine this possibility.

In addition to initial motor difficulties, research has shown that children prenatally exposed to opioids are at greater risk for problems with executive functioning and increased symptoms of an attention-deficit hyperactivity disorder (ADHD). Investigations have yielded results which suggest that approximately 5 % of exposed children received a diagnosis of ADHD by the time they were 3 years old (Palchik et al., 2013). Further, when compared to non-exposed children, children exposed to opioids were more likely to have increasing teacher ratings of ADHD symptoms, demonstrate decreased abilities in completing perceptual tasks associated with executive functioning, difficulty controlling their impulses, and challenges with mental planning and organization (Ornoy et al., 2001; Wahlsten & Sarman, 2013). Walhovd and colleagues (2007) found that exposure to opioids in utero was linked to a reduction in certain brain structures that are believed to be associated with behavioral responses to reward systems, which may also be related to symptoms of ADHD. While researchers have indicated that the association between prenatal exposure to opioids and later development of ADHD symptoms can be, in part, attributed to the effect of opioids on brain development (Ornoy et al., 2001), it is also possible that these findings are linked to lower birth weights that are also associated with prenatal exposure to opioids (Palchik et al., 2013).

Memory formation and retention is another area that may be impacted by in utero exposure to opioids. Research using adult rats that had been prenatally exposed to morphine found that they experienced difficulties related to hippocampal functioning, which affects memory (Villarreal, Derrick, & Vathy, 2008). Further, studies which tested memory abilities of exposed children found that opioid exposure was associated with decreased memory abilities, including working memory and short-term memory functioning (Wahlsten & Sarman, 2013). Difficulties with memory formation and retention represent a major area of concern for this population, as memory can have lasting effects on learning, academic performance, and daily functioning.

Similar to prenatal opioid exposure, in utero exposure to marijuana has also been shown to have an effect on memory abilities. For example, one study found that 13- to 16-year-olds who had experienced fetal exposure to marijuana exhibited greater difficulties remembering visual information, though less so with working memory functioning, than students with no exposure or exposure to other substances such as alcohol (Fried & Watkinson, 2001; Fried, Watkinson, & Gray, 2003). In addition to memory deficits, these same children were found to have more challenges in completing tasks that required them to sustain their attention over time and to analyze/integrate information (Fried et al., 2003; Fried & Watkinson, 2001). This may be related to additional evidence suggesting that prenatal marijuana exposure is associated with deficits in some aspects of executive functioning (Irner, 2012), such as response inhibition, attention, and visual analysis of information (Fried & Smith, 2001; Smith, Fried, Hogan, & Cameron, 2004). There is evidence to suggest that these effects are not short-term and may last well into adolescence (Fried & Smith, 2001; Smith et al., 2004).

Emotional and Behavioral Functioning

The effects of prenatal exposure to opioids on emotional and behavior functioning appear to involve behavioral regulation and potential associations with Autism Spectrum Disorders (ASD) based on research thus far. Assessments of 1 month old children prenatally exposed to opioids, combined with cocaine, indicated that infants in this group struggled to regulate behavioral responses to a visual attention task (Conradt et al., 2013). Palchick and colleagues (2013) found that 2- and 3-year-old children who had been exposed to opioids in utero exhibited some difficulties with behavioral regulation. Further, some of the children were experiencing symptoms of ASD (Palchik et al., 2013). While the authors indicate that these findings could also be related to the higher rate of preterm births among the exposed children, it is possible that prenatal exposure to opioids affects the ability of some children to appropriately regulate behaviors and emotions and/or demonstrate adequate social skills.

Recently, research has begun to shed some light on the effects of marijuana use during pregnancy on children's later emotional and behavioral functioning. Though research in the area is still in the initial stages, there is some evidence to suggest that prenatal exposure to marijuana is associated with depression and anxiety, as well as attention deficits, delinquent behaviors, and externalizing behaviors (Day, Leech, & Goldschmidt, 2011; Goldschmidt et al., 2004; Goldschmidt, Day, & Richardson, 2000). Research has shown that children whose mother had one or more marijuana joints per day during pregnancy were more likely to exhibit depressive symptoms, such as sadness and helplessness, at the age of 10 (Day et al., 2011). Further, the same researchers found that exposed children were more likely to exhibit delinquent behaviors, such as skipping school and rule breaking at age 14, though this relationship was mediated by reported symptoms of depression and attention difficulties at the age of 10. Another study found similar results, in that the effect of prenatal exposure to more than one joint per day on academic functioning was mediated by symptoms associated with depression and anxiety, which were also associated with marijuana use during pregnancy (Goldschmidt et al., 2004).

Similarly to these studies, investigators who examined the time in which prenatal exposure occurred in the pregnancy found that such exposure during the first and third trimester resulted in a greater chance that the child would exhibit delinquent behaviors at age 10 (Goldschmidt et al., 2000). However, once attention difficulties were taken into account, these effects were no longer present. Regarding internalizing behaviors, researchers found that exposure to marijuana during each of the trimesters during pregnancy increased the chance that the child would report depressive symptoms at age 10 (Goldschmidt et al., 2000).

Impact on Other Areas of Functioning

When assessed with the Bayley III, children 1–42 months old who were prenatally exposed to opioids showed decreased abilities in language, which included receptive (e.g., nonverbal, object identification), preverbal (e.g., babbling, gurgling), and expressive (e.g., naming objects, two-word utterances) skills when compared to children in the control condition (Beckwith & Burke, 2015). While only one study examined the influence of opiate exposure on children's language development, it represents a starting point from which to build future studies.

Specific Diagnostic Outcomes

One potential diagnostic outcome for prenatal opioid exposure is neonatal abstinence syndrome (NAS). A NAS diagnosis is provided when a newborn experiences withdrawal symptoms after birth due to a cessation of opioid exposure (Stanhope et al., 2013). These symptoms typically occur within the first 10 days and can last for up to 6 months after birth. Symptoms of NAS may include, but are not limited to, increased rates of crying, diarrhea, fever, irritability, seizures, and dehydration (Jansson et al., 2012; Stanhope et al., 2013). Research has found that children exposed to methadone and illicit forms of opioids were more likely to receive a diagnosis of NAS when compared to other forms (e.g., prescription drugs, buprenorphine) of opioids (Jansson et al., 2012; Stanhope et al., 2013). Long-term effects and implications of a NAS diagnosis have not been determined.

Prognosis and Moderating Factors

The immediate prognosis for newborns exposed to opioids is affected by the increased occurrence of certain risk factors. For example, prenatal exposure to opioids has been linked to lower birth weights (Harper, Solish, Feingold, Gersten-Woolf, & Sokal, 1977, Kandall et al., 1997), respiratory issues (Kandall et al., 1997), decreases in fetal heart rates (Jansson et al., 2012; Navaneethakrishnan, Tutty, Sinha, & Lindow, 2006; Ramirez-Cacho, Flores, Schrader, McKay, & Rayburn, 2006; Schmid et al., 2010), and preterm delivery (Jansson et al., 2012). However, some studies have indicated no difference between exposed and non-exposed children with regard to birth weight and overall neonatal functioning, as indicated by Apgar scores (Anyategbunam, Tran, Jadali, Randolph, & Mikhail, 1997). Further, it is unclear that withdrawal symptoms and complications immediately following birth have long term effects on child development and functioning.

One moderating factor that may influence the impact of prenatal opioid exposure is cigarette smoking during pregnancy. Researchers have found that opioid-dependent women may smoke more cigarettes during pregnancy when compared to other groups of pregnant women, confounding results examining effects of opioids as smoking is also linked to lower birth weight and concerns at birth (Winklbaur et al., 2009). Studies have shown that women who are heavy smokers (>20 cigarettes a day), in addition to participating in opiate maintenance programs, give birth to babies that were at greater risk for NAS and subsequent longer hospitalizations when compared to women who smoked less than ten cigarettes a day (Winklbaur et al., 2009).

Some of the long-term effects of opioid exposure may be attributed to factors outside of the changes caused by in utero exposure. These changes in development may be moderated by variables that are included in the child's environment and home life. For example, lower socioeconomic status appears to have an impact on the effect of prenatal opioid exposure (Baldacchino, Arbuckle, Petrie, & McCowan,

2014; Jones, 2013). Additional factors may include instability in the home (Jones, 2013; Wahlsten & Sarman, 2013), a lack of nutrition in the child's diet (Jones, 2013), and maternal depressive symptoms (Baldacchino et al., 2014; Smith, Costello, & Yonkers, 2015). Further, it is possible that certain parental diagnoses may put the fetus at increased risk of being exposed to opioids. Smith et al. (2015) found that pregnant women who were experiencing anxiety and panic disorders were more likely to use prescription opioids, illicit drugs, and smoke cigarettes, putting the fetus at greater risk. Researchers have also noted that the increase in hyperactivity, behavior problems, and inattention in opiate exposed children may be related to the higher rate of ADHD symptoms that their parents display (Ornoy et al., 2001). Interestingly, challenges with impulsivity and other symptoms associated with ADHD put these parents at greater risk for abusing substances and thus risking prenatal exposure to drugs for their children (Ornoy et al., 2001).

To date, there are no studies that investigated moderating variables in relation to prenatal marijuana exposure and subsequent outcomes for children. However, it is possible that influencing factors found in relation to opioids and other drugs (e.g., lower SES, cigarette smoking, maternal psychopathology) are relevant for studies investigating marijuana. Future research is needed to determine what environmental and risk factors may be present for children who were exposed to marijuana in utero.

Considerations for Intervention/Prevention and School Accommodations

There are some considerations for working with children who have been prenatally exposed to opioids and marijuana. The most important factor in decreasing the effects of in utero exposure to opioids would be prevention efforts. When working with opioid-dependent women, it is important for caregivers to be aware of the various effects of different forms of treatment on the developing fetus. There are currently three options for opioid maintenance for pregnant women: methadone, buprenorphine, and oral slow release morphine doses. Research has found that buprenorphine was associated with less severe NAS and withdrawal symptoms when compared to the other two forms of treatment (Fischer et al., 2006; Gyarmathy et al., 2009; Minozzi, Amato, Bellisario, Ferri, & Davoli, 2013; Winklbaur et al., 2009). However, additional studies have suggested that there are no differences in NAS diagnoses (Welle-Strand et al., 2013) between buprenorphine and methadone, with women in the methadone treatment groups demonstrating less drop out rates and women using slow release morphine reported less additional use of heroin (Minozzi et al., 2013). Further research is required to determine which of these three forms of treatment may be best in preventing the occurrence of NAS and other complications due to fetal exposure to opioids.

An additional factor may be the way in which treatment drugs are delivered. Studies have demonstrated that higher doses of methadone (>30 mg) were associated with moderate to severe withdrawal symptoms (Harper et al., 1977). Lower doses of methadone resulted in less withdrawal symptoms; however, lower doses did not result in no symptoms occurring in all newborns (Harper et al., 1977). Researchers have also reported that providing two smaller doses of methadone during the day, as opposed to one dose of the same amount, alleviated some of the concerning consequences of prenatal opioid exposure (Jansoon et al., 2009). Further, women who took part in methadone maintenance programs but continued to use additional illicit drugs were at great risk for complications and earlier delivery (Jansson et al., 2012). Despite these effects of opioid treatments, it may still be more beneficial than pure detoxification from opioids when pregnant. Studies have resulted in mixed findings regarding detox effects, with some reporting that doing so resulted in a greater risk of miscarriage and death of the infant, while others have indicated no increased risks during pregnancy or labor (Stanhope et al., 2013).

Some recommendations have been made regarding prevention and intervention for children exposed to opioids. These suggestions include providing family planning services (Ortigosa et al., 2012), a general curriculum increasing professional awareness of treatment and resource options for patients (Jones, 2013), limiting prescription refills of prescription opioids, and reserving opioid treatment drugs for women experiencing extreme opioid dependency (Stanhope et al., 2013). Intervention recommendations for exposed newborns include strategies for motor organization, neutral warmth, the use of a soothing pacifier, and parent provided infant massages (Conradt et al., 2013).

While recommendations have not been made for prenatal exposure to marijuana, many of the ones discussed in relation to opioid exposure might be beneficial. For example, physician and clinician increased awareness of identifying risk factors of marijuana use during pregnancy and treatment of potential side effects for the fetus would be helpful in reducing effects found in utero exposure to marijuana. Further, providing information and community resources for parents and guardians may help alleviate some of the noted concerns.

Regarding the school environment, there have been no systematic investigations into school integration and accommodations for children prenatally exposed to opioids and marijuana. Based on current literature, it is possible that accommodations for difficulties with motor control and behavioral regulation may be warranted in early childhood. Interventions and accommodations may be necessary for exposed children that focus on increasing executive functioning and short-term memory skills and decreasing behavior problems, such as those associated with ADHD. Based on the moderating influences of ecological factors, such as the home environment, parental psychosocial difficulties, and continued exposure to drug use, schools must take these factors into account when assessing children and providing interventions to address individual needs.

Conclusion

Research regarding prenatal exposure to opioids and marijuana is fairly sparse in the current literature. While there is some evidence to suggest that such exposure is related to difficulties in cognition, executive functioning, memory, and initial challenges due to withdrawal, the long-term effects have not been fully explored. This poses some challenges in determining direct effects of opioid and marijuana prenatal exposure and the impact such exposure may have on school performance. Recommendations for prevention include increased awareness both for clinicians and parents, restricted access to prescription opioids for pregnant women, and early intervention strategies for children experiencing withdrawal or NAS. Further, increased attention to in utero exposure to opioids and marijuana in the literature is warranted.

References

Anyategbunam, A., Tran, T., Jadali, D., Randolph, G., & Mikhail, M. (1997). Assessment of fetal well-being in methadone-maintained pregnancies: Abnormal nonstress tests. *Gynecologic and Obstetric Investigation, 43*, 25–28.

Azadi, A., & Dildy, G. (2008). Universal screening for substance abuse at the time of parturition. *American Journal of Obstetrics & Gynecology, 198*, 30–32. doi:10.1016/j/ajog.2007.10.780.

Baldacchino, A., Arbuckle, K., Petrie, D., & McCowan, C. (2014). Neurobehavioral consequences of chronic intrauterine opioid exposure in infants and preschool children: A systematic review and meta-analysis. *BMC Psychiatry, 14*, 104–116. doi:10.1186/1471-244X-14-104.

Beckwith, A., & Burke, S. (2015). Identification of early developmental deficits in infants with prenatal heroin, methadone, and other opioid exposure. *Clinical Pediatrics, 54*, 328–335. doi:10.1177/0009922814549545.

Cohen, M., Johnston, P., Ehlkes, T., Fulham, R., Ward, P., Thienel, R., … Schall, U. (2015). Functional magnetic resonance brain imaging of executive cognitive performance in young first episode schizophrenia patients and age-matched long-term cannabis users. *Neurology, Psychiatry, and Brain Research, 21*, 51–62. doi:10.1016/j.npbr.2014.09.002.

Conradt, E., Sheinkopf, S., Lester, B., Tronick, E., LaGasse, L., Shankaran, S., … Hammond, J. (2013). Prenatal substance exposure: Neurobiological organization at 1 month. *Journal of Pediatrics, 163*, 989–994. doi:10.1016/j.jpeds.2013.04.033.

Day, N., Leech, S., & Goldschmidt, L. (2011). The effects of prenatal marijuana exposure on delinquent behaviors are mediated by measures of neurocognitive functioning. *Neurotoxicology and Teratology, 33*, 129–136.

Desai, R., Hernandez-Diaz, S., Bateman, B., & Huybrechts, K. (2014). Increase in prescription opioid use during pregnancy among medicaid-enrolled women. *Obstetrics & Gynecology, 123*, 997–1002. doi:10.1097/AOG.0000000000000208.

Fischer, G., Ortner, R., Rohrmeister, K., Jagsch, R., Baewert, A., Langer, M., & Aschauer, H. (2006). Methadone versus buprenorphine in pregnant addicts: A double-blind, double-dummy comparison study. *Addiction, 101*, 275–281. doi:10.111/j.1360-0443.2006.01321.x.

Fried, P., & Smith, A. (2001). A literature review of the consequences of prenatal marihuana exposure: An emerging theme of a deficiency in aspects of executive function. *Neurotoxicology and Teratology, 23*, 1–11.

Fried, P., & Watkinson, B. (2001). Differential effects on facets of attention in adolescents prenatally exposed to cigarettes and marihuana. *Neurotoxicolgy and Teratology, 23*, 421–430.

Fried, P., Watkinson, B., & Gray, R. (2003). Differential effects on cognitive functioning in 12- to 16- year-olds prenatally exposed to cigarettes and marihuana. *Neurotoxicology and Teratology, 25*, 427–436.

Fried, P., Watkinson, B., & Siegel, L. (1997). Reading and language in 9- to 12-year olds prenatally exposed to cigarettes and marijuana. *Neurotoxicology and Teratology, 19*, 171–183.

Goldschmidt, L., Day, N., & Richardson, G. (2000). Effects of prenatal marijuana exposure on child behavior problems at age 10. *Neurotoxicology and Teratology, 22*, 325–336.

Goldschmidt, L., Richardson, G., Cornelius, M., & Day, N. (2004). Prenatal marijuana and alcohol exposure and academic achievement at age 10. *Neurotoxicology and Teratology, 26*, 521–532.

Goldschmidt, L., Richardson, G., Willford, J., & Day, N. (2008). Prenatal marijuana exposure and intelligence test performance at age 6. *Journal of the American Academy of Child & Adolescent Psychiatry, 47*, 254–263.

Gyarmathy, V., Giraduon, I., Hedrich, D., Montanari, L., Guarita, B., & Wiessing, L. (2009). Drug use and pregnancy: Challenges for public health. *Eurosurveillance, 14*, 33–36.

Harper, R., Solish, G., Feingold, E., Gersten-Woolf, N., & Sokal, M. (1977). Maternal ingested methadone, body fluid methadone, and the neonatal withdrawal syndrome. *American Journal of Obstetrics and Gynecology, 129*, 417–424.

Hart, C., & Ksir, C. (2015). *Drugs, society, and human behavior* (16th ed.). New York, NY: McGraw-Hill.

Hu, S., Sheng, W., Lokensgard, J., & Peterson, P. (2002). Morphine induces apoptosis of human microglia and neurons. *Neuropharmacology, 42*, 829–836.

Irner, T. (2012). Substance exposures in utero and developmental consequences in adolescence: A systematic review. *Child Neuropsychology, 18*, 521–549. doi:10.1080/09297049.2011.628309.

Jager, G., Kahn, R., Van Den Brink, W., Van Ree, J., & Ramsey, N. (2006). Long-term effects of frequent cannabis use on working memory and attention: An fMRI study. *Psychopharmacology, 185*, 358–369. doi:10.1007/s00213-005-0298-7.

Jansoon, L., DiPietro, J., Velez, M., Elko, A., Knauer, H., & Tivlighan, K. (2009). Maternal methadone dosing schedule and fetal neurobehaviour. *The Journal of Maternal-Fetal and Neonatal Medicine, 22*, 29–35. doi:10.1080/14767050802452291.

Jansson, L., DePietro, J., & Elko, A. (2005). Fetal response to maternal methadone administration. *American Journal of Obstetrics & Gynecology, 193*, 611–617. doi:10.1016/j.ajog.2005.02.075.

Jansson, L., Di Pietro, J., Elko, A., Williams, E., Milio, L., & Velez, M. (2012). Pregnancies exposed to methadone, methadone and other illicit substances, and poly-drugs without methadone: A comparison of fetal neurobehaviors and infant outcomes. *Drug and Alcohol Dependence, 122*, 213–219. doi:10.1016/j.drugalcdep.2011.10.003.

Jones, H. (2013). Treating opioid use disorders during pregnancy: Historical, current, and future directions. *Substance Abuse, 34*, 89–91. doi:10.1080/08897077.2012.752779.

Kandall, S., Albin, S., Gartner, L., Lee, K., Eidelman, A., & Lowinson, J. (1997). The narcotic-dependent mother: Fetal and neonatal consequences. *Early Human Development, 1*, 159–169.

Messinger, D., Bauer, C., Das, A., Seifer, R., Lester, B., Lagasse, L., … Poole, W. (2004). The maternal lifestyle study: Cognitive, motor, and behavioral outcomes of cocaine-exposed and opiate-exposed infants through three years of age. *Pediatrics, 113*, 1677–1685.

Minozzi, S., Amato, L., Bellisario, C., Ferri, M., & Davoli, M. (2013). Maintenance agonist treatments for opiate-dependent pregnant women. *The Cochrane Library, 12*, 1–53.

Navaneethakrishnan, R., Tutty, S., Sinha, C., & Lindow, S. (2006). The effect of maternal methadone use on the fetal heart pattern: A computerized CTG analysis. *BJOG, 113*, 948–950. doi:10.1111/j.1471-0528.2006.01020.x.

Ornoy, A., Segal, J., Bar-Hamburger, R., & Greenbaum, C. (2001). Developmental outcome of school-age children born to mothers with heroin dependency: Importance of environmental factors. *Developmental Medicine & Child Neurology, 43*, 668–675. doi:10.111/j.1469-8749.2001.tb00140.x.

Ortigosa, S., Friguls, B., Joya, X., Martinez, S., Marinoso, M., Alameda, F., … Garcia-Algar, O. (2012). Feto-placental morphological effects of prenatal exposure to drugs of abuse. *Reproductive Toxicology, 34*, 73–79. doi:10.1016.jreprotox.2012.04.002.

Palchik, A., Einspieler, C., Evstafeyeva, I., Talisa, V., & Marschik, P. (2013). Intra- uterine exposure to maternal opiate abuse and HIV: The impact on the developing nervous system. *Early Human Development, 89*, 229–235. doi:10.1016.j.earlhumdev.2013.02.004.

Ramirez-Cacho, W., Flores, F., Schrader, R., McKay, J., & Rayburn, W. (2006). Effect of chronic maternal methadone therapy on intrapartum fetal heart rate patterns. *Journal for the Society of Gynecological Investigation, 13*, 108–111. doi:10.1016/j.jsgi.2005.11.001.

Richardson, G., Ryan, C., Willford, J., Day, N., & Goldschmidt, L. (2002). Prenatal alcohol and marijuana exposure: Effects on neuropsychological outcomes at 10 years. *Neurotoxicology and Teratology, 24*, 309–320.

Schmid, M., Kuessel, L., Klein, K., Metz, V., Fischer, G., & Krampl-Bettelheim, E. (2010). First-trimester fetal heart rate in mothers with opioid addiction. *Addiction, 105*, 1265–1268. doi:10.1111/j.1360-0443.2010.02982.x.

Schoeler, T., & Bhattacharyya, S. (2013). The effect of cannabis use on memory function: An update. *Substance Abuse & Rehabilitation, 4*, 11–27. doi:10.2147/SAR.S25869.

Schrott, L., Franklin, L., & Serrano, P. (2008). Prenatal opiate exposure impairs radial arm maze performance and reduces levels of BDNF precursor following training. *Brain Research, 1198*, 132–140. doi:10.1016/j.brainres.2008.01.020.

Smith, M., Costello, D., & Yonkers, K. (2015). Clinical correlates of prescription opioid analgesic use in pregnancy. *Maternal Child Health, 19*, 548–556. doi:10.1007/s10995-014-1536-6.

Smith, A., Fried, P., Hogan, M., & Cameron, I. (2004). Effects of prenatal marijuana on response inhibition: An fMRI study of young adults. *Neurotoxiciology and Teratology, 26*, 533–542.

Stanhope, T., Gill, L., & Rose, C. (2013). Chronic opioid use during pregnancy: Maternal and fetal implications. *Clinics in Perinatology, 40*, 337–350. doi:10.1016/j.clp.2013.05.015.

Steingart, R., Abu-Roumi, M., Newman, M., Silverman, W., Slotkin, T., & Yanai, J. (2000). Neurobehavioral damage to cholinergic systems caused by prenatal exposure to heroin or phenobarbital: Cellular mechanisms and the reversal of deficits by neural grafts. *Developmental Brain Research, 122*, 125–133.

Substance Abuse and Mental Health Services Administration, Office of Applied Studies. (2009). *The NSDUH report: Substance use among women during pregnancy and following childbirth*. Rockville, MD: Substance Abuse and Mental Health Services Administration, Office of Applied Studies.

Villarreal, D., Derrick, B., & Vathy, I. (2008). Prenatal morphine exposure attenuates the maintenance of late LTP in lateral perforant path projections to the dentate gyrus and the CA3 region in vivo. *Journal of Neurophysiology, 99*, 1235–1242. doi:10.1152/jn.00981.2007.

Wahlsten, V., & Sarman, I. (2013). Neurobehavioral development of preschool-age children born to addicted mothers given opiate maintenance treatment with buprenorphine during pregnancy. *Acta Paediatrica, 102*, 544–549. doi:10.1111/apa.12210.

Walhovd, K., Moe, V., Slinning, K., Siquveland, T., Fjell, A., Bjornebekk, A., & Smith, L. (2009). Effects of prenatal opiate exposure on brain development – a call for attention. *Nature Reviews, 10*, 390. doi:10.1038/nrn2598-c1.

Walhovd, K., Slinning, V., Due-Tonnessen, P., Bjordnerud, A., Dale, A., vanderKowe, A., … Fischl, B. (2007). Volumetric cerebral characteristics of children exposed to opiates and other substances in utero. *Neuroimage, 36*, 1331–1344.

Walhovd, K., Westlye, L., Moe, V., Slinning, K., Due-Tonnessen, P., Bjornerud, A., … Fjell, A. (2010). White matter characteristics and cognition in prenatally opiate- and poly-substance exposed children: A diffusion tensor imaging study. *American Journal of Neuroradiology, 31*, 894–900. doi:10.3174/ajnr.A1957.

Welle-Strand, G., Skurtveit, S., Jones, H., Waal, H., Bakstad, B., Bjarko, L., & Ravndal, E. (2013). Neonatal outcomes following in utero exposure to methadone or buprenorphine: A national cohort study of opioid-agonist treatment of pregnant women in Norway from 1996 to 2009. *Drug and Alcohol Dependence, 127*, 200–206.

Winklbaur, B., Baewert, A., Jagsch, R., Rohrmeister, K., Metz, V., Jachmann, C., … Fischer, G. (2009). Association between prenatal tobacco exposure and outcomes of neonates born to opioid-maintained mothers. *European Addiction Research, 15*, 150–156. doi:10.1159/000216466.

Chapter 5
Neurodevelopmental Considerations with Antiepileptic Drug Use During Pregnancy

David W. Loring, Elizabeth E. Gerard, and Kimford J. Meador

Definitional Issues and Prevalence

Antiepileptic drugs (AEDs) are the primary therapeutic option for seizure control in patients with epilepsy. Women with epilepsy wanting to start families, however, face difficult decisions about how to best manage their epilepsy care while simultaneously minimizing risks to their unborn children from AED exposure. If a woman's epilepsy is mild (e.g., infrequent sensory seizures without altered awareness), she may choose to discontinue AEDs before attempting to become pregnant. For most women, however, AED discontinuation produces significant risks to both the mother (e.g., Sudden Unexplained Death in Epilepsy or SUDEP) and unborn child (e.g., fetal hypoxia; Edey, Moran, & Nashef, 2014; Viguera et al., 2007). For example, there is an approximate 10× mortality increase in pregnancy and the postpartum period in women with epilepsy compared to baseline population rates (Cantwell et al., 2011). The increase in mortality is assumed to be related to SUDEP (Edey et al., 2014). In addition to treating epilepsy, AEDs are also commonly used for psychiatric considerations

---

D.W. Loring, Ph.D., A.B.P.P. (✉)
Departments of Neurology and Pediatrics, Emory University,
12 Executive Park, Room 285, Atlanta, GA 30329, USA
e-mail: dloring@emory.edu

E.E. Gerard, M.D.
Feinberg School of Medicine, Northwestern University,
675 N. St. Clair, Galter 20-100, Chicago, IL 60611, USA
e-mail: e-gerard@northwestern.edu

K.J. Meador, M.D.
Department of Neurology & Neurological Sciences, Stanford University,
300 Pasteur Drive (Room A343), Stanford, CA 94305, USA
e-mail: kmeador@stanford.edu

C. Riccio, J. Sullivan (eds.), *Pediatric Neurotoxicology*, Specialty Topics in Pediatric Neuropsychology, DOI 10.1007/978-3-319-32358-9_5

(e.g., bipolar disorder, mood stabilization) and pain indications, and in fact, the number of AED prescriptions for non-epilepsy indications during pregnancy is higher than those for epilepsy (Bobo et al., 2012). Approximately 2 % of women during their pregnancy take AEDs for either psychiatric or neurologic indications (Bobo et al., 2012).

In utero AED risk has traditionally been operationalized by major congenital malformation risk, and it has been suggested that AED monotherapy doubles, and AED polytherapy triples, the risk of developing major congenital malformations (Hill, Wlodarczyk, Palacios, & Finnell, 2010). Although estimates vary based upon sampling characteristics, major congenital malformations are observed in 6.1 % of children born to women with epilepsy taking AEDs during pregnancy, and 2.8 % among children born to mothers with epilepsy who were not taking AEDs. This compares to 2.2 % in control mothers (Tomson & Battino, 2012). Valproate (VPA) has a higher major congenital malformation risk than either taking no AEDs or to other AEDs, with a 1–2 % risk of neural tube deficits, representing a 10–20× increase over the general population (Meador, Reynolds, Crean, Fahrbach, & Probst, 2008). Several AEDs including carbamazepine (CBZ), lamotrigine (LTG), phenytoin (PHT), or levetiracetam (LEV) have smaller risks of major congenital malformations (Campbell et al., 2014; Harden, 2014; Hernandez-Diaz et al., 2012; Mawhinney et al., 2013; Vajda, O'Brien, Lander, Graham, & Eadie, 2014). Phenobarbital and topiramate (TPM) exposures are associated with intermediate risks (Harden, 2014; Hernandez-Diaz et al., 2012; Margulis et al., 2012; Mines et al., 2014). In this chapter, we focus on cognitive and behavioral developmental outcomes of children exposed to AEDs during pregnancy that are necessary to inform treatment decision making, and briefly discuss the role of folate and breast feeding in these patients.

Impact on the Developing Child

Because AEDs have different mechanisms of action, neurodevelopmental risks of in utero exposure will vary. In this section, we review developmental impact across the medications for which adequate research and clinical data have been collected. Risks of AED exposure have only been partially described, however, and even when specific AED risks have been formally investigated, there are often methodological issues limiting the confidence of drug-specific findings including absence of assessor blinding during assessment, follow-up that begins at birth or later rather than during pregnancy, or failure to control for potential confounding factors such as maternal IQ, seizure type and frequency, or AED dose/blood levels.

Valproate (VPA)

Multiple studies have confirmed that among AEDs adequately studied, VPA is the AED associated with the greatest risk of cognitive and behavioral teratogenesis. VPA exposed children are more likely to miss developmental milestones and have decreased

IQ scores. In addition, verbal skills appear particularly vulnerable to VPA effects. VPA exposed children also have poorer adaptive skills, with increased risks of Attention Deficit Hyperactivity Disorder (ADHD) and Autism Spectrum Disorder (ASD).

Cognitive Effects

Despite a variety of methodological limitations, VPA exposure has consistently been associated with developmental delay and decreased general level of function. A meta-analysis of developmental outcomes of children of women with epilepsy estimates that VPA exposure is associated with a 6-point reduction in Full Scale IQ (Banach, Boskovic, Einarson, & Koren, 2010). Whether used as monotherapy or part of a polytherapy regimen, VPA exposure is associated with a higher likelihood of either intellectual disability (i.e., FSIQ < 70, 10 %) or borderline cognition (i.e., FSIQ = 70–79; 14 %) than other AEDs studied (Eriksson et al., 2005). Demonstrating the importance of potential confounds, mothers taking VPA in this study had lower FSIQ and also had lower levels of education ($p = 0.035$; Eriksson et al., 2005). A retrospective study controlling for maternal IQ demonstrated a lower verbal IQ (approximately ten points) in children exposed in utero to VPA ($n = 41$) versus other monotherapy groups and an unexposed group (Adab, Jacoby, Smith, & Chadwick, 2001) . The decrease in IQ in the VPA group was dose-dependent.

An alternative way of characterizing AED risk is the frequency of "additional educational needs" during schooling, which reflects the provision of additional assistance during mainstream education. Children exposed in utero to VPA had an odds ratio of 3.4 (95 % CI, 1.6–7.1) of being provided with additional educational services compared to unexposed children (Adab et al., 2001). VPA exposure has been associated with an increased risk of delayed early development in comparison to controls ($n = 230$; Bromley et al., 2010). In an observational cohort study, there was developmental delay in 40 % of VPA exposed children (OR 26.1, 95 % CI, 4.9–139; $p < 0.001$), 20 % for CBZ exposed children (OR 7.7, 95 % CI, 1.4–43.1; $p < 0.01$), but only 3 % for LTG exposure. This contrasts with 4.5 % in controls (Cummings, Stewart, Stevenson, Morrow, & Nelson, 2011).

The NEAD study (Neurodevelopmental Effects of Antiepileptic Drugs) characterized developmental outcomes of children exposed to either valproate (VPA), carbamazepine (CBZ), lamotrigine (LTG), or phenytoin (PHT) monotherapy during their mothers' pregnancy in a prospective patient cohort, controlling for multiple potential confounding factors. The NEAD study demonstrated increased risk of VPA exposure compared to other AEDs (Meador et al., 2009, 2013). When evaluated at age 6 years, children exposed to VPA had General Conceptual Ability (GCA) scores that were 7–10 points lower than children exposed to other AEDs demonstrating that additional time following exposure does not allow them to "catch up." This effect was seen in correlational analyses in which the strong relationship between maternal IQ and child GCA scores in all AED groups with the exception of VPA. VPA exposure was associated with decreased GCA, decreased memory, and decreased executive function. Of the various domains affected including GCA verbal abilities were most severely affected by VPA. A dose-dependent adverse effects across all cognitive domains assessed was also described.

Although risk of drug-induced major malformations are related to first trimester exposures, the risk for cognitive-behavioral problems, similar to alcohol, appears greatest during third trimester exposure. A dose relationship for VPA has been observed across trimesters, although this likely reflects that AED dose for epilepsy tends to be constant, with higher doses of VPA correlated with lower GCA, verbal and non-verbal indices, and also lower memory and executive function (Meador et al., 2013). This dose-relationship reflects VPA's neurodevelopmental toxicity, but does not indicate whether any fully safe VPA doses without any risk exists.

Because the behavioral risk of VPA occurs in the first trimester, women taking VPA often incur exposure risk since it will often occur prior to a woman knowing that she is pregnant. High dose VPA exposure (>800 mg/day) has been associated with an GCA that was nearly ten points lower than healthy controls, which was accompanied by an eightfold increased need of educational intervention (Baker et al., 2015). Lower VPA levels (≤800 mg/day) was not associated with reduced GCA, but it was associated with impaired verbal abilities and a sixfold increase in the need for educational intervention. Again, despite this dose-related effect, a completely safe dose of VPA has not been established.

Behavioral Effects

Early reports identified an association between autism and VPA exposure (Christianson, Chesler, & Kromberg, 1994; Rasalam et al., 2005; Williams et al., 2001; Williams & Hersh, 1997). In addition to ASD, 20 % of ASD affected children also experienced major congenital malformations (Rasalam et al., 2005). Even when excluding major congenital malformations, impaired social and adaptive functioning in VPA children has been described with an increased risk autism or ASD diagnosis (Christensen et al., 2013). The absolute risk was 2.5 % for autism and 4.4 % for ASD in the VPA exposed children cohort compared with 0.5 and 1.5 % in the general population. The rates of autism and ASD in children of mothers taking CBZ, clonazepam, oxcarbazepine (OXC), or lamotrigine (LTG) monotherapy were not increased.

When characterizing poor outcomes using a combined neurodevelopmental disorders (NDD) outcome to account for low incidence of specific events including autism, ASD, ADHD, or dyspraxia, a NDD was present in 6 of 50 (12 %) children exposed to VPA monotherapy and 3 of 20 (15 %) children exposed to VPA in polytherapy (33). These rates are higher than in 214 controls (1.9 %) (Bromley et al., 2013).

VPA exposed children have lower daily living and socialization skills than do children exposed to other AEDs. In the prospective NEAD cohort at both 3 and 6 years, VPA exposed children had poorer scores for adaptive functioning than children exposed to phenytoin or lamotrigine, but not carbamazepine (Cohen et al., 2011; Cohen et al., 2013). VPA exposed children were significantly more likely to receive poor scores for adaptive functioning compared to children exposed to phenytoin or lamotrigine, but not carbamazepine. VPA dose correlated with poorer scores for adaptive functioning, and VPA exposure correlated with a greater number of atypical (socially immature) behavior and inattention signs than did either PHT or LTG.

Carbamazepine (CBZ)

The evidence addressing CBZ exposure risks has been conflicting, although most reports describe no adverse cognitive or development effects (Adab et al., 2004; Gaily et al., 2004; Thomas, Sukumaran, Lukose, George, & Sarma, 2007; Vinten et al., 2005, 2009). Nevertheless, several studies describe increased rates of developmental delay (Cummings et al., 2011; Dean et al., 2002; Mawer, Clayton-Smith, Coyle, & Kini, 2002; Ornoy & Cohen, 1996). Although a meta-analysis surveying studies conducted before 2005 described adverse negative effects of CBZ exposure on Performance IQ, not all of these studies controlled for maternal IQ. A negative correlation between CBZ dose with verbal performance and motor functioning was observed in the NEAD study at 3 years but not when tested at 6 years (Cohen et al., 2011, 2013; Meador et al., 2009). No IQ difference for CBZ exposed children was described at age 6 years compared to controls, although the verbal index was 4.2 points lower (Baker et al., 2015). This was associated with an increased risk of having an IQ<85. Although CBZ is associated with a smaller risk of poor cognitive outcomes compared to VPA, there appears to be increased risk relative to controls. No increased risk of diagnosed neurodevelopmental disorders for CBZ exposed children was observed (Bromley et al., 2013).

CBZ exposed children may have decreased fine motor and social skills at 18 months, and have been characterized as having more aggressive behaviors at 36 months (Veiby et al., 2013). Adaptive scores for VPA exposed children at age 6 years in the NEAD study were significantly lower than that of children exposed to LTG or PHT but did not differ from CBZ exposed children (Cohen et al., 2013). CBZ exposure was also associated with an increased risk for ADHD by parental, but not teacher, behavior reports. A retrospective study found no difference between parentally reported adaptive behavior of CBZ exposed children age 6–16 years compared with unexposed children (Vinten et al., 2009). In summary, although there are some inconsistencies in the literature, CBZ appears to have less cognitive and behavioral risk than VPA, and appears comparable to controls regarding overall level of general function.

Lamotrigine (LTG)

Risks of LTG exposure appear low, with developmental outcomes that do not differ from controls (Bromley et al., 2010; Cummings et al., 2011). The NEAD study described GCA scores in LTG exposed children that did not differ from either CBZ or PHT exposed children, while being significantly higher than children exposed to VPA (Cohen et al., 2011; Meador et al., 2009, 2013). In the 6-year-old NEAD cohort, both VPA and LTG exposure were associated with poorer verbal indices than non-verbal indices, and both had higher incidence of atypical handedness (Meador et al., 2013) raising the possibility of the AEDs altering the process of normal cerebral language development and lateralization. In contrast to the NEAD findings, an independent report described no IQ score differences between VPA and LTG exposed children (Rihtman, Parush, & Ornoy, 2013). However, LTG and VPA were both associated with poorer non-verbal IQs compared with controls, although the non-verbal IQ in the control group was seven points higher than verbal IQ.

In one study, LTG exposure has been reported to be associated with increased frequency of autistic traits based on a parental questionnaire (Veiby et al., 2013). Parents of children exposed to LTG in the NEAD study rated children as being at increased risk for ADHD, although this pattern was not reported by teachers (Cohen et al., 2013). This pattern of neurodevelopmental disorders has not been observed, however, in other reports (Bromley et al., 2013).

Levetiracetam (LEV)

In a subset from the UK pregnancy register, 51 children exposed to levetiracetam were found not to differ from controls at either 3–24 months or 36–54 months, but were better than VPA exposed children (Shallcross et al., 2011, 2014). The developmental scores of the exposed children did not differ from those of controls at either time point, but were better than VPA. This is the only current report of developmental outcomes for LEV exposure.

Phenobarbital (PB)

In several prospective studies, phenobarbital exposure is associated with lower IQ scores (Reinisch, Sanders, Mortensen, & Rubin, 1995) which appears primarily reflected with decreased verbal IQ. Exposure during the third trimester appears to be associated with the greatest negative effect. This relationship has been described in a separate prospective study (Thomas et al., 2007). Retrospective studies, however, have produced inconsistent results (Dean, Colantonio, Ratcliff, & Chase, 2000; Dessens et al., 2000; van der Pol, Hadders-Algra, Huisjes, & Touwen, 1991). Although phenobarbital is infrequently prescribed in North America and Europe, its low cost makes phenobarbital a common first-line treatment option in less well developed regions (Zhang, Zeng, & Li, 2011).

Phenytoin (PHT)

Several reports of PHT exposure have noted no differential cognitive outcome compared to controls (Adab et al., 2004; Koch et al., 1999; Thomas et al., 2007; Wide, Winbladh, Tomson, Sars-Zimmer, & Berggren, 2000). Even in the absence of generalized cognitive impairment, decreased locomotor performance has been observed

(Wide et al., 2000). One study describing decreased FSIQ associated with PHT exposure (Scolnik et al., 1994) was criticized due to significant differences in maternal IQs across groups (Loring, Meador, & Thompson, 1994). Other reports have described increased risk of developmental delay in children exposed to PHT, but also associated with VPA and CBZ exposure (Dean et al., 2002). The NEAD study reported no differences between PHT exposed children from either CBZ or LTG exposed children on FSIQ or verbal IQ, with PHT scores higher than with VPA exposure. No differences in adaptive behavior following PHT exposure as reported by parents compared to controls have been noted (Vinten et al., 2009).

Topiramate (TPM)

TPM exposure was associated with lower IQ scores in a very small sample of nine children, which was accompanied by poorer motor and visual spatial skills, and high rates of speech, occupational or physical therapy (Rihtman, Parush, & Ornoy, 2012).

Other AEDs

There is little or no information on the developmental outcomes associated with exposure to other AEDs including benzodiazepines, eslicarbazepine, ezogabine, felbamate, gabapentin, lacosamide, oxcarbazepine, perampanel, pregabalin, rufinamide, vigabatrin, or zonisamide.

Polytherapy

Multiple studies described an increased risk of poor developmental outcomes for children exposed to multiple AEDs during pregnancy (Adab et al., 2001; Dean et al., 2002; Dessens et al., 2000; Gaily et al., 2004; Koch et al., 1999; Nadebaum, Anderson, Vajda, Reutens, & Wood, 2012; Thomas et al., 2007; Veiby et al., 2013), although several reports have not found an increased risk (Adab et al., 2004; Bromley et al., 2010; Gaily, Kantola-Sorsa, & Granstrom, 1988; Wide et al., 2000). This discrepancy likely reflects different polytherapy combinations examined. When polytherapy combinations include VPA, an increased cognitive risk is described whereas polytherapy combinations with AEDs other than VPA are not associated with a similar risk. Polytherapy exposures including VPA are associated with lower FSIQ and verbal scores compared with either VPA monotherapy or polytherapy combinations with AEDs other than VPA (Baker et al., 2015; Nadebaum et al., 2012). Nevertheless, the effects of various polytherapy AED combinations remain uncertain and need to be more fully established.

Prognosis and Moderating Factors

Long-term studies of developmental outcomes have not been performed. Unfortunately, there is no research as yet that has identified specific moderating factors or long term outcomes. At the same time, there is no reasons to suspect that children with neurodevelopmental deficits or ASD from AED exposure in untero would differ from others with similar neurobehavioral disorders simply as a function of etiology.

Possible Mechanisms of Action

AED-induced cognitive and behavioral deficits have been described in the animal literature at dosages lower than what is necessary to increase risks of physical malformation (Adams, Vorhees, & Middaugh, 1990). Phenobarbital, for example, produces neuronal deficits, reduces brain weight and brain catecholamine levels, and impairs development of normal behaviors (Forcelli, Janssen, Vicini, & Gale, 2012). Prenatal phenytoin has been associated with dose-dependent impairment of coordination and learning (Ogura et al., 2002). Behavioral deficits have been described not only with older AEDs (e.g., PB, PHT, VPA), but also impaired rotorod performance for adult rats with neonatal-exposure to lamotrigine (Forcelli et al., 2012). Behavioral and anatomical defects likely involve different mechanisms—anatomical risks are related to first trimester exposure, and functional deficits appear primarily related to third trimester exposure. Third trimester exposure association interferes with the development of functional properties and connectivity, and susceptible to AED-induced apoptosis and altered synaptogenesis (Forcelli et al., 2012). Possible mechanisms associated with functional AED teratogenicity include folate deficiency, reactive intermediates (e.g. epoxides or free radicals), ischemia, apoptosis-related mechanisms, and neuronal suppression (Gedzelman & Meador, 2012).

The leading hypothesis for the mechanism behind behavioral/cognitive dysfunction involves AED induced apoptosis and altered synaptogenesis. Similar to alcohol, exposure of the immature brain to some AEDs is associated with widespread neuronal apoptosis (Turski & Ikonomidou, 2012). NMDA antagonist and GABA mimetic traits of ethanol have been postulated to produce apoptogenic action since other drugs that block NMDA glutamate receptors also trigger apoptosis in the developing brain. This may be clinically relevant because many AEDs used therapeutically in humans have NMDA antagonist or GABA mimetic properties (e.g., barbiturates and benzodiazepines; Olney et al., 2002). The associated cognitive deficits are likely more related to dysfunction in the surviving neurons than to the actual neuronal loss; exposure of the immature brain to AEDs impairs synaptic maturation in neurons that survive the initial exposure (Forcelli et al., 2012). Genetic predisposition likely also plays a role involving interaction of teratogens with multiple liability genes (Finnell, Shields, Taylor, & Chernoff, 1987). Genetic predisposition may explain the observed individual variability.

Considerations to Minimize Risk and Maximize Cognitive Outcome

Folate

Folate supplementation for women of reproductive age is now standard of care based on population studies demonstrating decreased neural tube defect risk (Blencowe, Cousens, Modell, & Lawn, 2010), although the optimal dose has not yet been established (Aguglia et al., 2009; Kjaer et al., 2008; Wilson et al., 2003). Several studies have demonstrated a similar relationship between folate levels or supplementation and decreased major congenital malformations in women with epilepsy although larger studies are needed (Harden et al., 2009; Kaaja, Kaaja, & Hiilesmaa, 2003; Kjaer et al., 2008).

In the NEAD study, children whose mothers reported periconception folate supplementation had higher Developmental Abilities Scale (DAS) GCA scores at 6 years of age than children whose mother did not take folate during their pregnancy (Meador et al., 2013). When excluding VPA, there was a dose-related effect of folate on conceptual abilities scores. This suggests that folate may have a positive effect on cognitive development, although others have failed to observe a similar beneficial effect of folate supplementation on cognitive outcome (Baker et al., 2015). Whether there is a more general beneficial effect of folate on cognitive outcome is unknown since, in the case of the NEAD study, the positive effect may simply have occurred from mitigating the negative AED effects. However, other studies report a beneficial effect of periconceptional folic acid supplementation for cognitive and behavioral outcomes in the general population (Chatzi et al., 2012; Roth et al., 2011; Schmidt et al., 2012; Suren et al., 2013). There is presently insufficient evidence to conclude that folate supplementation mitigates the structural or developmental teratogenic effects of AEDs, but it appears to provide a more general benefit and should be used in women of childbearing age being treated with AEDs.

Breast Feeding

Breast feeding provides important health benefits for both mother and child (Ip, Chung, Raman, Trikalinos, & Lau, 2009) that may include improved cognitive development (Heikkila, Kelly, Renfrew, Sacker, & Quigley, 2014; Kramer et al., 2008; Quigley et al., 2012). This benefit also appears to be present in children exposed to AEDs who are breast-fed. In the NEAD study, AED exposed children who were breast-fed had higher DAS GCA scores and Verbal Scores when tested at age 6 years than children who were not breast-fed (Meador et al., 2014). Although a similar pattern was described in a separate cohort of children when tested up to age 18 months, the benefit was no longer observed when tested at age 36 months (Veiby et al., 2013). Importantly, however, both studies indicate an absence of increased cognitive risk for children being breast-fed by mothers taking AEDs. Breast feeding by women taking AEDs has often been discouraged due to concerns that the child will be exposed to AED through breast milk. Unlike in utero exposure, in which the fetal levels are similar to maternal plasma concentrations, AEDs are differentially secreted into human milk. Although additional studies are needed, the current data suggest that the theoretical concern of infant breast milk AED exposure likely does not outweigh the known long-lasting benefits of breast feeding.

School Accommodations

There has been no systematic research demonstrating the specific benefit of school accommodations in this group of children. However, as with other developmental disorders, children with AED induced language delay or attentional impairment will likely benefit based upon their specific needs from modification of assignment length, the provision of extended time for assignments and tests, the assistant of a peer tutor/study partner, and private location for testing as needed. Similarly, children with ASD related to AED exposure may benefit from strategies to develop social skills and teaching social rules, with small group (or one-to-one) instruction and interventions generally appropriate for those with ASD.

Conclusions

Women of reproductive age taking AEDs for any indication should be counseled about exposure risks. These risks should also be discussed with teens and preteens and their parents before the girls become sexually active. Because roughly half of pregnancies in women with epilepsy are unplanned (Davis, Pack, Kritzer, Yoon, & Camus, 2008), not discussing risks until a woman is planning pregnancy is often too late. Contraceptive counseling is also extremely important for all women taking AEDs since they have significant drug–drug interactions with hormonal contraception (Gaffield, Culwell, & Lee, 2011).

Even with effective contraception, however, medication management of a reproductive-age woman should involve AEDs with lowest teratogenic risk that effectively manage their epilepsy. Thus, VPA is a poor first choice for females of child-bearing potential. Unfortunately, some women will have inadequate control of seizures or mood symptoms with medications other than VPA. In these cases, the smallest effective dose of VPA should be employed. Although the dose-related exposure risks appear to be the greatest for VPA, women taking other AEDs should be managed with the smallest effective doses as well. Polytherapy should be avoided if possible. Finally, it may also be necessary to establish that AEDs are appropriately indicated since some patients with non-AED responsive seizures or atypical histories may have non-epileptic seizures, and appropriate monitoring in an epilepsy unit may be necessary to establish this diagnosis.

An area of debate is whether AED changes should ever be contemplated during pregnancy. When characterization of AED teratogenesis was limited to major congenital malformations, this was generally not considered since by the time pregnancy was confirmed, the risks of cross-titrating AEDs was thought to simply expose the fetus to polytherapy and increased the risk of seizures after the major congenital malformation risk had already occurred. We now know that cognitive AED risks likely occur throughout pregnancy and, in particular, during the third trimester. Consequently, some have suggested that it is reasonable to consider AED changes during pregnancy, particularly if the woman is taking VPA. This consideration should include seizure history or severity of her mood disorder, history of prior medication trials and effectiveness, likelihood of responding to a different medication, and the ability to closely monitor her and her child. This is strictly a clinical consideration since there is insufficient evidence to argue for or against this approach.

Women taking AEDs should receive folate supplementation since it decreases risk of neural tube defects, may reduce the risk of other malformations, and may have a positive effect on cognitive development. Although it is unclear if folate provides benefit to women taking AEDs beyond that seen in the general population, supplementation is recommended by multiple professional organizations.

Most women taking AEDs should not be discouraged from breast-feeding their child. For women taking CBZ, LTG, PHT, or VPA in monotherapy, there is no evidence to suggest risk to the child. Women taking other AEDs or being treated with polytherapy may consider the risks vs. benefits of breast feeding since the AED risks remain primarily theoretical. Further, pediatricians treating children exposed to AEDs in utero should also monitor the child's development closely and consider early intervention for children exposed to AEDs (especially VPA) who demonstrate any signs of developmental delay.

References

Adab, N., Jacoby, A., Smith, D., & Chadwick, D. (2001). Additional educational needs in children born to mothers with epilepsy. *Journal of Neurology, Neurosurgery & Psychiatry, 70*, 15–21.

Adab, N., Kini, U., Vinten, J., Ayres, J., Baker, G., Clayton-Smith, J., … Chadwick, D. W. (2004). The longer term outcome of children born to mothers with epilepsy. *Journal of Neurology, Neurosurgery & Psychiatry, 75*(11), 1575–1583.

Adams, J., Vorhees, C. V., & Middaugh, L. D. (1990). Developmental neurotoxicity of anticonvulsants: human and animal evidence on phenytoin. *Neurotoxicology & Teratology, 12*(3), 203–214.

Aguglia, U., Barboni, G., Battino, D., Cavazzuti, G. B., Citernesi, A., Corosu, R., … Verrotti, A. (2009). Italian consensus conference on epilepsy and pregnancy, labor and puerperium. *Epilepsia, 50 Suppl 1*, 7–23.

Baker, G. A., Bromley, R. L., Briggs, M., Cheyne, C. P., Cohen, M. J., Garcia-Finana, M., … Clayton-Smith, J. (2015). IQ at 6 years after in utero exposure to antiepileptic drugs: A controlled cohort study. *Neurology, 84*(4), 382–390.

Banach, R., Boskovic, R., Einarson, T., & Koren, G. (2010). Long-term developmental outcome of children of women with epilepsy, unexposed or exposed prenatally to antiepileptic drugs: A meta-analysis of cohort studies. *Drug Safety, 33*(1), 73–79.

Blencowe, H., Cousens, S., Modell, B., & Lawn, J. (2010). Folic acid to reduce neonatal mortality from neural tube disorders. *International Journal of Epidemiology, 39*(Suppl 1), i110–i121.

Bobo, W. V., Davis, R. L., Toh, S., Li, D. K., Andrade, S. E., Cheetham, T. C., … Cooper, W. O. (2012). Trends in the use of antiepileptic drugs among pregnant women in the US, 2001–2007: A medication exposure in pregnancy risk evaluation program study. *Paediatric and Perinatal Epidemiology, 26*(6), 578–588.

Bromley, R. L., Mawer, G. E., Briggs, M., Cheyne, C., Clayton-Smith, J., Garcia-Finana, M., … Baker, G. A. (2013). The prevalence of neurodevelopmental disorders in children prenatally exposed to antiepileptic drugs. *Journal of Neurology, Neurosurgery & Psychiatry, 84*(6), 637–643.

Bromley, R. L., Mawer, G., Love, J., Kelly, J., Purdy, L., McEwan, L., … Baker, G. A. (2010). Early cognitive development in children born to women with epilepsy: a prospective report. *Epilepsia, 51*(10), 2058–2065.

Campbell, E., Kennedy, F., Russell, A., Smithson, W. H., Parsons, L., Morrison, P. J., … Morrow, J. (2014). Malformation risks of antiepileptic drug monotherapies in pregnancy: updated results from the UK and Ireland Epilepsy and Pregnancy Registers. *Journal of Neurology, Neurosurgery & Psychiatry, 85*(9), 1029–1034.

Cantwell, R., Clutton-Brock, T., Cooper, G., Dawson, A., Drife, J., Garrod, D., … Springett, A. (2011). Saving mothers' lives: Reviewing maternal deaths to make motherhood safer: 2006-2008. The eighth report of the confidential enquiries into maternal deaths in the United Kingdom. *BJOG, 118 Suppl 1*, 1–203.

Chatzi, L., Papadopoulou, E., Koutra, K., Roumeliotaki, T., Georgiou, V., Stratakis, N., … Kogevinas, M. (2012). Effect of high doses of folic acid supplementation in early pregnancy on child neurodevelopment at 18 months of age: the mother-child cohort 'Rhea' study in Crete, Greece. *Public Health Nutrition, 15*(9), 1728–1736.

Christensen, J., Gronborg, T. K., Sorensen, M. J., Schendel, D., Parner, E. T., Pedersen, L. H., & Vestergaard, M. (2013). Prenatal valproate exposure and risk of autism spectrum disorders and childhood autism. *JAMA, 309*(16), 1696–1703.

Christianson, A. L., Chesler, N., & Kromberg, J. G. (1994). Fetal valproate syndrome: Clinical and neuro-developmental features in two sibling pairs. *Developmental Medicine & Child Neurology, 36*(4), 361–369.

Cohen, M. J., Meador, K. J., Browning, N., Baker, G. A., Clayton-Smith, J., Kalayjian, L. A., … Loring, D. W. (2011). Fetal antiepileptic drug exposure: motor, adaptive, and emotional/behavioral functioning at age 3 years. *Epilepsy & Behavior, 22*(2), 240–246.

Cohen, M. J., Meador, K. J., Browning, N., May, R., Baker, G. A., Clayton-Smith, J., … Loring, D. W. (2013). Fetal antiepileptic drug exposure: Adaptive and emotional/behavioral functioning at age 6 years. *Epilepsy Behav, 29*(2), 308–315.

Cummings, C., Stewart, M., Stevenson, M., Morrow, J., & Nelson, J. (2011). Neurodevelopment of children exposed in utero to lamotrigine, sodium valproate and carbamazepine. *Archives of Disease in Childhood, 96*(7), 643–647.

Davis, A. R., Pack, A. M., Kritzer, J., Yoon, A., & Camus, A. (2008). Reproductive history, sexual behavior and use of contraception in women with epilepsy. *Contraception, 77*(6), 405–409.

Dean, S., Colantonio, A., Ratcliff, G., & Chase, S. (2000). Clients' perspectives on problems many years after traumatic brain injury. *Psychological Reports, 86*(2), 653–658.

Dean, J. C., Hailey, H., Moore, S. J., Lloyd, D. J., Turnpenny, P. D., & Little, J. (2002). Long term health and neurodevelopment in children exposed to antiepileptic drugs before birth. *Journal of Medical Genetics, 39*(4), 251–259.

Dessens, A. B., Cohen-Kettenis, P. T., Mellenbergh, G. J., Koppe, J. G., van De Poll, N. E., & Boer, K. (2000). Association of prenatal phenobarbital and phenytoin exposure with small head size at birth and with learning problems. *Acta Paediatrica, 89*(5), 533–541.

Edey, S., Moran, N., & Nashef, L. (2014). SUDEP and epilepsy-related mortality in pregnancy. *Epilepsia, 55*(7), e72–e74.

Eriksson, K., Viinikainen, K., Monkkonen, A., Aikia, M., Nieminen, P., Heinonen, S., & Kalviainen, R. (2005). Children exposed to valproate in utero—population based evaluation of risks and confounding factors for long-term neurocognitive development. *Epilepsy Research, 65*(3), 189–200.

Finnell, R. H., Shields, H. E., Taylor, S. M., & Chernoff, G. F. (1987). Strain differences in phenobarbital-induced teratogenesis in mice. *Teratology, 35*(2), 177–185.

Forcelli, P. A., Janssen, M. J., Vicini, S., & Gale, K. (2012). Neonatal exposure to antiepileptic drugs disrupts striatal synaptic development. *Annals of Neurology, 72*(3), 363–372.

Gaffield, M. E., Culwell, K. R., & Lee, C. R. (2011). The use of hormonal contraception among women taking anticonvulsant therapy. *Contraception, 83*(1), 16–29.

Gaily, E., Kantola-Sorsa, E., Hiilesmaa, V., Isoaho, M., Matila, R., Kotila, M., … Granstrom, M. L. (2004). Normal intelligence in children with prenatal exposure to carbamazepine. *Neurology, 62*(1), 28–32.

Gaily, E., Kantola-Sorsa, E., & Granstrom, M. L. (1988). Intelligence of children of epileptic mothers. *Journal of Pediatrics, 113*(4), 677–684.

Gedzelman, E. R., & Meador, K. J. (2012). Neurological and psychiatric sequelae of developmental exposure to antiepileptic drugs. *Frontiers in Neurology, 3*, 182.

Harden, C. L. (2014). Pregnancy and epilepsy. *Continuum (Minneap, MN), 20*(1 Neurology of Pregnancy), 60–79.

Harden, C. L., Hopp, J., Ting, T. Y., Pennell, P. B., French, J. A., Hauser, W. A., … Le Guen, C. (2009). Practice parameter update: management issues for women with epilepsy—focus on pregnancy (an evidence-based review): obstetrical complications and change in seizure frequency: Report of the Quality Standards Subcommittee and Therapeutics and Technology Assessment Subcommittee of the American Academy of Neurology and American Epilepsy Society. *Neurology, 73*(2), 126–132.

Heikkila, K., Kelly, Y., Renfrew, M. J., Sacker, A., & Quigley, M. A. (2014). Breastfeeding and educational achievement at age 5. *Maternal & Child Nutrition, 10*(1), 92–101.

Hernandez-Diaz, S., Smith, C. R., Shen, A., Mittendorf, R., Hauser, W. A., Yerby, M., & Holmes, L. B. (2012). Comparative safety of antiepileptic drugs during pregnancy. *Neurology, 78*(21), 1692–1699.

Hill, D. S., Wlodarczyk, B. J., Palacios, A. M., & Finnell, R. H. (2010). Teratogenic effects of antiepileptic drugs. *Expert Review of Neurotherapeutics, 10*(6), 943–959.

Ip, S., Chung, M., Raman, G., Trikalinos, T. A., & Lau, J. (2009). A summary of the agency for healthcare research and quality's evidence report on breastfeeding in developed countries. *Breastfeeding Medicine, 4*(Suppl 1), S17–S30.

Kaaja, E., Kaaja, R., & Hiilesmaa, V. (2003). Major malformations in offspring of women with epilepsy. *Neurology, 60*(4), 575–579.

Kjaer, D., Horvath-Puho, E., Christensen, J., Vestergaard, M., Czeizel, A. E., Sorensen, H. T., & Olsen, J. (2008). Antiepileptic drug use, folic acid supplementation, and congenital abnormalities: A population-based case-control study. *BJOG, 115*(1), 98–103.

Koch, S., Titze, K., Zimmermann, R. B., Schroder, M., Lehmkuhl, U., & Rauh, H. (1999). Long-term neuropsychological consequences of maternal epilepsy and anticonvulsant treatment during pregnancy for school-age children and adolescents. *Epilepsia, 40*(9), 1237–1243.

Kramer, M. S., Aboud, F., Mironova, E., Vanilovich, I., Platt, R. W., Matush, L., … Shapiro, S. (2008). Breastfeeding and child cognitive development: new evidence from a large randomized trial. *Archives of General Psychiatry, 65*(5), 578–584.

Loring, D. W., Meador, K. J., & Thompson, W. O. (1994). Neurodevelopment after in utero exposure to phenytoin and carbamazepine. *JAMA, 272*(11), 850–851.

Margulis, A. V., Mitchell, A. A., Gilboa, S. M., Werler, M. M., Mittleman, M. A., Glynn, R. J., & Hernandez-Diaz, S. (2012). Use of topiramate in pregnancy and risk of oral clefts. *American Journal of Obstetrics & Gynecology, 207*(5), 405.e401–405.e407.

Mawer, G., Clayton-Smith, J., Coyle, H., & Kini, U. (2002). Outcome of pregnancy in women attending an outpatient epilepsy clinic: Adverse features associated with higher doses of sodium valproate. *Seizure, 11*(8), 512–518.

Mawhinney, E., Craig, J., Morrow, J., Russell, A., Smithson, W. H., Parsons, L., … Hunt, S. J. (2013). Levetiracetam in pregnancy: results from the UK and Ireland epilepsy and pregnancy registers. *Neurology, 80*(4), 400–405.

Meador, K.J., Baker, G.A., Browning, N., Clayton-Smith, J, Combs-Cantrell, D.T., Cohen, M., … Loring, D.W. (2009). Cognitive function at 3 years of age after fetal exposure to antiepileptic drugs. *New England Journal of Medicine, 360*(16), 1597–1605.

Meador, K. J., Baker, G. A., Browning, N., Cohen, M. J., Bromley, R. L., Clayton-Smith, J., … Loring, D. W. (2014). Breastfeeding in children of women taking antiepileptic drugs: Cognitive outcomes at age 6 years. *JAMA Pediatrics, 168*(8), 729–736.

Meador, K. J., Baker, G. A., Browning, N., Cohen, M J., Bromley, R. L., Clayton-Smith, J. , … Loring, D. W. (2013). Fetal antiepileptic drug exposure and cognitive outcomes at age 6 years (NEAD study): A prospective observational study. *The Lancet Neurology, 12*(3), 244–252.

Meador, K., Reynolds, M. W., Crean, S., Fahrbach, K., & Probst, C. (2008). Pregnancy outcomes in women with epilepsy: A systematic review and meta-analysis of published pregnancy registries and cohorts. *Epilepsy Research, 81*(1), 1–13.

Mines, D., Tennis, P., Curkendall, S. M., Li, D. K., Peterson, C., Andrews, E. B., … Chan, K. A. (2014). Topiramate use in pregnancy and the birth prevalence of oral clefts. *Pharmacoepidemiology & Drug Saftey, 23*(10), 1017–1025.

Nadebaum, C., Anderson, V., Vajda, F., Reutens, D., & Wood, A. (2012). Neurobehavioral consequences of prenatal antiepileptic drug exposure. *Developmental Neuropsychology, 37*(1), 1–29.

Ogura, H., Yasuda, M., Nakamura, S., Yamashita, H., Mikoshiba, K., & Ohmori, H. (2002). Neurotoxic damage of granule cells in the dentate gyrus and the cerebellum and cognitive deficit following neonatal administration of phenytoin in mice. *Journal of Neuropathology and Experimental Neurology, 61*(11), 956–967.

Olney, J. W., Wozniak, D. F., Jevtovic-Todorovic, V., Farber, N. B., Bittigau, P., & Ikonomidou, C. (2002). Drug-induced apoptotic neurodegeneration in the developing brain. *Brain Pathology, 12*(4), 488–498.

Ornoy, A., & Cohen, E. (1996). Outcome of children born to epileptic mothers treated with carbamazepine during pregnancy. *Archives of Disease in Childhood, 75*(6), 517–520.

Quigley, M. A., Hockley, C., Carson, C., Kelly, Y., Renfrew, M. J., & Sacker, A. (2012). Breastfeeding is associated with improved child cognitive development: A population-based cohort study. *Journal of Pediatrics, 160*(1), 25–32.

Rasalam, A. D., Hailey, H., Williams, J. H., Moore, S. J., Turnpenny, P. D., Lloyd, D. J., & Dean, J. C. (2005). Characteristics of fetal anticonvulsant syndrome associated autistic disorder. *Developmental Medicine & Child Neurology, 47*(8), 551–555.

Reinisch, J. M., Sanders, S. A., Mortensen, E. L., & Rubin, D. B. (1995). In utero exposure to phenobarbital and intelligence deficits in adult men. *JAMA, 274*(19), 1518–1525.

Rihtman, T., Parush, S., & Ornoy, A. (2012). Preliminary findings of the developmental effects of in utero exposure to topiramate. *Reproductive Toxicology, 34*(3), 308–311.

Rihtman, T., Parush, S., & Ornoy, A. (2013). Developmental outcomes at preschool age after fetal exposure to valproic acid and lamotrigine: Cognitive, motor, sensory and behavioral function. *Reproductive Toxicology, 41*, 115–125.

Roth, C., Magnus, P., Schjolberg, S., Stoltenberg, C., Suren, P., McKeague, I. W., … Susser, E. (2011). Folic acid supplements in pregnancy and severe language delay in children. *JAMA, 306*(14), 1566–1573.

Schmidt, R. J., Tancredi, D. J., Ozonoff, S., Hansen, R. L., Hartiala, J., Allayee, H., … Hertz-Picciotto, I. (2012). Maternal periconceptional folic acid intake and risk of autism spectrum disorders and developmental delay in the CHARGE (CHildhood Autism Risks from Genetics and Environment) case-control study. *American Journal of Clinical Nutrition, 96*(1), 80–89.

Scolnik, D., Nulman, I., Rovet, J., Gladstone, D., Czuchta, D., Gardner, H. A., … Einarson, T. (1994). Neurodevelopment of children exposed in utero to phenytoin and carbamazepine monotherapy. *JAMA, 271*(10), 767–770.

Shallcross, R., Bromley, R. L., Cheyne, C. P., Garcia-Finana, M., Irwin, B., Morrow, J., & Baker, G. A. (2014). In utero exposure to levetiracetam vs valproate: Development and language at 3 years of age. *Neurology, 82*(3), 213–221.

Shallcross, R., Bromley, R. L., Irwin, B., Bonnett, L. J., Morrow, J., & Baker, G. A. (2011). Child development following in utero exposure: Levetiracetam vs sodium valproate. *Neurology, 76*(4), 383–389.

Suren, P., Roth, C., Bresnahan, M., Haugen, M., Hornig, M., Hirtz, D., ... Stoltenberg, C. (2013). Association between maternal use of folic acid supplements and risk of autism spectrum disorders in children. *JAMA, 309*(6), 570–577.

Thomas, S. V., Sukumaran, S., Lukose, N., George, A., & Sarma, P. S. (2007). Intellectual and language functions in children of mothers with epilepsy. *Epilepsia, 48*(12), 2234–2240.

Tomson, T., & Battino, D. (2012). Teratogenic effects of antiepileptic drugs. *The Lancet Neurology, 11*(9), 803–813.

Turski, C. A., & Ikonomidou, C. (2012). Neuropathological sequelae of developmental exposure to antiepileptic and anesthetic drugs. *Frontiers in Neurology, 3*, 120.

Vajda, F. J., O'Brien, T. J., Lander, C. M., Graham, J., & Eadie, M. J. (2014). The teratogenicity of the newer antiepileptic drugs: An update. *Acta Neurologica Scandinavica, 130*(4), 234–238.

van der Pol, M. C., Hadders-Algra, M., Huisjes, H. J., & Touwen, B. C. (1991). Antiepileptic medication in pregnancy: Late effects on the children's central nervous system development. *American Journal of Obstetrics & Gynecology, 164*(1 Pt 1), 121–128.

Veiby, G., Daltveit, A. K., Schjolberg, S., Stoltenberg, C., Oyen, A. S., Vollset, S. E., ... Gilhus, N. E. (2013). Exposure to antiepileptic drugs in utero and child development: a prospective population-based study. *Epilepsia, 54*(8), 1462–1472.

Viguera, A. C., Whitfield, T., Baldessarini, R. J., Newport, D. J., Stowe, Z., Reminick, A., ... Cohen, L. S. (2007). Risk of recurrence in women with bipolar disorder during pregnancy: prospective study of mood stabilizer discontinuation. *American Journal of Psychiatry, 164*(12), 1817–1824.

Vinten, J., Adab, N., Kini, U., Gorry, J., Gregg, J., & Baker, G. A. (2005). Neuropsychological effects of exposure to anticonvulsant medication in utero. *Neurology, 64*(6), 949–954.

Vinten, J., Bromley, R. L., Taylor, J., Adab, N., Kini, U., & Baker, G. A. (2009). The behavioral consequences of exposure to antiepileptic drugs in utero. *Epilepsy & Behavior, 14*(1), 197–201.

Wide, K., Winbladh, B., Tomson, T., Sars-Zimmer, K., & Berggren, E. (2000). Psychomotor development and minor anomalies in children exposed to antiepileptic drugs in utero: A prospective population-based study. *Developmental Medicine & Child Neurology, 42*(2), 87–92.

Williams, P. G., & Hersh, J. H. (1997). A male with fetal valproate syndrome and autism. *Developmental Medicine & Child Neurology, 39*(9), 632–634.

Williams, G., King, J., Cunningham, M., Stephan, M., Kerr, B., & Hersh, J. H. (2001). Fetal valproate syndrome and autism: Additional evidence of an association. *Developmental Medicine & Child Neurology, 43*(3), 202–206.

Wilson, R. D., Davies, G., Desilets, V., Reid, G. J., Summers, A., Wyatt, P., & Young, D. (2003). The use of folic acid for the prevention of neural tube defects and other congenital anomalies. *Journal of Obstetrics and Gynaecology Canada, 25*(11), 959–973.

Zhang, L. L., Zeng, L. N., & Li, Y. P. (2011). Side effects of phenobarbital in epilepsy: A systematic review. *Epileptic Disorders, 13*(4), 349–365.

Chapter 6
Psychotropic Medication in Pregnancy: Focus on Child Outcomes

Josephine Power, Megan Galbally, and Andrew Lewis

Definitional Issues and Prevalence

Research specifically in pregnancy has shown rates of antidepressant use have more than doubled in the USA, Denmark and the Netherlands (Andrade et al., 2008; Bakker, Kölling, van den Berg, de Walle, & de Jong van den Berg, 2008; Cooper, Willy, Pont, & Ray, 2007). This rise in the prescription of psychotropic medications, including for pregnant women, has at times outstripped our understanding of their side effects and longer term impacts and in no area is this more acute than the field of perinatal psychiatry, in which the balance between the risks presented by treatment must be weighed against the risks inherent in the illness itself. At present there is a relative paucity of research into the impact of psychotropic medication to guide clinicians assisting patients to make decisions regarding psychotropic medication use in pregnancy, a problem compounded by the inherent difficulties of performing research in this area: patients are difficult to recruit and there are numerous

J. Power, M.B.B.S., M.P.M., F.R.A.N.Z.C.P. (✉)
Department of Perinatal Mental Health, Mercy Hospital for Women, Melbourne, VIC, Australia

General Hospital Mental Health, Austin Health, Melbourne, VIC, Australia
e-mail: JPower@mercy.com.au

M. Galbally, M.B.B.S., F.R.A.N.Z.C.P., Ph.D.
Foundation Chair in Perinatal Psychiatry, Murdoch University, University of Notre Dame and Fiona Stanley Hospital, Murdoch, WA, Australia
e-mail: M.Galbally@murdoch.edu.au

A. Lewis, Ph.D.
School of Psychology, Deakin University, Waurn Ponds, VIC, Australia
e-mail: andrew.lewis@deakin.edu.au

C. Riccio, J. Sullivan (eds.), *Pediatric Neurotoxicology*, Specialty Topics in Pediatric Neuropsychology, DOI 10.1007/978-3-319-32358-9_6

confounding variables that are difficult to control for. Separating medication effects from illness effects is enormously challenging, with ethical limitations to study design preventing use of gold standard double-blind randomised controlled trial methodology. Most published research is in the form of prospective case–control studies and the majority suffer from small numbers of recruits, lack of power and limited follow-up. The larger observational population studies are often based on approximate data, and are unable to examine complicated questions relating to the interaction of illness and treatment with psychosocial circumstances. Of the studies that are published, few follow up exposed children beyond the first year of life.

Psychotropic medication is a broad term referring to drugs acting on the central nervous system to induce a change in mood, psychiatric symptoms or behaviour. The psychotropic medications of focus in this chapter are those that are used almost exclusively for treatment of mental disorders: antidepressants, antipsychotics and lithium carbonate. It should be noted that all of these medications cross the placenta (Hendrick et al., 2003) and therefore all have potential to influence fetal neurodevelopment. Given the increasing use of psychotropic medication in the general population, it is inevitable that unintentional exposure will occur. Fifty percentage of pregnancies are unplanned, and this figure may be higher among individuals with certain mental illnesses. Newer psychotropics also have fewer propensities to impair fertility (Miller & Finnerty, 1996) therefore the possibility of pregnancy must be considered in all women of childbearing age. The broad categories of psychotropic medications are considered separately.

Antidepressants

Indication and Rates of Use in Pregnancy

Antidepressant medication is one of the most commonly prescribed psychotropics in pregnancy. They are used to treat depression and anxiety disorders, and include the older tricyclic antidepressants (TCAs), serotonin-specific reuptake inhibitors (SSRIs) such as sertraline and citalopram, serotonin–noradrenaline reuptake inhibitors (SNRIs) such as venlafaxine, and a range of other agents such as mirtazapine and agomelatine. These agents have a range of therapeutic targets as well as pharmacokinetic differences that may be important; however in many reported studies in the literature they are examined as a group.

Depression is a significant illness affecting pregnant women. Approximately 7.2 % of pregnant women will experience depression (Gaynes et al., 2005), and for many medication will form part of recommended treatment. Studies in various jurisdictions have shown a range of prescription rates, but all agree that the figure appears to be rising. From US data, one study showed 8 % of pregnant women were prescribed an antidepressant with an increase during the study period (Andrade et al., 2008); another in Tennessee found an increase from 5.7 to 13.4 % from 1999 to 2003 (Cooper et al., 2007); and a further study from British Colombia showed an increase in SSRI use from 2.3 to 5 % (Oberlander, Warburton, Misri, Aghajanian, & Hertzman, 2006). In Europe the prevalence of antidepressant use tends to be lower at around 1–2 % (Kieler et al., 2012; Ververs et al., 2006), but it does appear to be increasing there as well (Bakker et al., 2008), and most women continue use throughout pregnancy therefore exposure is prolonged and continues across times of neurodevelopmental vulnerability.

The effects of antidepressant discontinuation in pregnancy are important. Approximately 50 % of women will cease antidepressant medication without consulting their treating doctor (Battle & Salisbury, 2010), placing themselves at an elevated risk of relapse. In one study 70 % of those women who ceased antidepressant medication relapsed as opposed to 26 % of those who continued treatment (Cohen et al., 2006).

Antipsychotics

Indications and Rates of Use in Pregnancy

Antipsychotic medications were developed to treat psychotic disorders such as schizophrenia but some have found uses outside of these indications, most importantly as mood stabilisers in Bipolar Affective Disorder (BPAD). Increasingly, however, they are used for a range of other psychiatric and behavioural conditions. Again, they are a disparate group, but broadly speaking they comprise the first-generation agents (FGAs) such as chlorpromazine and haloperidol that are less frequently used due to elevated rates of extra-pyramidal side effects (EPSEs) in particular, and the second-generation medications (SGAs) such as olanzapine and risperidone that are less likely to provoke EPSEs but that have been associated with other problematic side effects such as type II diabetes and the metabolic syndrome. Schizophrenia has been associated with numerous poor pregnancy outcomes including low birth weight, prematurity and intrauterine growth restriction (IUGR). This group of mothers has also been observed to display less maternal sensitivity with consequent impaired infant attachment, and has a high risk of relapse in the postpartum period. These relapses may also be of high risk to the infant and mother: children of mothers with schizophrenia are at greater risk of dying throughout infancy and into childhood (Webb, Avel, Pickles, & Appleby, 2005).

Prescription rates of antipsychotics, lithium and anticonvulsant mood stabilisers are increasing. In the Tennessee Medicaid population there has been an increase from nearly 14 to almost 31 per 1000 pregnancies with a significant increase in atypical antipsychotic prescriptions and a decrease in typical antipsychotic prescriptions likely reflecting a wider change in prescribing practices (Epstein et al., 2013). In the period 2001–2007 in the USA a study of 585,615 deliveries observed a 2.5-fold increase in atypical antipsychotic use from 0.33 to 0.82 % of pregnancies. The use of typical antipsychotics remained stable. The most common mental health diagnosis for which an atypical antipsychotic was prescribed was depression (63 %), followed by BPAD (43 %) and schizophrenia (13 %) (Toh et al., 2013).

Lithium

Indications and Rates of Use in Pregnancy

Lithium carbonate is a mood stabiliser medication prescribed to treat BPAD or to augment therapy in other psychiatric conditions. It is a salt that was discovered in 1949 by Australian psychiatrist Dr. John Cade to be effective for the management of mania. There have been numerous studies over the years since showing efficacy for treatment of BPAD when compared with anti-epileptic medications, antipsychotics and other treatments. Its role in pregnancy is for the ongoing management of BPAD: to prevent relapse or to treat a manic episode. Importantly it has also been found to be one of the most effective treatments for postpartum psychosis.

Data regarding prescription rates in pregnancy are limited. One European study found that of the drugs prescribed to 41,293 pregnant women during pregnancy, only five were prescribed lithium (Egen-Lappe & Hasford, 2004). Prescription rates are likely to be low given the reported association of lithium prescription with Ebstein's anomaly, a cardiac defect, initially published in the *Lancet* (Nora, Nora, & Toews, 1974). More recent evaluations of the association have suggested that the risk may have been overstated (Cohen, Friedman, & Jeffereson, 1994) and that lithium is not an important teratogen (Jacobsen et al., 1992).

BPAD is a severe, chronic condition that often relapses and remits but may follow a more enduring, progressive course with poor outcomes and psychosocial disability. This disorder often has an onset during the childbearing years, and mood stabiliser medication is frequently a prominent component of the long term management plan. The interaction of BPAD and pregnancy is important and has significant potential ramifications for mother and infant. A prospective study showed that the risk of relapse in pregnancy is greatly elevated when women cease mood stabiliser medication: 85.5 % as opposed to 37 % (Viguera et al., 2000) with those women who ceased medication spending a greater period of time unwell. Increased symptom burden may also result in increased pharmacotherapy with higher doses and combination therapy required to induce remission but at the cost of additional fetal exposure. The postpartum period is also a time of particular risk for women with BPAD (Yonkers et al., 2004). The evidence suggests that rapid discontinuation is a particular problem, as can happen when women elect to do so precipitously and potentially without medical advice in response to diagnosis of pregnancy. Lithium has also been shown to be of benefit to women with a history of puerperal psychosis, with significant reduction in risk of relapse achieved by commencing treatment immediately postpartum (Bergink et al., 2012).

Impact on the Developing Child

Intellectual Functioning

Antidepressants

There are limited published studies that examine neurodevelopment outcomes following fetal exposure to antidepressants. For the most part, this body of literature examines SSRIs, with some including TCAs, and most of these use inadequate measures in children under 12 months of age. Eight studies have used more robust measures of development, and three have tested children beyond the first year of life. The majority have found no association with poorer child development. More reassuringly, of the available reports, none have found an association with poorer global cognition and this includes now four that have followed children to 4 years of age and undertaken the Wechsler tests—the most robust measures across childhood for cognition (Galbally, Lewis, & Buist, 2015; Klinger et al., 2011; Mattson, Eastvold, Jones, Harris, & Chambers, 1999; Nulman et al., 2012). The largest study examining exposure to antidepressants in pregnancy has followed exposed infants to early school age, and has noted that it is exposure to maternal depression rather than antidepressants that predicts future development (Nulman et al., 2012).

The results of these studies must be interpreted with caution: the methodology and exposures are highly variable between studies, and they are prone to bias and uncontrolled confounding. However, there have not, to date, been reports of an association between in utero exposure to antidepressants and intellectual impairment in children to early school age. It is impossible to comment about outcomes beyond this, as there is no data available, and it is possible that more subtle deficits may not be apparent until later in life.

Antipsychotics

Published studies examining the neurodevelopmental effects of antipsychotics are very limited. This lack of information regarding the impact of antipsychotics is important as the children of mothers with schizophrenia have long been recognised as being at risk of developmental delay and neurocognitive deficits. The first publication examining this issue was published in 1977 (Fish, 1977) and since then there have been many reports of developmental delay, learning difficulties and cognitive deficits (Niemi et al., 2003; Wan et al., 2008).

Most of the available information is from case reports, case series and retrospective studies, the majority of which rely on parental report rather than independent, validated testing as a measure of development, and none with follow-up beyond 12 months. A number of such case reports have described no developmental problems for infants exposed to antipsychotics (Duran et al., 2008; Gupta & Grover, 2004; Lin et al., 2010); however there is a published report of an infant exposed to clozapine who had delayed language development up to 5 years of age (Mendhekar, 2007). Older reviews, in which women were more likely to have been prescribed FGAs, have not found differences in IQ scores up to the age of 5 (Altshuler et al., 1996; Thiels, 1987).

Of the studies that used a prospective design, few use specific measures of infant neurodevelopment. Johnson, LaPrairie, Brennan, Stowe, and Newport (2012) found an association with lower scores on a standardised test of neuromotor performance at 6 months of age with exposure to antipsychotics as a fetus, when compared to no or antidepressant exposure. One recent case-controlled, prospective study administered the Bayley Scales of Infant and Toddler Development, third edition (BSID-III) to infants up to 12-months of age who were exposed to atypical antipsychotics in utero (Peng et al., 2013). The study found that a higher percentage of exposed infants had low birth weight (13.2 % vs. 2.6 %) although mean height and weight measured throughout the study did not differ between the groups. At 2 months of age, a higher percentage of antipsychotic-exposed infants met criteria for delayed development in cognitive, motor, social-emotional and adaptive behaviour scales with lower mean composite scores in these domains as well. There was no difference in language scale. At 12 months of age there was no significant difference between the two groups in these measures. Lower scores were also associated with no breastfeeding, but the association with atypical antipsychotic exposure was stronger. This study was not able to separate possible illness effects.

It would be reasonable to conclude that there is no strong evidence for persistent poor cognitive function in infants exposed to antipsychotics, but the evidence in this area is sorely lacking.

Lithium

Lithium has been in clinical use for many years, but there are only three studies addressing the neurodevelopmental outcomes of children exposed in utero. The earliest publication, using data from a birth registry, followed 60 exposed children up to 7 years of age, using unexposed siblings as the control group. Based on maternal reports, 10 of the exposed group and 6 of the unexposed group had developmental abnormalities, some of which were confirmed (Schou, 1976). Jacobsen et al. (1992) and van der Lugt et al. (2012) have found no difference in neurodevelopmental outcome between exposed and non-exposed children. The study by van der Lugt et al. (2012) used the WISC or WPPSI and BSID-III and found no neurodevelopmental concerns, however it was limited by being a retrospective cohort study that examined only 15 children at a wide range of ages (3–15 years).

Academic Functioning

There are no studies that specifically examine academic function following fetal exposure to antidepressants, antipsychotics or lithium. This is largely attributable to the length of follow-up of studies examining exposure to psychotropic medication in pregnancy on child developmental outcomes with none to date following children beyond 6 years of age. This is an important unresolved question, as the evidence is clear that the offspring of parents with severe mental illness are more likely to have poorer clinical and social outcomes. As an example, Niemi et al. (2003) report that of 145 children of mothers with psychosis, 15 % were found to have a severe academic problem vs. 8 % of controls.

Neuropsychological Functioning

Antidepressants

A finding of delayed motor development has been found in clinical studies of children exposed to antidepressants in utero as compared with controls, but this finding is not consistent. The available research is limited by small sample size, heterogeneous exposure and differences in methodology that make comparison unfeasible, however four prospective, case-controlled studies have now reported a deficit in motor development when children over 12-months of age are tested using a validated research tool (Casper et al., 2003, 2011; Galbally, Lewis, & Buist, 2011; Hanley, Brain, & Oberlander, 2013). This finding is supported by one birth register study showing an association with delayed motor milestones (Mortensen et al., 2003).

These findings are contradicted by another birth register study that found no delay in motor milestones between the ages of 6 and 19 months (Pederson, Henriksen, & Olsen, 2010), and a recent study by Austin et al. (2013) up to 18 months of age has not found an association with motor delay or cognitive impairment using the BSID-III. It is difficult to interpret the meaning of these findings at present: it is unclear whether they will be validated by future research but certainly there is a plausible mechanism whereby delayed motor development may occur. In addition to an important role in brain maturation in utero (Whitaker-Azmitia, 2001), the serotonin system is known to regulate muscle tone and motor function in the central nervous system, therefore may be vulnerable to the influence of serotonergic drugs.

Several studies have demonstrated no impact of prenatal antidepressant exposure with neuropsychological deficits. Weikum et al. (2013) have shown that exposed children do not perform more poorly on tests of executive function when compared with controls at 6 years of age. Similarly, Galbally et al. (2015) found no effect of antidepressant exposure on cognition.

Antipsychotics

Concerning the impact of antipsychotics, there is some evidence of poorer outcomes among infants exposed to antipsychotics, but the evidence is generally scant and compromised by uncontrolled confounding factors. In a case–control study Johnson et al. (2012) found that at 6 months of age infants exposed to antipsychotics in utero scored lower on a standard test of neuromotor function when compared with those exposed to antidepressants and a control group without exposure. This study was unable to distinguish between the effects of pharmacotherapy and the effects of maternal mental illness, and must be interpreted with caution, as there is evidence that maternal psychosis has an impact on neuropsychological function in offspring. Wan et al. (2008) reviewed the literature concerning the children of mothers with psychosis, and found that they are more likely to have impairment in verbal ability, executive function and processing speed.

Lithium

One study that used validated testing to assess children exposed to lithium in utero did not find any deficits (van der Lugt et al., 2012). As previously mentioned, this study was very small in size and it is difficult to be reassured that there is no possibility of any deficits on its strength alone.

Emotional and Behavioural Functioning

Antidepressants

Studies into in utero exposure to antidepressants and future emotional or behavioural difficulties are scant, but to date have not found an association that can be clearly attributed to medication rather than the effects of maternal anxiety or depression. There has been no reported increase in difficult infant temperament (Mattson et al., 1999; Nulman et al., 1997) or externalising or internalising disorders in preschool children (Misri et al., 2006; Oberlander et al., 2007; Pedersen et al., 2013). Oberlander et al. (2010) have explored the interaction between maternal mood, prenatal SSRI exposure and behavioural outcomes in offspring, and have suggested that the relationship may be mediated through a genetic variation in a serotonin transporter gene.

Of importance is that maternal mood has been more consistently associated with poor emotional and behavioural outcomes for children. A number of studies have demonstrated an association with externalising disorders at preschool age (Oberlander et al., 2010); internalising disorders (Misri et al., 2006; Oberlander et al., 2010) and child behaviour problems at early school age (Nulman et al., 2012; Pedersen et al., 2013).

Antidepressant exposure in utero has been explored in relation to affect expression and self-regulation in infants. Reebye, Morison, Panikkar, Misri, and Grunau (2002) assessed mother–infant dyads for evidence of positive or negative interactions between the pairs. They found that mother–infant pairs exposed to SSRIs alone showed a similar profile of interaction when compared with a control group without maternal depression. This was supported by similar findings at 8 months postpartum (Reebye, Ng, Misri, & Stikarovska, 2012), where there was no evidence of altered maternal-child relationship or capacity for infant self-regulation among those mothers who took an SSRI during pregnancy as compared with healthy controls.

Antipsychotics

There are very limited studies examining the emotional and behavioural impact of prenatal antipsychotic use. In part, this is because it is not ethical to leave mothers with psychosis untreated during pregnancy, therefore separating the effects of illness from pharmacotherapy is problematic. Mothers that have untreated psychosis in pregnancy may also be a group less likely to have adequate antenatal care and more likely to have other lifestyle behaviours known to be damaging to the developing fetus, such as smoking or other substance use.

In one study of 52 children exposed to chlorpromazine in utero, Kris (1965) found no impact on social, emotional or cognitive development. Similarly Stika et al. (1990) found no difference in behaviour or cognition in a cohort of 66 school age children exposed to typical antipsychotics. Little data exist to guide the use of atypical antipsychotics during pregnancy: there have been case reports of developmental delay following exposure to some atypical agents, but no other data (McKenna et al., 2005).

Lithium

There have been no reports published that associated lithium with poorer emotional or behavioural outcomes among exposed offspring, however specific investigation of this is lacking.

Impact on Other Areas of Functioning

Antidepressants

Poor Neonatal Adaptation

There is evidence that antidepressant exposure has an early, measurable impact on the central nervous system. Poor neonatal adaptation syndrome (PNAS) is diagnosed in neonates exposed to an SSRI in late pregnancy (Moses-Kolko et al., 2005). The syndrome consists of CNS, motor, respiratory and GI signs: most commonly crying, jitteriness, tremor, feeding difficulties, sneezing and sleep dysregulation (Galbally, Lewis, Lum, & Buist, 2009). It occurs in 30 % of exposed infants (Levinson-Castiel, Merlob, Linder, Sirota, & Klinger, 2006), and is generally mild and transient. It has been hypothesised that PNAS represents a drug withdrawal or toxicity, but ceasing SSRI use in the immediate period prior to delivery has not been shown to alter outcomes (Warburton, Hertzman, & Oberlander, 2010). The longer term impact of PNAS is unknown, but it has not been associated with detrimental outcomes at this stage.

It is possible that PNAS may be a neurobiological disturbance relating to SSRI exposure and/or the underlying maternal mental illness, and a study has shown that there are immediate neurobehavioral changes in SSRI-exposed infants following delivery when compared with healthy controls (Zeskind & Stephens, 2004), suggesting an early alteration in neurobiological function. A further study that may support this has shown altered pain reactivity in neonates exposed to SSRIs that persists to 2 months postpartum (Oberlander et al., 2005). SSRI exposure in utero may alter HPA response patterns as suggested by a study examining salivary cortisol levels in 3-month old infants (Oberlander et al., 2008); however there was a major contribution from maternal mood and breastfeeding.

Language

Studies have examined TCAs, SSRIs and venlafaxine (Nulman et al., 1997, 2002, 2012) and found no impact on language development in preschool and early school age children. These studies did show, however, an association with untreated maternal depression and poorer language outcomes. In contrast, a study by Weikum, Oberlander, Hensch, and Werker (2012) has suggested that there is an impact of SSRI exposure on early language development when maternal depression is controlled for in infants at 6 and 10 months. Once again the literature in this area is incomplete: antidepressants are studied as disparate groups, it is difficult to address all confounders, and children have only been followed for a limited time.

Antipsychotics

There have been several reported cases of neonatal extrapyramidal syndrome following exposure to FGAs (Gentile, 2010). The FDA issued a warning in 2011 advising that clinicians be alert to the possibility of EPSEs in exposed neonates.

Lithium

Neonatal toxicity may occur in situations where the mother is toxic at delivery. A lithium level must be checked in the infant immediately postpartum, ideally using cord blood. Exposure to lithium in later pregnancy has been associated with a neonatal adaptation syndrome with variable features of hypotonia, muscle twitching, feeding difficulties, lethargy, cardiac arrhythmias, cyanosis and breathing difficulties (Kozma, 2005; Simard, Gumbiner, Lee, Lewis, & Norman, 1989). It is usually self-limiting and resolves without intervention in most cases.

Specific Diagnostic Outcomes

Antidepressants and Autism

The association with prenatal antidepressants and autism spectrum disorder (ASD) is unclear at present. A few studies have now reported an association between maternal antidepressant use and autism, although none have been able to control for the effects of maternal mood. This has been postulated to be related to the impact of antidepressants on the developing serotonergic system, as a number of studies have suggested that abnormalities in serotonin levels and serotonergic pathways are present in ASD (Pardo & Eberhart, 2007). These studies include those looking at serotonin synthesis (Chandana et al., 2005; Chugani et al., 1999), receptor binding (Murphy et al., 2006), and studies of pharmacotherapy (Kolevzon, Mathewson, & Hollander, 2006), but it should be noted that a recent Cochrane review has concluded that there is no evidence that SSRIs are of benefit for children with ASD, on the contrary there is some evidence of harm (Williams, Wheeler, Silove, & Hazell, 2010). Some studies of serotonin genes have suggested an association with ASD, although the findings are inconclusive at this stage (Anderson et al., 2009; Devlin et al., 2005).

In terms of research findings, in a case control study, Croen, Grether, Yoshida, Odouli, and Hendrick (2011) found that mothers of children with ASD were more likely to have been prescribed an antidepressant in the year before delivery than mothers of children without ASD. Rai et al. (2013) have reported an association between a history of maternal depression and ASD, with the effect confined to women who used antidepressants during pregnancy where that information was available. The association was only apparent for autism without intellectual disability, but this study was not able to distinguish between medication and illness effects, and could not differentiate between types of antidepressant used. Despite this, assuming a causal, unconfounded relationship, maternal antidepressant use only explained 0.6% of autism diagnoses. Harrington, Lee, Crum, Zimmerman, and Hertz-Picciotto (2014) found an association between prenatal SSRI exposure and ASD or developmental delay that was strongest for boys exposed in the first trimester of pregnancy. Two population-based cohort studies, using the same database, showed conflicting results. The first (Sorensen et al., 2013) did not find an association between prenatal antidepressant exposure and autism when confounding factors were controlled for. The second (Hviid, Melbye, & Pasternak, 2014), while not detecting a significant association, could not rule out an increased relative risk (1.61) and suggested that further study was necessary. A meta-analysis (Man et al., 2015) noted that while the available studies for review lacked heterogeneity, usually a criteria for undertaking a meta-analysis, based on their analysis there was evidence to support an increased risk of ASD following in utero exposure to SSRIs, but given the methodologies of existing studies causality could not be established as yet. A further concern is repeated studies which have found autism to be associated with a family history of mental illness (Larsson et al., 2004) and given antidepressants are prescribed for women with depression, anxiety and for some with bipolar disorder and schizoaffective disorder the influence of maternal mental illness and hence family history on a child's risk of developing autism needs to be fully accounted for as a key confounding variable.

Antidepressants and ADHD

There has been some research interest into examining an association between in utero exposure to antidepressants and Attention Deficit Hyperactivity Disorder (ADHD). It is important to note that there is an increased risk of ADHD with maternal anxiety and depression (Lesesne, Visser, & White, 2003), but this has been difficult to control for experimentally. To date, the findings are inconclusive. A Danish birth cohort study did not show an association between maternal antidepressant use during pregnancy and ADHD (Laugesen, Olsen, Telen Andersen, Froslev, & Sorensen, 2013). This finding is supported by a study by Weikum et al. (2013) in which there was no increase in diagnosis of ADHD among their cohort of 6-year-olds exposed to SSRIs. Clements et al. (2014) used data from children diagnosed with ASD or ADHD, and found that they could not support an association with ASD and prenatal antidepressant exposure, but there was a small increase in ADHD risk after controlling for maternal depression. However, they could not exclude the possibility that this result may be due to uncontrolled confounders.

Prognosis and Moderating Factors

In considering the important factors affecting prognosis and outcome for those offspring exposed to psychotropic medication in utero, it must be emphasised again that research in this area is generally lacking and existing research is confounded by the effects of psychiatric illnesses and their sequelae. Even in the case of antenatal antidepressant use, the most extensively studied, the evidence remains patchy and incomplete, and there is no consensus opinion regarding outcomes and prognosis.

At this stage, in light of the risks associated with untreated mental illness in pregnancy, women should be counselled to balance these with the unknown effects of psychotropics on the developing fetus. More research is evidently needed to guide clinicians and their patients in this decision-making process.

Considerations for Prevention/Intervention/School Accommodations and School Reintegration

The most important intervention in addressing the neurodevelopmental effects of psychotropic medication occurs prior to conception where planning can occur. Where possible, women should be offered preconception counselling to discuss the risks and benefits of the treatment options appropriate in her particular situation and to optimise mental health care along with physical health, nutritional status, substance use and psychosocial supports.

Given that the majority of pregnancies are unplanned, in most cases decisions regarding psychotropic use will be made after unintentional exposure has already occurred. At this stage the woman should be counselled that abrupt withdrawal of medication is more likely to present risks, and she should be given current, comprehensive information about the risks and benefits of psychotropic use in pregnancy. These must be weighed against risks that may arise if medication is withdrawn, and the known impact of relapse in pregnancy and the postpartum period.

The general paucity of research into developmental outcomes following antenatal psychotropic exposure makes it difficult to make broad recommendations about school interventions and integration for this group. At this stage, the most pragmatic approach is a high index of suspicion and early assessment when developmental difficulties are suspected, with a focus on interventions tailored to individual strengths and challenges as opposed to a more generic programme.

Recommendations

1. The pregnancies of women with severe mental illness must be treated as high-risk from an obstetric point of view. Ideally there should be early involvement of an obstetric team with experience managing high-risk pregnancies, and in a setting with resources to detect and respond to pregnancy complications.
2. Neonates must be observed for evidence of PNAS with antidepressant exposure, drug toxicity in the case of lithium, and for antipsychotic exposure: extrapyramidal side effects or sedation, with a low threshold for paediatric review if there are concerns. Observation should continue for the first 48–72 h postpartum.
3. Maternal mental health should be monitored throughout pregnancy, preferably by clinicians with experience in issues relating to perinatal mental health. Evidence of relapse should be responded to promptly, to circumvent the use of combination or high-dose psychopharmacotherapy as can occur when relapses are severe or detected late.
4. Support should be provided to the parents in decision-making regarding psychotropic use in pregnancy, with current, relevant literature presented in a clear and comprehensible format. Opportunity should be given for both parents to ask questions, and the family should be supported in pursuing other treatment modalities that may reduce or alleviate the need for pharmacotherapy, while providing adequate supervision and support if medication is necessary.
5. Psychiatric mother–baby units can provide specialist, intensive care to mothers with mental illness, and assist them in developing attachment relationships with their infants.
6. Social support programmes may help families integrate into the community.
7. In light of the unresolved concerns about the impact of psychotropic medication, attention must be paid to developmental milestones from birth. This is particularly important as this group of children, particularly those with parents with severe mental illness, are known to be at risk of poor developmental outcomes, whatever

the cause, and are a group that need special attention. Their vulnerabilities appear to be present throughout childhood and adolescence and most likely beyond, and they require early referral for specialist assessment and intervention if there are concerns about developmental delay, poor academic performance or behavioural or psychiatric concerns.

Conclusion

Psychotropic medications play a central role in management for many mental disorders, particularly relapsing illnesses with moderate to severe symptoms and associated impairment of functioning. When women are of a childbearing age the consideration of choice of agent with regards to risks in pregnancy and alternative treatment options, such as psychological therapy, should be part of routine care. Currently for all psychotropic medications there is only limited knowledge of longer term effects from exposure in pregnancy on child developmental outcomes. However, this must be balanced against potential risks from untreated mental disorders. This makes decisions about treatment challenging for women and clinicians alike.

References

Altshuler, L., Cohen, L., Martin, S., Burt, V.K., Gitlin, M., Mintz, J. (1996). Pharmacological management of psychiatric illness during pregnancy: Dilemmas and guidelines. *American Journal of Psychiatry, 153*, 592–596.

Anderson, B. M., Schnetz-Boutaud, N. C., Bartlett, J., Wotawa, A. M., Wright, H. H., Abramson R.K., ... Haines J. (2009). Examination of association of genes in the serotonin system to autism. *Neurogenetics, 10*(3), 209–216.

Andrade, S. E., Raebel, M. A., Brown, J., Lane, K., Livingston, J., Boudreau, D., ... Platt, R. (2008). Use of antidepressant medications during pregnancy: A multisite study. *American Journal of Obstetrics and Gynecology*, 198, 194–195.

Austin, M. P., Karatas, J. C., Mishra, P., Christl, B., Kennedy, D., & Oei, J. (2013). Infant neurodevelopment following in utero exposure to antidepressant medication. *Acta Paediatrica, 102*, 1054–1059.

Bakker, M. K., Kölling, P., van den Berg, P. B., de Walle, H. E. K., & de Jong van den Berg, L. T. (2008). Increase in use of selective serotonin reuptake inhibitors in pregnancy during the last decade, a population-based cohort study from the Netherlands. *British Journal of Clinical Pharmacology, 65*(4), 600–606.

Battle, C. L., & Salisbury, A. L. (2010). Treatment of antenatal depression. *Journal of Midwifery and Women's Health, 55*, 479.

Bergink, V., Bouvy, P. F., Vervoort, J. S. P., Koorengevel, K. M., Steegers, E. A. P., & Kushner, S. A. (2012). Prevention of postpartum psychosis and mania in women at high risk. *American Journal of Psychiatry, 169*(6), 609–615.

Casper, R. C., Fleisher, B. E., Lee-Ancajas, J. C., Gilles, A., Gaylor, E., DeBattista, A., Hoymne, H. E. (2003). Follow-up of children of depressed mothers exposed or not exposed to antidepressant drugs during pregnancy. *Journal of Pediatrics*, 142, 402–408.

Casper, R. C., Gilles, A. A., Fleisher, B. E., Baran, J., Enns, G., & Lazzeroni, L. C. (2011). Length of prenatal exposure to selective serotonin reuptake inhibitor (SSRI) antidepressants: Effects on neonatal adaptation and psychomotor development. *Psychopharmacology, 217*, 211–219.

Chandana, S. R., Behen, M. E., Juhász, C., Muzik, O., Rothermel, R. D., Mangner, T. J., Chakraborty, P. K., Chugani, H. T., Chugani, D. C. (2005). Significance of abnormalities in developmental trajectory and asymmetry of cortical serotonin synthesis in autism. *International Journal of Developmental Neuroscience*, 23(2–3), 171–182.

Chugani, D. C., Muzik, O., Behen, M., Rothermel, R., Janisse, J. J., Lee, J., Chugani, H. T. (1999). Developmental changes in brain serotonin synthesis capacity in autistic and nonautistic children. *Annals of Neurology*, 45(3), 287–295.

Clements, C. C., Castro, V. M., Blumenthal, S. R., Rosenfield, H. R., Murphy, S. N., Fava, M., Erb, J. L., Churchill, S. E., Kaimal, A. J., Doyle, A. E., Robinson, E. B., Smoller, J. W., Kohane, I. S., Perlis, R. H. (2014). Prenatal antidepressant exposure is associated with risk for attention-deficit hyperactivity disorder but not autism spectrum disorder in a large health system. *Molecular Psychiatry*, 20, 727–734.

Cohen, L. S., Altshuler, L. L., Harlow, B. L., Nonacs, R., Newport, D. J., Viguera, A. C., Suri R., Burt, V. K., Hendrick, V., Reminick, A. M., Loughead, A., Vitonis, A. F., Stowe, Z. N. (2006). Relapse of major depression during pregnancy in women who maintain or discontinue antidepressant treatment. *JAMA*, 295, 499–507.

Cohen, L. S., Friedman, J. M., & Jeffereson, J. W. (1994). A re-evaluation of risk of in-utero exposure to lithium. *JAMA, 271*, 146–150.

Cooper, W. O., Willy, M. E., Pont, S. J., & Ray, W. A. (2007). Increasing use of antidepressants in pregnancy. *American Journal of Obstetrics and Gynecology, 196*, 544–545.

Croen, L. A., Grether, J. K., Yoshida, C. K., Odouli, R., & Hendrick, V. (2011). Antidepressant use during pregnancy and childhood autism spectrum disorders. *Archives of General Psychiatry, 68*(11), 1104–1112.

Devlin, B., Cook, E. H. Jr, Coon, H., Dawson, G., Grigorenko, E. L., ... C.P.E.A. Genetics Network (2005). Autism and the serotonin transporter: The long and short of it. *Molecular Psychiatry, 10*(12), 1110–1116.

Duran, A., Ugur, M.M., Turan, S., Emuk, M. (2008). Clozapine use in two women with schizophrenia during pregnancy. *Journal of Psychopharmacology, 22*, 111–113.

Egen-Lappe, V., & Hasford, J. (2004). Drug prescription in pregnancy: Analysis of a large statutory sickness fund population. *European Journal of Clinical Pharmacology, 60*, 659–666.

Epstein, R. A., Bobo, W. V., Shelton, R. C., Arbogast, P. G., Morrow, J. A., Wang, W., ... Cooper, W. O. (2013). Increasing use of atypical antipsychotics and anticonvulsants during pregnancy. *Pharmacoepidemiology and Drug Safety*, 22(7), 794–801.

Fish, B. (1977). Neurobiologic antecedents of schizophrenia in children. Evidence for an inherited, congenital neurointegrative defect. *Archives of General Psychiatry, 34*(11), 1297–313.

Galbally, M., Lewis, A. J., Lum, J., & Buist, A. (2009). Serotonin discontinuation syndrome following in utero exposure to antidepressant medication: Prospective controlled study. *Australian and New Zealand Journal of Psychiatry, 43*, 846–854.

Galbally, M., Lewis, A. J., & Buist, A. (2011). Developmental outcomes of children exposed to antidepressants in pregnancy. *Australian and New Zealand Journal of Psychiatry, 45*, 393–399.

Galbally, M., Lewis, A., & Buist, A. (2015). Child developmental outcomes in preschool children following antidepressant exposure in pregnancy. *Australian and New Zealand Journal of Psychiatry, 49*(7), 642–650.

Gaynes, B.N., Gavin, N., Meltzer-Brody, S., Lohr, K. N., Swinson, T., Gartlehner, G., ... Miller, W.C. (2005). Perinatal depression: prevalence, screening accuracy, and screening outcomes. *Evidence Report/Technology Assessment,* 119, 1–8.

Gentile, S. (2010). Antipsychotic therapy during early and late pregnancy. A systematic review. *Schizophr Bulletin, 36*, 518–544.

Gupta, N., Grover, S. (2004). Safety of clozapine in 2 successive pregnancies. *Canadian Journal of Psychiatry, 49*, 863.

Hanley, G. E., Brain, U., & Oberlander, T. F. (2013). Infant developmental outcomes following prenatal exposure to antidepressants, and maternal depressed mood and positive affect. *Early Human Development, 89*(8), 519–524.

Harrington, R. A., Lee, L.-C., Crum, R. M., Zimmerman, A. W., & Hertz-Picciotto, I. (2014). Prenatal SSRI use and offspring with autism spectrum disorder or developmental delay. *Pediatrics, 133*(5), 1241–1248.

Hendrick, V., Smith, L. M., Suri, R., Hwang, S., Haynes, D., & Altshuler, L. (2003). Birth outcomes after prenatal exposure to antidepressant medication. *American Journal of Obstetrics and Gynecology, 188*, 812–815.

Hviid, A., Melbye, M., & Pasternak, B. (2014). Use of selective serotonin reuptake inhibitors during pregnancy and risk of autism. *New England Journal of Medicine, 369*, 2406–2415.

Jacobsen, S.J., Jones, K., Johnson, K., Ceolin, L., Kaur, P., Sahn, D., … Santelli, R. (1992). Prospective multi-centre study of pregnancy outcome after lithium exposure during first trimester. *Lancet*, 339, 530–533.

Johnson, K. C., LaPrairie, J. L., Brennan, P. A., Stowe, Z. N., & Newport, J. (2012). Prenatal antipsychotic exposure and neuromotor performance during infancty. *Archives of General Psychiatry, 69*(8), 787–794.

Kieler, H., Artama, M., Engeland, A., Ericsson, O., Furu, K., Gissler, M.,… Haglund, B. (2012) Selective serotonin reuptake inhibitors during pregnancy and risk of persistent pulmonary hypertension in the newborn: population based cohort study from the five Nordic countries. *British Medical Journal 344*, d8012.

Klinger, G., Frankenthal, D., Merlob, P., Diamond, G., Sirota, L., Levinson-Castiel, R., … Inbar, D. (2011). Long-term outcome following selective serotonin reuptake inhibitor induced neonatal abstinence syndrome. *Journal of Perinatology*, 31, 615–620.

Kolevzon, A., Mathewson, K. A., & Hollander, E. (2006). Selective serotonin reuptake inhibitors in autism: A review of efficacy and tolerability. *Journal of Clinical Psychiatry, 67*(3), 407–414.

Kozma, C. (2005). Neonatal toxicity and transient neurodevelopmental deficits following prenatal exposure to lithium: Another clinical report and a review of the literature. *American Journal of Medical Genetics, 132*, 441–444.

Kris, E. B. (1965). Children of mothers maintained on pharmacotherapy during pregnancy and postpartum. *Current Therapeutic Research, 7*, 785–789.

Larsson, H. J., Eaton, W. W., Madsen, K. M., Vestergaard, M., Olesen, A. V., Agerbo, E., … Mortensen, P. B. (2004). Risk factors for autism: perinatal factors, parental psychiatric history, and socioeconomic status. *American Journal of Epidemiology*, 161(10), 916–925.

Laugesen, K., Olsen, M. S., Telen Andersen, A. B., Froslev, T., & Sorensen, H. T. (2013). In utero exposure to antidepressant drugs and risk of attention deficit hyperactivity disorder: A nationwide Danish cohort study. *BMJ Open, 2*, 3(9).

Lesesne, C. A., Visser, S. N., & White, C. P. (2003). Attention-deficit/hyperactivity disorder in school-aged children: Association with maternal mental health and use of health care resources. *Pediatrics, 111*(1), 1232–1237.

Levinson-Castiel, R., Merlob, P., Linder, N., Sirota, L., & Klinger, G. (2006). Neonatal abstinence syndrome after in utero exposure to selective serotonin reuptake inhibitors in term infants. *Archives of Pediatric and Adolescent Medicine, 160*, 173–176.

Lin, H., Chen, I., Chen, Y., Lee, H., Wu, F. (2010). Maternal schizophrenia and pregnancy outcome: does the use of antipsychotics make a difference? *Schizophr Research, 116*, 55–60.

Man, K. K., Ton, H. H., Wong, L. Y., Chan, E. W., Simonoff, E., & Wong, I. C. (2015). Exposure to selective serotonin reuptake inhibitors during pregnancy and risk of autism spectrum disorder in children: A systematic review and meta-analysis of observational studies. *Neuroscience and Biobehaviour Review, 49C*, 82–89.

Mattson, S., Eastvold, A., Jones, K., Harris, J., & Chambers, C. (1999). Neurobehavioral follow-up of children prenatally exposed to fluoxetine. *Teratology, 59*, 376.

McKenna, K., Koren, G., Tetelbaum, M., Wilton, L., Shakir, S., Diav-Citrin, O., … Einarson, A. (2005). Pregnancy outcome of women using atypical antipsychotic drugs: A prospective comparative study. *Journal of Clinical Psychiatry*, 66, 444–449.

Mendhekar, D.N. (2007). Possible delayed speech acquisition with clozapine therapy during pregnancy and lactation. *Journal of Neuropsychiatry and Clinical Neuroscience, 19*, 196–197.

Miller, L. J., & Finnerty, M. (1996). Sexuality, pregnancy, and childrearing among women with schizophrenia-spectrum disorders. *Psychiatric Services, 47*, 502–506.

Misri, S., Reebye, P., Kendrick, K., Carter, D., Ryan D., Grunau, R.E., & Oberlander, T. F. (2006). Internalizing behaviors in 4-year-old children exposed in utero to psychotropic medications. *American Journal of Psychiatry*, 163, 1026–1032.

Mortensen, J. T., Olsen, J., Larsen, H., Bendsen, J., Obel, C., & Sorensen, H. T. (2003). Psychomotor development in children exposed in utero to benzodiazepines, antidepressants, neuroleptics, and anti-epileptics. *European Journal of Epidemiology, 18*, 769–771.

Moses-Kolko, E. L., Bogen, D., Perel, J., Bregar, A., Uhl, K., Levin, B., & Wisner, K. L. (2005). Neonatal signs after late in utero exposure to serotonin reuptake inhibitors: Literature review and implications for clinical applications. *JAMA*, 293, 2372–2383.

Murphy, D. G. M., Daly, E., Schmitz, N., Toal, F., Murphy, K., Curran, S., … Travis, M. (2006). Cortical serotonin 5-HT2A receptor binding and social communication in adults with Asperger's syndrome: An in vivo SPECT study. *American Journal of Psychiatry*, 163(5), 934–936.

Niemi, L.T., Suvisaari, J.M., Tuulio-Henriksson, A., Lonnqvist, J.K. (2003). Childhood developmental abnormalities in schizophrenia: evidence from high risk studies. *Schizophrenia Research, 602*, 239–258.

Nora, J. J., Nora, A. H., & Toews, W. H. (1974). Lithium, Ebstein's anomaly and other congenital heart defects. *Lancet, 2*, 594–595.

Nulman, I., Koren, G., Rovet, J., Barrera, M., Pulver, A., Streiner, D., & Feldman, B. (2012). Neurodevelopment of children following prenatal exposure to venlafaxine, selective serotonin reuptake inhibitors, or untreated maternal depression. *American Journal of Psychiatry*, 169, 1165–1174.

Nulman, I., Rovet, J., Stewart, D.E., Wolpin, J., Gardner, H. A., Theis, J. G., … Koren, G. (1997). Neurodevelopment of children exposed in utero to antidepressant drugs. *New England Journal of Medicine*, 336, 258–262.

Nulman, I., Rovet, J., Stewart, D. E., Wolpin, J., Pace-Asciak, P., Shuhaiber, S., & Koren, G. (2002). Child development following exposure to tricyclic antidepressants or fluoxetine throughout fetal life: A prospective, controlled study. *American Journal of Psychiatry*, 159, 1889–1895.

Oberlander, T. F., Grunau, R. E., Fitzgerald, C., Papsdorf, M., Rurak, D., & Riggs, W. (2005). Pain reactivity in 2-month-old infants after prenatal and postnatal serotonin reuptake inhibitor medication exposure. *Pediatrics, 115*, 411–425.

Oberlander, T. F., Grunau, R., Mayes, L., Riggs, W., Rurak, D., Papsdorf, M., & Misri, S., Weinberg, J. (2008). Hypothalamic-pituitary-adrenal (HPA) axis function in 3-month old infants with prenatal selective serotonin reuptake inhibitor (SSRI) antidepressant exposure. *Early Human Development*, 84, 689–697.

Oberlander, T. F., Papsdorf, M., Brain, U. M., Misri, S., Ross, C., & Gruneau, R. E. (2010). Prenatal effects of selective serotonin reuptake inhibitor antidepressants, serotonin transporter promoter genotype (SLC6A4), and maternal mood on child behavior at 3 years of age. *Archives of Pediatric and Adolescent Medicine, 164*, 444–451.

Oberlander, T. F., Reebye, P., Misri, S., Papsdorf, M., Kim, J., & Grunau, R. E. (2007). Externalizing and attentional behaviors in children of depressed mothers treated with a selective serotonin reuptake inhibitor antidepressant during pregnancy. *Archives of Pediatrica and Adolescent Medicine, 161*, 22–29.

Oberlander, T. F., Warburton, W., Misri, S., Aghajanian, J., & Hertzman, C. (2006). Neonatal outcomes after prenatal exposure to selective serotonin reuptake inhibitor antidepressants and maternal depression using population-based linked health data. *Archives of General Psychiatry, 63*, 898–906.

Pardo, C. A., & Eberhart, C. G. (2007). The neurobiology of autism. *Brain Pathology, 17*(4), 434–447.

Pedersen, L. H., Henriksen, T. B., Bech, B. H., Licht, R. W., Kjaer, D., & Olsen, J. (2013). Prenatal antidepressant exposure and behavioral problems in early childhood—A cohort study. *Acta Psychiatrica Scandinavia, 127*, 126–135.

Pederson, L., Henriksen, T. B., & Olsen, J. (2010). Fetal exposure to antidepressants and normal milestone development at 6 and 19 months of age. *Pediatrics, 125*, e600–e608.

Peng, M., Gao, K., Ding, Y., Ou, J., Calabrese, J., Wu, R., Zhao, J. (2013). Effects of prenatal exposure to atypical antipsychotics on postnatal development and growth of infants: a case-controlled, prospective study. *Psychopharmacology, 228*, 577–584.

Rai, D., Lee, B., Dalman, C., Golding, J., Lewis, G., & Magnusson, C. (2013). Parental depression, maternal antidepressant use during pregnancy, and risk of autism spectrum disorders: Population based case-control study. *British Medical Journal, 346*, f2059.

Reebye, P. N., Morison, S. J., Panikkar, H., Misri, S., & Grunau, R. E. (2002). Affect expression in prenatally psychotropic exposed and nonexposed mother–infant dyads. *Infant Mental Health Journal, 23*, 403–416.

Reebye, P. N., Ng, T. W. C., Misri, S., & Stikarovska, I. (2012). Affect expression and self-regulation capacities of infants exposed in utero to psychotropics. *Frontiers in Psychiatry, 3*, 11.

Schou, M. (1976). What happened later to the lithium babies? A follow-up study of children born without malformations. *Acta Psychiatrica Scandinavia, 54*, 193–197.

Simard, M., Gumbiner, B., Lee, A., Lewis, H., & Norman, D. (1989). Lithium carbonate intoxication. A case report and review of the literature. *Archives of Internal Medicine, 149*, 36–46.

Sorensen, M. J., Gronborg, T. K., Christensen, J., Parner, E. T., Vestergaard, M., Schendel, D., & Pedersen, L. H. (2013) Antidepressant exposure in pregnancy and risk of autism spectrum disorders. *Clinical Epidemiology*, 5, 449–459.

Stika, L., Elisova, K., Honzakova, L., Hrochova, H., Plechatova, H., Strnadova, J., … Vinar, O. (1990). Effects of drug administration in pregnancy on children's school behaviour. *Pharmaceutisch Weekblad*, 12, 252–255.

Thiels, C. (1987). Pharmacotherapy of psychiatric disorder in pregnancy and during breastfeeding: a review. *Psychopharmacology, 20*, 133–146.

Toh, S., Li, Q., Cheetham, T. C., Cooper, W. O., Davis, R. L., Dublin, S., Hammad, T. A., … Andrade, S. E. (2013). Prevalence and trends in the use of antipsychotic medications during pregnancy in the US, 2001-2007: A population-based study of 585,615 deliveries. *Archives of Women's Mental Health*, 16(2), 149–157.

van der Lugt, N. M., van de Matt, J. S., van Kamp, I. L., Knoppert-van der Klein, E. A., Hovens, J. G., & Walther, F. J. (2012). Fetal, neonatal and developmental outcomes of lithium exposed pregnancies. *Early Human Development, 88*, 375–378.

Ververs, T., Kaasenbrood, H., Visser, G., Schobben, F., De Jong-Van Den Berg, L., & Egberts, T. (2006). Prevalence and patterns of anti-depressant drug use during pregnancy. *European Journal of Clinical Pharmacology, 62*, 863–870.

Viguera, A. C., Nonacs, R., Cohen, L. S., Tondo, L., Murray, A., & Baldessarini, R. J. (2000). Risk of recurrence of bipolar disorder in pregnant and nonpregnant women after discontinuing lithium maintenance. *American Journal of Psychiatry, 157*(2), 179–184.

Wan, M.W., Abel, K.M., Green, J. (2008). The transmission of risk to children from mothers with schizophrenia: a developmental psychopathology model. *Clinical Psychology Review, 28*(4), 613–637.

Warburton, W., Hertzman, C., & Oberlander, T. F. (2010). A register study of the impact of stopping third trimester selective serotonin reuptake inhibitor exposure on neonatal health. *Acta Psychiatrica Scandinavia, 121*, 471–479.

Webb, R., Avel, K., Pickles, A., & Appleby, L. (2005). Mortality in offspring of parents with psychotic disorders: A critical review and meta-analysis. *American Journal of Psychiatry, 162*(6), 1045–1056.

Weikum, W. M., Oberlander, T. F., Hensch, T. K., & Werker, J. F. (2012). Prenatal exposure to antidepressants and depressed maternal mood alter trajectory of infant speech perception. *Procedures of the National Academy of Sciences (USA), 109*(2), 17221–17227.

Whitaker-Azmitia, P. (2001). Serotonin and brain development: Role in human developmental diseases. *Brain Research Bulletin, 56*(5), 479–485.

Weikum, W.M., Brain, U., Chau, C.M.Y., Grunau, R.E., Boyce, W.T., Diamond, A., Oberlander, T.F. (2013). Prenatal serotonin reuptake inhibitor antidepressant exposure and serotonin transporter promoter geneotype (SLC6A4) influence executive functions at 6 years of age. *Frontiers in Cellular Neuroscience, 7*, 120–131.

Williams, K., Wheeler, D. M., Silove, N., & Hazell, P. (2010). Selective serotonin reuptake inhibitors (SSRIs) for autism spectrum disorders (ASD). *Cochrane Database Systematic Review, 8*(8), CD004677.

Yonkers, K. A., Wisner, K. L., Stowe, Z., Leibenluft, E., Cohen, L., Miller, L., Manber, R., Viguera, A., Suppes, T., Altshuler, L. (2004). Management of bipolar disorder during pregnancy and the postpartum period. *American Journal of Psychiatry*, 161(4), 608–620.

Zeskind, P. S., & Stephens, L. E. (2004). Maternal selective serotonin reuptake inhibitor use during pregnancy and newborn neurobehavior. *Pediatrics, 113*, 368–375.

Chapter 7
Neurocognitive Effects of Pesticides in Children

Genny Carrillo, Ranjana K. Mehta, and Natalie M. Johnson

Definitional Issues and Prevalence

Humans are constantly exposed to complex environmental mixtures in air, food, and water, including pesticides. Pesticides in the USA are commonly used in homes (Berkowitz et al., 2003; Biehler, 2009). In urban rental units, pesticide treatment may be done by professionals according to a regular schedule, while in owner-occupied homes pesticide use may be on an as-needed basis (Julien et al., 2008). In agricultural and rural areas, pesticides are often applied without the proper safety procedures and used in the wrong environments due to lack of knowledge.

In ancient times, Romans killed insect pests by burning sulfur and controlled weeds with salt. In the 1600s, ants were controlled with mixtures of honey and arsenic. By the late nineteenth century, US farmers were using calcium arsenate, nicotine sulfate, and sulfur to control insect pests in field crops, with poor results due to primitive chemistry and application methods. After World War II the discovery

G. Carrillo, M.D., Sc.D., M.P.H., M.S.P.H. (✉)
Department of Environmental and Occupational Health, School of Public Health, Texas A&M Health Science Center, College Station, TX, USA
e-mail: gcarrillo@tamhsc.edu

R.K. Mehta, Ph.D., M.S.
Department of Environmental and Occupational Health, School of Public Health, Texas A&M Ergonomics Center, College Station, TX, USA

Faculty of the Texas A&M Institute for Neuroscience, College Station, TX, USA
e-mail: rmehta@tamu.edu

N.M. Johnson, Ph.D.
Department of Environmental and Occupational Health, School of Public Health, Texas A&M Health Science Center, College Station, TX, USA

Faculty Member of the Texas A&M Interdisciplinary Faculty of Toxicology, College Station, TX, USA
e-mail: natalie.johnson@tamhsc.edu

C. Riccio, J. Sullivan (eds.), *Pediatric Neurotoxicology*, Specialty Topics in Pediatric Neuropsychology, DOI 10.1007/978-3-319-32358-9_7

of DDT, BHC, aldrin, dieldrin, endrin, and 2,4-D was introduced to the market. These new chemicals were inexpensive, effective, and enormously popular. Due to their neurological toxicity, many of them have been removed from the market in the USA, but are still available in some other countries (US Environmental Protection Agency, 2014). In the USA, the Environmental Protection Agency (EPA) regulates pesticides at the national level under the authority of the Federal Insecticide, Fungicide and Rodenticide Act (FIFRA) and other laws. They work cooperatively with state agencies to register pesticides, educate applicators, monitor compliance, and investigate pesticide problems. Other federal agencies such as the Food and Drug Administration (FDA) also work with the EPA to ensure food safety, and US Department of Agriculture (USDA) and the US Fish and Wildlife Service (USFWS) assess the risk of pesticides to wildlife or the environment.

A pesticide is any substance or mixture of substances intended for preventing, destroying, repelling, or mitigating pests; however, the term pesticide also applies to herbicides, fungicides, and various other substances used to control pests. US law states that a pesticide is also any substance, or mixture of substances, intended for use as a plant regulator, defoliant, or desiccant (US Environmental Protection Agency, 2014).

Types of Pesticides

Pesticides are identified depending on the type of pests they control. Another way to think about pesticides is to consider those that are chemical pesticides, or derived from a common source or production method. Other categories of pesticides include biopesticides, antimicrobials, and pest control devices. Among the most used pesticides are organophosphates (OP) pesticides, carbamate pesticides, organochlorine (OC) insecticides, and pyrethoid pesticides (US Environmental Protection Agency, 2014).

Organophosphate Pesticides (OP)

These pesticides affect the nervous system by disrupting the enzyme that regulates acetylcholine, a neurotransmitter. Most OP are pesticides that are formulated to kill, harm, repel, or mitigate one or more species of insect or insecticides. Insecticides work in different ways. Some insecticides disrupt the nervous system, whereas others may damage their exoskeletons, repel them or control them by some other means. They can also be packaged in various forms including sprays, dusts, gels, and baits. Because of these factors, each insecticide can pose a different level of risk to non-target insects, people, pets, and the environment (US Environmental Protection Agency, 2014). Those pesticides were developed in Germany in the 1940s and soon became an important defense against agricultural pests. A serious downside, however, is that they also happen to be extremely toxic, and some are very poisonous (they were used in World War II as nerve agents). However, they are usually not permanent in the environment.

Carbamate Pesticides

Carbamate is a derivative of carbamic acid and most often used as surface sprays or baits in the control of household pests. They affect the nervous system by disrupting an enzyme that regulates acetylcholine, a neurotransmitter. Acetylcholinesterase is an enzyme found in the nervous system, red blood cells, and blood plasma. These pesticides damage nerve function by acting as acetylcholinesterase inhibitors in the nervous system. Carbamates are esters of *N*-methyl carbamic acid. Aldicarb, carbaryl, propoxur, oxamyl, and terbucarb are carbamates. The enzyme effects are usually reversible (Agency for Toxic Substances and Disease Registry, 2008).

Organochlorine Insecticides (OC)

OC insecticides were once commonly used to protect crops, livestock, buildings, and households from the damaging effects of insects, but many have been removed from the market due to their detrimental health and environmental effects, and their persistence (e.g., DDT and chlordane). These are compounds that contain carbon, chlorine, and hydrogen. Their chlorine–carbon bonds are very strong, which means they do not break down easily. They are highly insoluble in water, but are attracted to fats causing them to be readily stored and accumulated in the fatty tissue of any animal ingesting them, including humans. OCs also may affect humans if they drink milk of a dairy cow that has ingested the chemical because it is excreted in its milk fat (Qu, Suri, Bi, Sheng, & Fu, 2010).

Pyrethroid Pesticides

The pyrethroid pesticides were developed as a synthetic version of the naturally occurring pesticide pyrethrin, which is one of the oldest known insecticides and comes from the dried and crushed flower heads of two species of asters: *Chrysanthemum cinerariifolium* and *C. coccineum*. Purified pyrethrum, called pyrethrins, has been very useful in insect control. It kills a variety of insects and mites, knocking them off plants very quickly. For this reason, as well as its relatively low toxicity to people, pyrethrins remain very popular today (e.g., Raid® Flying Insect Killer). Pyrethrins also have the desirable environmental characteristic in that they break down quickly (minutes to hours) in the outdoor environment; however, from a pest control perspective, this might be an advantage to killing unwanted insects.

Pesticides and Our Children

Children encounter pesticides daily through the environment in which they live, e.g., home, school, playgrounds, hospitals, and in many public buildings and parks. Pesticides can enter a child's body through four possible routes: the skin, lungs, mouth, and eyes. The skin is the largest organ in the body; however, for its size, a child's skin surface is twice that of an adult per unit of body weight (Hoppin, Adgate, Eberhart, Nishioka, & Ryan, 2006; Kofman, Berger, Massarwa, Friedman, & Jaffar, 2006). When skin is wet, cut, or irritated, pesticides can penetrate even faster. Pesticides applied as foggers, bombs, and aerosols generally have the smallest particle size and thus are the most readily inhaled. Children also ingest pesticide residue from contaminated food, drinking water, and by accidentally ingesting dust (Driver et al., 2013).

There are many published studies referring to the potential health effects of pesticides on the developing fetus and in childhood (Campbell, 2013; Garry, 2004; Harari et al., 2010). Depending on stage of development, the fetus is selectively sensitive to particular chemical toxicants. Studies have shown that children who live near agricultural communities may be exposed more frequently to pesticides as a result of drift or residue tracked into their homes, via shoes and clothing (Freeman et al., 2004; Shalat et al., 2003). A 2004 study conducted in South Texas reported that pesticides were detected frequently and at relatively high concentrations in house dust and hand-rinse samples in relation to outside samples. It should be noted that none of the pesticides detected in house dust or hand-rinse samples are considered acceptable for indoor use (Carrillo-Zuniga et al., 2004).

Although there is evidence of the effects of OPs on neurodevelopment and behavior in adults, limited information is available about their effects in children who might be more vulnerable to neurotoxic compounds (Bouchard, Bellinger, Wright, & Weisskopf, 2010; Perera et al., 2006). Organophosphate exposure at levels common among US children may contribute to ADHD prevalence (Bouchard et al., 2010; Rauh et al., 2006), and higher concentrations of OP metabolites in the urine of pregnant women have been found to be associated with increased odds of attention problems and poorer attention scores in their young children (Marks et al., 2010).

Impact on the Developing Child: Biological Basis for Increased Susceptibility

The adage "children are not little adults" is very relevant in regard to children's increased likelihood of exposure to pesticides due to behavioral patterns, increased respiratory rate, and surface area of skin for dermal absorption. From a developmental viewpoint, fetuses and infants are at high risk for adverse neurodevelopmental effects caused by environmental exposures, including pesticides (Grandjean & Landrigan, 2014). Neural development is a precisely coordinated process that begins early in gestation under control from specific hormones and neurotransmitters, such as the above-mentioned acetylcholine. Over a period of 9 months from when embryonic nerve cells first begin dividing, the newly formed fetal brain will resemble its classical contoured structure, per the gyri and sulci, and consist of tens of billions of neurons (Stiles & Jernigan, 2010). Therefore, pesticide exposure during this window of susceptibility can be devastating on the developing fetal brain.

For instance, pesticides inhibiting cholinesterase function directly affect the regulatory action of acetylcholine on synapse formation (Augusti-Tocco, Biagioni, & Tata, 2006). The placenta does not offer protection against all of these insults, and a variety of pesticides have been detected in umbilical cord blood indicating fetal circulation (Aylward et al., 2014).

In addition, the physiologic immaturity of the developing metabolic system increases the vulnerability of infants and children to the effects of pesticide exposure. For instance, infant levels and activity of paraoxygenase 1 (PON1), an enzyme that detoxifies OPs, are low in early infancy (Chen et al., 2004; Holland et al., 2006). Huen et al. (2009) showed the effects of PON1 polymorphisms could affect expression of the PON1 enzyme as late as 7 years of age, indicating increased susceptibility to organophosphate pesticides extend beyond early infant years. Overall, increased absorption and decreased elimination due to lower renal clearance rates place children at heightened risk for the neurotoxic effects of pesticides. Pesticides have caused severe damage to the unborn children of pregnant women who are exposed to them. For this reason, topics related to different neuropsychological, emotional, and behavioral functioning will be reviewed based upon various types of pesticides.

Neurocognitive Functioning

Organophosphate Pesticides (OP) Exposure and Neurocognitive Functioning

In adults, the effects of OP following chronic occupational exposure has been consistent adverse neurobehavioral effects such as deficits reported in motor speed and coordination, information processing speed, executive functioning, attention, and short-term memory, which are indicative of CNS dysfunction (Rohlman, Anger, & Lein, 2011). Exposure to OP pesticides has been consistently linked to neurobehavioral deficits in children and adolescents as well. Abdel Rasoul et al. (2008) reported a dose–effect relationship between increased years of exposure to OP pesticides and cognitive deficits in adolescent Egyptian agricultural workers. The study employed serum acetylhydrolase (AChE) due to its more rapid response to chlorpyrifos exposure. An Arabic version of the Wechsler Adult Intelligence Scale (WAIS) was used to assess neurobehavioral function. Across all ages, ranging from 9 to 18 years, OP exposure was associated with decrements in general intellectual functioning and neuropsychological functioning (i.e., abstract thinking, attention, spatial relations, short-term auditory, visual memory, visual conception, and perceptual memory speed assessed using 30 general information questions for children (Abdel Rasoul et al., 2008). Using the Eysenck Personality Questionnaire, Abdel Rasoul et al. also reported neurological symptoms and higher scores on the personality traits of psychoticism and neuroticism in adolescents with greater OP exposure. While results from this study corroborated findings reported in other studies with adult workers

(Farahat et al., 2003; Kamel & Hoppin, 2004), the dose–response relationship presented here lacks an explanation regarding potential neurotoxicity mechanisms through which cognitive functions are impacted by OP pesticides.

In contrast, Bouchard et al. (2010) reported that prenatal, but not postnatal exposure to OP pesticides measured using maternal urinary dialkyl phosphate (DAP) concentrations during pregnancy, and from children at 6 months, 1, 2, 3.5, and 5 years, were associated with poorer intellectual development by age 7. Cognitive abilities of 7-year-olds participating in the study were assessed using the Wechsler Intelligence Scale for Children—Fourth Edition (WISC-IV). Strong negative associations between urinary DAP metabolites during pregnancy were found with cognitive scores on all subtests in children at age 7. These associations were most strongly associated with Verbal Comprehension and Full Scale IQ. Postnatal DAP concentrations at 6 months, 2, 3.5, and 5 years were not associated with cognitive scores (Bouchard et al., 2010). Bouchard et al. argued that in utero exposure to OP pesticides may substantially impact fetal development processes such as cell division, migration, formation of synapses, and myelination (Tau & Peterson, 2009) when compared to postnatal pesticide exposure.

Rauh et al. (2006) examined the relationship between prenatal exposure to chlorpyrifos on the neurodevelopment and behavior of a 3-year-old (Rauh et al., 2006). Chlorpyrifos levels were measured in umbilical cord blood at delivery as the dosimetric measure of prenatal exposure. The Bayley Scales of Infant Development II (BSID-II) were used to generate a continuous Mental Development Index (MDI) and a corresponding Psychomotor Development Index (PDI) at 12, 24, and 36 months of age. Behavior problems were measured through maternal responses on the 99-item Child Behavior Checklist (CBCL) for ages 1.5–5 years, which collects information on child behaviors occurring in the 2 months prior to application of the questionnaire (Achenbach & Rescorla, 2000). Children exposed to higher levels of chlorpyrifos were found to have significantly lower PDI scores at 36 months of age than those with lower chlorpyrifos levels. In addition, at 36 months there were significantly greater proportions of children with cognitive and psychomotor delays among those exposed prenatally to high levels of chlorpyrifos. The MDI and PDI scores indicated a confirmed trend of adverse cognitive and psychomotor effects increasing over time. Finally, children who were exposed prenatally to high levels of pesticides were significantly more likely to score in the clinical range for attention problems, attention-deficit/hyperactivity disorder (ADHD) problems, and pervasive developmental disorder (PDD) problems, than were children with lower levels of chlorpyrifos exposure at 36 months.

Overall, there is substantial evidence that prenatal exposure to OP pesticide can adversely impact neuropsychological functioning and behavioral outcomes in children. In contrast, findings from studies that investigated the link between postnatal exposures to OP pesticides to impaired neurocognitive functioning are comparatively inconsistent.

Pyrethroid Pesticides (PP) Exposure and Neurocognitive Functioning

Horton et al. (2011) investigated the impact of prenatal exposure to pyrethroid insecticides on neurodevelopment among children at 36-months. Prenatal exposure to Permethrin (a common pyrethroid) was analyzed using umbilical cord plasma at delivery, and maternal plasma collected within 48 h of delivery. Both MDI and PDI scores were obtained using the BSID-II among children aged 36 months. No significant associations between prenatal exposure to Permethrin and MDI or PDI were observed at 36 months. Horton et al. (2011) acknowledged that methodological limitations with measuring Permethrin exposure could potentially have impacted the study findings. Pyrethroid insecticides, including permethrin, are rapidly metabolized; however, uncontrolled exposures to other pesticides or neurodevelopmental toxicants may have confounded these results. Indeed, the study did report a negative association of piperonyl butoxide (PBO) measured in personal air collection during the third trimester of pregnancy, and MDI scores in children at 36 months. PBO is the most common pyrethroid insecticide synergist, and was collected to determine maternal pesticide exposure using personal air samples. Despite the common use of pyrethroids, particularly as a replacement to OP pesticides, this is the only epidemiological study that provided some evidence linking pyrethroids exposure to delayed mental development in children at 36 months.

Organochlorine Insecticide (OC) Exposure and Neurocognitive Functioning

In adults, long-term occupational exposure to DDT is associated with neurobehavioral dysfunctions and impaired performance with increasing years of DDT application (van Wendel de Joode et al., 2001). Exposure to OC can occur both in utero and early life because of their lipophilicity via breastfeeding (Ribas-Fitó et al., 2005). Using cord serum levels of DDT, Ribas-Fitó et al., 2006, followed newborns to 4 years of age. Neuropsychological testing of the children at this age included assessment of intellectual abilities, attention, and social competence (Ribas-Fitó et al., 2006). The Spanish version of the McCarthy Scales of Children's Abilities (McCarthy, 1972) was used to assess verbal memory, working memory, memory span or short-term memory, and executive functioning. The study reported a dose–response relationship between higher prenatal exposure of DDT levels and impairments in verbal and memory performance. More important, the study reported a strong association between DDT exposure at birth with decreases in verbal, memory, quantitative and perceptual performance skills among preschoolers, even at low doses. Similar neurocognitive decrements with DDT exposure were found when children were followed longitudinally from 6 to 24 months (Eskenazi et al., 2006). In this study, levels of maternal serum DDT were found to be negatively associated with mental development on the BSID assessed at 12 and 24 months, but not at 6 months. Scores on the PDI were consistently negatively correlated to DDT exposure; however, decrements in psychomotor performance were greater at the 6 and 12 month visit when compared to the 24-month visit.

The study by Ribas-Fitó et al. (2006) discussed earlier did not find a link between cognitive impairments and prenatal dichlorodiphenyldichloroethene (DDE) exposure. These findings aligned with results reported in Gladen et al. (1988) and Rogan and Gladen (1991). Both of these studies found no association between in utero or postnatal DDE exposure, nor in children's scores on the MDI or PDI during subsequent assessments occurring at 12, 18, and 24 months (Gladen et al., 1988; Rogan & Gladen, 1991). However, Gladen et al. (1988) reported a positive association between in utero exposure to DDE and the mental development of infants at 6 months. In children over 3 years of age, Ribas-Fitó et al. (2006) found that in utero DDE exposure was associated with decrements in the memory domain from the MSCA; however, no differences were observed across other cognitive domains. This finding was corroborated by Rogan and Gladen (1991), who found no dose–response relationship between DDE exposure and any cognitive ability.

In general, there are few studies that have addressed in utero exposure to OC insecticides, particularly DDT and DDE, to neurocognitive development in infants and children. While these studies emphasize the negative relationship between serum DDT and DDE and neurodevelopment, the association is stronger with DDT than with DDE.

Although research is limited, a few recent epidemiologic studies have reported associations between in utero OP exposure and adverse effects on neurobehavioral development (Engel et al., 2011; Eskenazi et al., 2010; Rauh et al., 2006). These studies found that biomarkers of prenatal OP exposure are associated with an increased number of abnormal neonatal reflexes, as measured by the Brazelton Scales of Neonatal Development (Engel et al., 2011; Rauh et al., 2006); and poorer mental development in early childhood as measured on the Bayley Scales of Infant Development (Eskenazi et al., 2010; Rauh et al., 2006). According to the National Academy of Sciences, concern about children's exposure to pesticides is valid because "exposure to neurotoxic compounds at levels believed to be safe for adults could result in permanent loss of brain function in children if it occurred during the prenatal and early childhood period of brain development" (National Research Council, 1993, p. 61).

Academic Functioning

Kofman et al. (2006) studied 26 children aged 6–12 at Soroka Medical Center who were hospitalized for acute OP poisoning before age 3 and treated with standard emergency procedures. Children from the unexposed control group were recruited through friends and relatives of the exposed children in the same community, and then matched according to age and sex. All children in this study were native speakers of Arabic from the Bedouin population of the Negev region of Israel, and attended regular schools. All children underwent a battery of neuropsychological testing limited to the areas of memory, attention, and inhibitory control, as these behavioral functions have been found to be related to the cholinergic system in animal and human studies (Kofman et al., 2006). The structured interview did not reveal any conduct disorders, health, or academic problems. One boy who had swallowed paint thinner (solvent) and one girl who had swallowed kerosene (hydrocarbon used as a cooking fuel) repeated first grade. Academic difficulties in school were not reported by the parents except for two children in each group. None of the children took medication, and only one child had been hospitalized since the poisoning incident. Poisonings involving the CNS in infancy and early childhood are not uncommon (Eskenazi, Bradman, & Castorina, 1999; Lifshitz, Shahak, Bolotin, & Sofer, 1997; Ruckart, Kakolewski, Bove, & Kaye, 2004). There was only one long-term follow-up study, which occurred after 1–2 years of age (Ruckart et al., 2004). It was initially believed that the children participating in this study had overcome an acute one-time OP exposure, and all attended regular schools. However, a finer assessment of specific cognitive abilities indicated impairment on the verbal learning and motor inhibition tasks in the exposed children compared with matched control children. Additional follow-up studies would be required to determine whether these mild developmental delays are long-lasting or if they will be overcome with continued maturation.

Specific Diagnostic Outcomes

The increasing incidences of pesticide poisoning in developing countries as reported by Konradsen et al. (2003) confirmed that pesticide poisoning is linked to the use of acutely toxic pesticides that is often accompanied with a weak or absent legislative framework regulating pesticide use. While regulatory practices around the use of pesticides are improving, efforts are lacking to develop specific regulatory practices pertaining to special education eligibility due to pesticide-related cognitive impairments. While cost estimates pertaining to pesticide-related special education programs are not available, it is likely that the link between pesticide use and Autism and ADHD related behavior places a substantial economic burden on the education system. The total estimated costs for special education for children with autism spectrum disorder in the USA were more than $5.7 billion in 2011 (Lavelle et al., 2014). Little research has been done in developing and testing diagnostic outcomes specific to pesticide use, particularly those that can be employed by community or school counselors to identify pesticide-related decrements in a child's academic and cognitive performance. A review of existing special education programs and/or eligibility criteria did not reveal any specific educational programs pertaining to pesticide-related cognitive impairments as it relates to a student's academic progress. Future work is warranted both at the basic clinical level to develop diagnostic outcomes to identify at-risk children, as well as at the policy level to implement policies in school systems to accommodate the changing cognitive capabilities of children affected by pesticide use.

Prognosis and Moderating Factors

Based upon published studies, the prognosis of children exposed to OP, including those who had prenatal exposure, has been shown to negatively affect child neurobehavioral development (Sánchez Lizardi, O'Rourke, & Morris, 2008). Children exposed to OC will have poorer mental development than those exposed to chlorpyrifos (CPF), as issues related to Working Memory Index and Full-Scale IQ will show. Due to prenatal exposure, problems of longer-term educational implications of early cognitive deficits will show up later in the life. These development challenges will cause the child to likely have some disability related to learning. Exposure to chemicals in the environment may decrease the attentiveness of every child, but for vulnerable children the exposure could cause symptoms and impairment that warrant an ADHD diagnosis. Disability has been defined in many ways and it is important to identify a definition that is adequate and maintained over time (Currie & Kahn, 2012).

There is education available related to Healthy Homes on how to avoid the use of hazardous chemicals in households. These practices will avoid or limit the exposure of dangerous pesticides to pregnant women and their fetuses, as well as young children. The Healthy Homes curriculum, which was developed by the National Healthy Homes Training Center and Network, has been used in a holistic manner with chronic diseases, such as asthma (Carrillo-Zuniga et al., 2012), and focuses on the Seven Principles of Healthy Homes (how to keep a home dry, clean, ventilated, pest free, safe, contaminant free, improving the indoor environment, and decreasing hazardous exposures within the home).

Considerations for Prevention and Intervention

Utilizing the Healthy Homes Curriculum to educate parents and caregivers is important so that they can learn how to avoid the use and misuse of chemicals pesticides that are dangerous. Furthermore, new green alternative safe products can be used for households and the environment to decrease exposure or eliminate chemicals that could be dangerous. In order to avoid exposure in other places, since September 1, 1995, all school districts in Texas have been required to use integrated pest management (IPM) practices. Another requirement is all pesticide applications on school grounds and in buildings be made only when students are not expected to be present for normal academic instruction or organized extracurricular activities for at least 12 h after the application (Institute of North America, 2014). IPM is an effective and environmentally sensitive approach to pest management that relies on a combination of common-sense practices. IPM programs use current, comprehensive information on the life cycles of pests and their interaction with the environment. The IPM approach can be applied to both agricultural and non-agricultural settings, such as the home, garden, and workplace (US Environmental Protection Agency, 2014).

This information, in combination with available pest control methods, is used to manage pest damage by the most economical means, and with the least possible hazard to people, property, and the environment. However, it is important for families living in agricultural surroundings to learn when aerial fumigation is conducted so that they know when to close all windows, as well as avoid being outdoors while it is occurring. Moreover, it is important for families to be informed about the advantages of buying organic vegetables and fruits whenever possible, which are free of pesticides.

Interventions in schools and childcare centers that eliminate pesticide use can have a large impact on reducing childhood exposure since children spend a large percentage of their time in these settings when away from their homes. In fact, infants may spend as many as 50 h per week in daycare, representing a major source of potential exposure (Tulve, Suggs, McCurdy, Cohen Hubal, & Moya, 2002). While the National Health and Safety Performance standards for childcare recommend use of an integrated pest control program (American Academy of Pediatrics, American Public Health Association, & National Resource Center for Health and Safety in Child Care and Early Education, 2011) research has shown a majority of centers currently rely on pesticides for pest control and prevention. For example, Bradman, Dobson, Leonard, and Messenger (2010) found that out of 637 childcare centers randomly selected in California, 55 % of the centers reported using pesticides. Specifically, 47 % reported using insecticide sprays or foggers, which have the potential to leave residues on the ground and other surfaces (Bradman et al., 2010).

For children with cognitive, academic, or behavioral concerns in conjunction with pesticide exposure, established procedures for obtaining appropriate supports through early childhood centers and schools should be followed. In agricultural areas, early screening for appropriate early intervention efforts (i.e., universal screening) may be appropriate. If indicated, comprehensive evaluation can be helpful in identifying specific areas in need of remediation and can inform systematic intervention planning (Riccio & Reynolds, 2013).

Conclusion

Pesticides create hazardous exposures for everyone, especially children and pregnant women. Recent investigations have emphasized the adverse effects of both prenatal and postnatal exposure to pesticides on mental and psychomotor development, memory and executive functioning, as well as behavioral outcomes. The degree to which neurocognitive development is negatively impacted has shown to be by pesticide type, prenatal or postnatal, and dose-dependent. While the negative associations between pesticide exposure and cognitive abilities are evident across several epidemiological studies, the link between some pesticide types such as DDE and PP, and their impact on specific neurocognitive functioning are less clear. In order to have a better understanding of the complexity of this problem, more prospective studies are needed pre-uterus, and after the delivery, to identify and correlate the child's exposure, as well as the relationship with intellectual, neuropsychological, and emotional and behavioral functioning.

References

Abdel Rasoul, G. M., Abou Salem, M. E., Mechael, A. A., Hendy, O. M., Rohlman, D. S., & Ismail, A. A. (2008). Effects of occupational pesticide exposure on children applying pesticides. *NeuroToxicology, 29*(5), 833–838. doi:10.1016/j.neuro.2008.06.009.

Achenbach, T. M., & Rescorla, L. A. (2000). *Manual for the ASEBA preschool forms and profiles: Child behavior checklist & profile for ages 1.5–5*. Burlington, VT: University of Vermont, Research Center for Children, Youth, and Families. English.

Agency of Toxic Substances and Disease Registry. (2008). *Toxic substances portal*. Retrieved March 6, 2015, from http://www.atsdr.cdc.gov/substances/toxchemicallisting.asp?sysid=39

American Academy of Pediatrics, American Public Health Association, & National Resource Center for Health and Safety in Child Care and Early Education. (2011). *Caring for our children: National health and safety performance standards; Guidelines for early care and education programs*. Elk Grove Village, IL: American Academy of Pediatrics.

Augusti-Tocco, G., Biagioni, S., & Tata, A. (2006). Acetylcholine and regulation of gene expression in developing systems. *Journal of Molecular Neuroscience, 30*(1-2), 45–47. doi:10.1385/JMN:30:1:45.

Aylward, L. L., Hays, S. M., Kirman, C. R., Marchitti, S. A., Kenneke, J. F., English, C., … Becker, R. A. (2014). Relationships of chemical concentrations in maternal and cord blood: A review of available data. *Journal of Toxicology and Environmental Health, Part B, 17*(3), 175–203. doi:10.1080/10937404.2014.884956.

Berkowitz, G. S., Obel, J., Deych, E., Lapinski, R., Godbold, J., Liu, Z., … Wolff, M. S. (2003). Exposure to indoor pesticides during pregnancy in a multiethnic, urban cohort. *Environmental Health Perspectives, 111*(1), 79–84.

Biehler, D. D. (2009). Permeable homes: A historical political ecology of insects and pesticides in US public housing. *Geoforum, 40*(6), 1014–1023. doi:10.1016/j.geoforum.2009.08.004.

Bouchard, M. F., Bellinger, D. C., Wright, R. O., & Weisskopf, M. G. (2010). Attention-deficit/hyperactivity disorder and urinary metabolites of organophosphate pesticides. *Pediatrics, 125*(6), e1270–e1277. doi:10.1542/peds.2009-3058.

Bradman, A., Dobson, C., Leonard, V., & Messenger, B. (2010). *Pest management and pesticide use in California child care centers, Vol 239*. Berkeley, CA: Center for Children's Environmental Health Research, UC Berkeley School of Public Health.

Campbell, A. W. (2013). Pesticides: Our children in jeopardy. *Alternative Therapies in Health And Medicine, 19*(1), 8–10.

Carrillo-Zuniga, G., Coutinho, C., Shalat, S. L., Freeman, N. C. G., Black, K., Jimenez, W., … Donnelly, K. C. (2004). Potential sources of childhood exposure to pesticides in an agricultural community. *Journal of Children's Health, 2*(1), 29–39. doi:10.1080/15417060490463181.

Carrillo-Zuniga, G., Kirk, S., Mier, N., Garza, N. I., Lucio, R. L., & Zuniga, M. A. (2012). The impact of asthma health education for parents of children attending head start centers. *Journal of Community Health, 37*, 1296–1300. doi:10.1007/s10900-012-9571-y.

Centers for Disease Control and Prevention. (1999). *Autism spectrum disorders (Factshet)*.

Chen, D., Hu, Y., Chen, C., Yang, F., Fang, Z., Wang, L., & Li, J. (2004). Polymorphisms of the paraoxonase gene and risk of preterm delivery. *Epidemiology, 15*((4), 466–470.

Currie, J., & Kahn, R. (2012). Children with disabilities: Introducing the issue. *Future of Children, 22*(1), 3–11.

Driver, J., Ross, J., Pandian, M., Assaf, N., Osimitz, T., & Holden, L. (2013). Evaluation of predictive algorithms used for estimating potential postapplication, nondietary ingestion exposures to pesticides associated with children's hand-to-mouth behavior. *Journal of Toxicology and Environmental Health, Part A, 76*(9), 556–586. doi:10.1080/15287394.2013.785347.

Engel, S. M., Wetmur, J., Chen, J., Zhu, C., Barr, D. B., Canfield, R. L., & Wolff, M. S. (2011). Prenatal exposure to organophosphates, paraoxonase 1, and cognitive development in childhood. *Environmental Health Perspectives, 119*(8), 1182–1188. doi:10.1289/ehp.1003183.

Eskenazi, B., Bradman, A., & Castorina, R. (1999). Exposures of children to organophosphate pesticides and their potential adverse health effects. *Environmental Health Perspectives Supplements, 107*, 409.

Eskenazi, B., Huen, K., Marks, A., Harley, K. G., Bradman, A., Barr, D. B., & Holland, N. (2010). PON1 and neurodevelopment in children from the CHAMACOS study exposed to organophosphate pesticides in utero. *Environmental Health Perspectives, 118*(12), 1775–1781. doi:10.1289/ehp.1002234.

Eskenazi, B., Marks, A. R., Bradman, A., Fenster, L., Johnson, C., Barr, D. B., & Jewell, N. P. (2006). In utero exposure to dichlorodiphenyltrichloroethane (DDT) and dichlorodiphenyldichloroethylene (DDE) and neurodevelopment among young Mexican American children. *Pediatrics, 118*(1), 233–241. doi:10.1542/peds.2005-3117.

Farahat, T. M., Abdelrasoul, G. M., Amr, M. M., Shebl, M. M., Farahat, F. M., & Anger, W. K. (2003). Neurobehavioural effects among workers occupationally exposed to organophosphorous pesticides. *Occupational and Environmental Medicine, 60*(4), 279–286. doi:10.1136/oem.60.4.279.

Freeman, N. C. G., Shalat, S. L., Black, K., Jimenez, M., Donnelly, K. C., Calvin, A., & Ramirez, J. (2004). Seasonal pesticide use in a rural community on the US/Mexico border. *Journal of Exposure Analysis and Environmental Epidemiology, 14*(6), 473–478.

Garry, V. F. (2004). Pesticides and children. *Toxicology and Applied Pharmacology, 198*(2), 152–163. doi:10.1016/j.taap.2003.11.027.

Gladen, B. C., Rogan, W. J., Hardy, P., Thullen, J., Tingelstad, J., & Tully, M. (1988). Development after exposure to polychlorinated biphenyls and dichlorodiphenyl dichloroethene transplacentally and through human milk. *The Journal of Pediatrics, 113*(6), 991–995. doi:10.1016/S0022-3476(88)80569-9.

Grandjean, P., & Landrigan, P. J. (2014). Neurobehavioural effects of developmental toxicity. *The Lancet Neurology, 13*(3), 330–338. doi:10.1016/S1474-4422(13)70278-3.

Harari, R., Julvez, J., Murata, K., Barr, D., Bellinger, D. C., Debes, F., & Grandjean, P. (2010). Neurobehavioral deficits and increased blood pressure in school-age children prenatally exposed to pesticides. *Environmental Health Perspectives, 118*(6), 890–896. doi:10.1289/ehp.0901582.

Holland, N., Furlong, C., Bastaki, M., Richter, R., Huen, K., …Eskenazi, B. (2006). Paraoxonase polymorphisms, haplotypes, and enzyme activity in Latino mothers and newborns. *Environmental Health Perspectives, 114*(7), 985–991.

Hoppin, J. A., Adgate, J. L., Eberhart, M., Nishioka, M., & Ryan, P. B. (2006). Environmental exposure assessment of pesticides in farmworker homes. *Environmental Health Perspectives, 114*(6), 929–935.

Horton, M. K., Rundle, A., Camann, D. E., Boyd Barr, D., Rauh, V. A., & Whyatt, R. M. (2011). Impact of prenatal exposure to piperonyl butoxide and permethrin on 36-month neurodevelopment. *Pediatrics, 127*(3), e699–e706. doi:10.1542/peds.2010-0133.

Huen, K., Harley, K., Brooks, J., Hubbard, A., Bradman, A., Eskenazi, B., & Holland, N. (2009). Developmental changes in PON1 enzyme activity in young children and effects of PON1 polymorphisms. *Environmental Health Perspectives, 117*(10), 1632–1638. doi:10.1289/ehp.0900870.

Institute of North America. (2014). School IPM 2020. Reducing pest problems and pesticides hazards in our nation's schools. Retrived March 7, 2015, from http://www.ipminstitute.org/school_ipm_2015/resources.htm#Model_Manuals

Julien, R., Levy, J. I., Adamkiewicz, G., Hauser, R., Spengler, J. D., Canales, R. A., & Hynes, H. P. (2008). Pesticides in urban multiunit dwellings: hazard identification using classification and regression tree (CART) analysis. *Journal of the Air & Waste Management Association (1995), 58*(10), 1297–1302.

Kamel, F., & Hoppin, J. A. (2004). Association of pesticide exposure with neurologic dysfunction and disease. *Environmental Health Perspectives, 112*(9), 950–958. doi:10.1289/ehp.7135.

Kofman, O., Berger, A., Massarwa, A., Friedman, A., & Jaffar, A. A. (2006). Motor inhibition and learning impairments in school-aged children following exposure to organophosphate pesticides in infancy. *Pediatric Research, 60*(1), 88–92.

Konradsen, F., van der Hoek, W., Cole, D. C., Hutchinson, G., Daisley, H., Singh, S., & Eddleston, M. (2003). Reducing acute poisoning in developing countries—Options for restricting the availability of pesticides. *Toxicology, 192*(2–3), 249–261. doi:10.1016/S0300-483X(03)00339-1.

Lavelle, T. A., Weinstein, M. C., Newhouse, J. P., Munir, K., Kuhlthau, K. A., & Prosser, L. A. (2014). Economic burden of childhood autism spectrum disorders. *Pediatrics, 133*(3), e520–e529.

Lifshitz, M., Shahak, E., Bolotin, A., & Sofer, S. (1997). Carbamate poisoning in early childhood and in adults. *Journal of Toxicology Clinical Toxicology, 35*, 25–27.

Marks, A. R., Harley, K., Bradman, A., Kogut, K., Barr, D. B., Johnson, C., … Eskenazi, B. (2010). Organophosphate pesticide exposure and attention in young Mexican-American children: the CHAMACOS study. *Environmental Health Perspectives, 118*(12), 1768–1774. doi:10.1289/ehp.1002056.

McCarthy, D. (1972). *Manual for the McCarthy Scales of children's abilities (Spanish adaptation: Madrid, Spain: TEA Ediciones, S.A., 1996)*. New York, NY: Psychological Corporation.

National Research Council. (1993). *Pesticides in the diets of infants and children*. Washington, DC: National Academy Press.

Perera, F. P., Rauh, V., Whyatt, R. M., Tsai, W., Tang, D., Diaz, D., … Kinney, P. (2006). Effect of prenatal exposure to airborne polycyclic aromatic hydrocarbons on neurodevelopment in the first 3 years of life among inner-city children. *Environmental Health Perspectives, 114*(8), 1287–1292.

Qu, W., Suri, R. P., Bi, X., Sheng, G., & Fu, J. (2010). Exposure of young mothers and newborns to organochlorine pesticides (OCPs) in Guangzhou, China. *Science of the Total Environment, 408*(16), 3133–3138. doi:10.1016/j.scitotenv.2010.04.023.

Rauh, V. A., Garfinkel, R., Perera, F. P., Andrews, H. F., Hoepner, L., Barr, D. B., … Whyatt, R. W. (2006). Impact of prenatal chlorpyrifos exposure on neurodevelopment in the first 3 years of life among inner-city children. *Pediatrics, 118*(6), e1845–e1859. doi:10.1542/peds.2006-0338.

Ribas-Fitó, N., Grimalt, J. O., Marco, E., Sala, M., Mazón, C., & Sunyer, J. (2005). Breastfeeding and concentrations of HCB and p, p′-DDE at the age of 1 year. *Environmental Research, 98*, 8–13.

Ribas-Fitó, N., Torrent, M., Carrizo, D., Muñoz-Ortiz, L., Júlvez, J., Grimalt, J. O., & Sunyer, J. (2006). In utero exposure to background concentrations of DDT and cognitive functioning among preschoolers. *American Journal of Epidemiology, 164*(10), 955–962. doi:10.1093/aje/kwj299.

Riccio, C. A., & Reynolds, C. R. (2013). Principles of neuropsychological assessment in children and adolescents. In D. Saklofske, V. L. Schwean, & C. R. Reynolds (Eds.), *Oxford handbook of psychological assessment of children and adolescents* (pp. 331–346). Oxford: Oxford University Press.

Rogan, W. J., & Gladen, B. C. (1991). PCBs, DDE, and child development at 18 and 24 months. *Annals of Epidemiology, 1*(5), 407–413. doi:10.1016/1047-2797(91)90010-A.

Rohlman, D. S., Anger, W. K., & Lein, P. J. (2011). Correlating neurobehavioral performance with biomarkers of organophosphorous pesticide exposure. *NeuroToxicology, 32*(2), 268–276. doi:10.1016/j.neuro.2010.12.008.

Ruckart, P. Z., Kakolewski, K., Bove, F. J., & Kaye, W. E. (2004). Long-term neurobehavioral health effects of methyl parathion exposure in children in Mississippi and Ohio. *Environmental Health Perspectives, 112*(1), 46–51.

Sánchez Lizardi, P., O'Rourke, M. K., & Morris, R. J. (2008). The effects of organophosphate pesticide exposure on Hispanic children's cognitive and behavioral functioning. *Journal of Pediatric Psychology, 33*(1), 91–101. doi:10.1093/jpepsy/jsm047.

Shalat, S. L., Donnelly, K. C., Freeman, N. C. G., Calvin, J. A., Ramesh, S., Jimenez, M., … Ramirez, J. (2003). Nondietary ingestion of pesticides by children in an agricultural community on the US/Mexico border: preliminary results. *Journal of Exposure Analysis and Environmental Epidemiology, 13*(1), 42–50.

Stiles, J., & Jernigan, T. L. (2010). The basics of brain development. *Neuropsychology Review, 20*(4), 327–348. doi:10.1007/s11065-010-9148-4.

Tau, G. Z., & Peterson, B. S. (2009). Normal development of brain circuits. *Neuropsychopharmacology, 35*(1), 147–168.

Tulve, N. S., Suggs, J. C., McCurdy, T., Cohen Hubal, E. A., & Moya, J. (2002). Frequency of mouthing behavior in young children. *Journal of Exposure Analysis and Environmental Epidemiology, 12*(4), 259–264.

United States Environmental Protection Agency (2014). *Pesticides*. Retrieved March 6, 2015, from http://www.epa.gov/pesticides/about/types.htm

United States Environmental Protection Agency. (2015). *Integrated pest management (IPM) principles*. Retrieved March 6, 2015 from http://www.epa.gov/pesticides/factsheets/ipm.htm#what

van Wendel de Joode, B., Wesseling, C., Kromhout, H., Monge, P., Garcia, M., & Mergler, D. (2001). Chronic nervous-system effects of long-term occupational exposure to DDT. *The Lancet, 357*(9261), 1014–1016. doi:10.1016/S0140-6736(00)04249-5.

Chapter 8
Exposure to Lead and Other Heavy Metals: Child Development Outcomes

Victor Villarreal and Maria J. Castro

Definition and Brief History

A heavy metal is a member of a subset of elements that exhibit metallic properties. Some heavy metals (e.g., iron, cobalt, copper, and zinc) serve as nutrients at low concentration levels and are essential for human health, but they can be toxic in high concentration. Other heavy metals have no known vital or beneficial effects on humans; moreover, exposure to certain heavy metals (e.g., cadmium, mercury, arsenic, chromium, and lead) can be toxic even in low concentration. The study of the effects of lead is particularly important because humans have been exposed to high levels of lead for centuries, exposure to lead has occurred on global scale, high lead exposure continues today, and established research suggests that exposure to lead can have particularly detrimental effects on children.

Lead—chemical symbol *Pb*—is a silvery metal with a slightly blue color. It has a low melting point, is easily molded and shaped, is resistant to corrosion, and can be combined with other metals to form alloys. For these and other reasons, lead has been used by humans for millennia. For example, the Romans used lead in pots, dishes, coins, cosmetics, weights, and pipes that still exist (Reddy & Braun, 2010). Today, lead is used in products as diverse as batteries, glazes and paints, solder,

---

V. Villarreal, Ph.D. (✉)
Department of Educational Psychology, The University of Texas at San Antonio, 501 W. Cesar E. Chavez Blvd., San Antonio, TX 78207, USA
e-mail: victor.villarreal@utsa.edu

M.J. Castro, M.A.
Department of Educational Psychology, The University of Texas at San Antonio, 501 W. Cesar E. Chavez Blvd., San Antonio, TX 78207, USA
e-mail: mcastr2@gmail.com

C. Riccio, J. Sullivan (eds.), *Pediatric Neurotoxicology*, Specialty Topics in Pediatric Neuropsychology, DOI 10.1007/978-3-319-32358-9_8

cable covers, shot and ammunition, roofing materials, and radiation shielding. Lead also continues to be used as an additive in gasoline in several countries (United Nations Environment Programme [UNEP], 2014).

The detrimental effects of lead have been known for centuries (Reddy & Braun, 2010), but the first "modern" clinical description of lead poisoning (i.e., high concentration of lead in the body) appeared in 1839 and included descriptions of abdominal and neurological aspects of lead exposure (Hernberg, 2000). Reports over the following century further associated lead exposure to hematological effects (e.g., anemia), joint and muscle pain, kidney problems, and risk of abortions and stillbirths (Hernberg, 2000). Although these early reports were based on observations and examinations of adult samples, specific awareness of the effects of lead poisoning in children was reported in the early twentieth century. In 1904, Turner and Gibson (as cited in Rabin, 1989) described lead poisoning in a sample of Australian children, and they attributed the disease to flaking lead-based paint from homes. One of the first published accounts of lead poisoning in children in the USA came one decade later, in 1914, and child lead poisoning as a common childhood disease continued to gain wider recognition in the 1920s (Rabin, 1989).

After the slow realization of the detrimental effects of lead, efforts were made to decrease lead contamination and subsequent exposure. The earliest attempts to do this were in Europe, where lead-based paint was banned in many countries—including Sweden, Czechoslovakia, Austria, Poland, Spain, Finland, and Norway—in the early 1910s and 1920s (Silbergeld, 1997). Attempts to limit lead exposure in the USA were not enacted until much later; in the USA, lead was banned in paint in 1978, in pipes in 1986, and in gasoline in 1995 (Environmental Protection Agency [EPA], 1998). Most recently, in 2000, leaded gasoline was banned by the European Union. Notably, environmental lead from these sources has not been eliminated and, along with the previously reported current uses of lead, it continues to contribute to lead exposure.

Sources of Lead Exposure

Environmental Exposure

Lead constitutes only 0.002 % of the Earth's crust and has become widely distributed almost entirely as the result of human activity (World Health Organization [WHO], 2010). Although lead has been used for centuries, the largest contributor to global lead contamination has been through the relatively recent use of lead as an additive in gasoline (Landrigan, Schechter, Lipton, Fahs, & Schwartz, 2002; Mielke, Laidlaw, & Gonzales, 2011; UNEP, 1999). Lead released in exhaust fumes from leaded gasoline contributed greatly to increased airborne lead concentrations and high lead deposits in water, soil, and dust. Although the use of lead in gasoline has been phased out over the preceding decades, resulting in dramatic decreases in environmental lead concentration (EPA, 1995), as of 2014 it continued to be used in gasoline in six countries (UNEP, 2014). After lead in gasoline, lead in paint is one of the largest sources of global lead contamination and of human lead exposure. Lead-based paint is especially likely to be found in older homes (i.e., homes built before 1978 in the USA); in these homes, leaded paint may be deteriorating and flaking or it may still be found under layers of new paint. Other sources of lead contamination include lead in plumbing, lead in food and animal products, and lead in toys and various other products (Akkus & Ozdenerol, 2014; Edwards, 2008; Margai & Oyana, 2010).

Regardless of the source of lead, ingestion is the most common route of adult and childhood lead exposure; it has been estimated that more than 80 % of the daily intake of lead is derived from the ingestion of food, dirt, and dust (WHO, 2010). Among children, their age-appropriate hand-to-mouth behavior results in greater likelihood of their bringing lead-containing objects or substances (e.g., contaminated soil, flaking lead-based paint) to their mouth, thus greatly increasing their risk of exposure (Akkus & Ozdenerol, 2014). Moreover, the onset of pica—the persistent eating of nonnutritive substances (which includes paint and soil) (American Psychiatric Association, 2013)—is commonly reported in childhood, further contributing to a greater likelihood of lead exposure through ingestion in children rather than in adults. Exposure to other types of heavy metals (e.g., cadmium, manganese, mercury, cadmium) also regularly occurs through ingestion (Caldwell, Mortensen, Jones, Caudill, & Osterloh, 2009; Carvalho et al., 2014; Davidson, Myers, Weiss, Shamlaye, & Cox, 2006). Remarkably, exposure to dangerous amounts of aluminum has occurred through the ingestion of standard intravenous feeding solutions typically given to infants (Bishop, Morley, Day, & Lucas, 1997). After ingestion, inhalation is the most common route of exposure to lead and other heavy metals. Although inhalation represents a greater risk for adults, as it regularly occurs in facilities such as metal processing plants where adults may be employed, it is a risk to children that are exposed to lead from car exhausts (in countries that still use leaded gasoline), as well as smoke from the open burning of waste and of lead contaminated materials in and near homes (Carvalho et al., 2014; WHO, 2010).

Maternal Exposure

Maternal exposure to heavy metals represents another significant source of exposure to developing children because of the placental transfer that occurs during the prenatal period (Hinwood et al., 2013; Röllin, Sandanger, Hansen, Channa, & Odland, 2009; Shirai, Suzuki, Yoshinaga, & Mizumoto, 2010; Silbernagel et al., 2011). During fetal development, the placenta offers some protection against unwanted chemical exposure; for example, cadmium does not readily transfer across the placenta (Odland, Nieboer, Romanova, Thomassen, & Lund, 1999; Salpietro et al., 2002). However, the placenta is not an effective barrier against all chemicals, as it is known that blood mercury and lead readily transfer to the developing fetus (Al-Saleh, Shinwari, Mashhour, Mohamed, & Rabah, 2011; Costa,

Aschner, Vitalone, Syversen, & Soldin, 2004; Röllin et al., 2009; Shannon, 2003). Moreover, the concentration of metals in umbilical cord blood has been shown to be substantially higher than that in maternal blood (Grandjean & Landrigan, 2006), suggesting increased risk of exposure for developing children.

Several longitudinal studies have found associations between prenatal exposure to heavy metals (typically determined by examining concentration of metals in cord blood) and detrimental effects in children in a variety of domains (e.g., Boucher et al., 2012; Grandjean et al., 1997; Lanphear et al., 2005; Sagiv, Thurston, Bellinger, Amarasiriwardena, & Korrick, 2012; Sioen et al., 2013). Although some research suggests that postnatal exposure to heavy metals may be more influential than prenatal exposure (Bellinger, 1994; Leviton et al., 1993), it should be noted that it is difficult to differentiate between the relative magnitude of the effects of prenatal and postnatal heavy metal exposure. This is the case because of the high likelihood of postnatal environmental exposure of children that have been exposed to metals during the prenatal period (Burns, Baghurt, Sawyer, McMichael, & Tong, 1999; Needleman, McFarland, Ness, Fienberg, & Tobin, 2002; Wasserman, Staghezza-Jaramillo, Shrout, Popovac, & Graziano, 1998). For example, prenatal lead exposure may be associated with high lead concentrations in maternal blood caused by maternal exposure to lead-based paint in a home; an infant raised in that home will subsequently be exposed to the same lead-based paint that contributed to the prenatal lead exposure.

Diagnosis and Prevalence

Diagnosis

In the 1960s, elevated childhood lead level was defined by the US Centers for Disease Control and Prevention (CDC) as a blood lead level (BLL) concentration of at least 60 micrograms per deciliter (μg/dl). Increased recognition of the effects of lead exposure at lower BLLs led the CDC to repeatedly reduce the threshold that defines elevated BLLs to 40 μg/dl in the 1970s, 25 μg/dl in the 1980s, and 10 μg/dl in the 1990s (WHO, 2010). This was the standard for nearly two decades; however, recent studies have provided evidence of detrimental effects at even lower BLLs (i.e., 3–10 μg/dl), suggesting that there is no minimal threshold for the toxicity of lead exposure (Chiodo, Jacobson, & Jacobson, 2004; Cho et al., 2010; Gilbert & Weiss, 2006; Kim et al., 2010; Lanphear et al., 2005; Nigg et al., 2008; Wang et al., 2008). Thus, in 2012, the CDC placed at 5 μg/dl the goal for lead exposure prevention in children (CDC, 2012).

The manifestations of lead poisoning are dose-dependent. High BLLs (>100 μg/dl) are life-threatening; they can cause potentially fatal encephalopathy in children (WHO, 2010). Other well-recognized and often observed symptoms of particularly high BLLs involve the gastrointestinal and central nervous systems and may include symptoms such as abdominal pain, vomiting, clumsiness, ataxia, alternating periods of hyperirritability and stupor, coma, and seizures (Lidsky & Schneider, 2006; WHO, 2010). The combination of such symptoms and affirmative responses to questions about lead exposure should raise the suspicion of lead poisoning. However, lead poisoning is primarily a subclinical disease and the overt symptoms previously noted are not typically present in children exposed to lead; rather, the effects of lead exposure normally manifest as deficits in intellectual functioning, academic achievement, and other areas that are reviewed in this chapter. Regardless of the manifestation of lead exposure and lead poisoning, BLL measurements are ultimately required to make an accurate diagnosis (Markowitz, 2000).

Prevalence

Due in large part to the ban of lead as an additive in gasoline, childhood BLLs have been falling over the preceding decades. For example, data from the USA from 1976 to 1980 indicated that approximately 88 % of children ages 1–5 years had BLLs ≥ 10 μg/dl. Since then, the percentage has decreased sharply, to 4.4 % from 1991 to 1994, 1.6 % from 1999 to 2002, and 0.8 % from 2007 to 2010 (Wheeler & Brown, 2013). Despite progress in reducing BLLs among children, long-standing disparities exist. In the USA, the BLLs of younger children, those belonging to poor families and those enrolled in Medicaid, and African-American children are significantly higher than those of older, more affluent, and either European American or Mexican American children (Wheeler & Brown, 2013). Moreover, BLLs vary from country to country. Globally, 16 % of all children in 2004 were estimated to have BLLs > 10 μg/dl (WHO, 2009); however, it is estimated that 90 % of children with BLLs > 10 μg/dl live in low-income countries (WHO, 2010) and in those where there are substantial industrial uses of lead and where leaded gasoline is still permitted.

Impact on the Developing Child

A discussion of the impact of exposure to heavy metals is incomplete without an understanding of the unique vulnerability of children. As previously noted, toxic chemicals can pass through the placental barrier (Al-Saleh et al., 2011; Costa et al., 2004; Röllin et al., 2009; Shannon, 2003) and easily access the developing brain, interfering with important processes (e.g., rapid brain growth, development of different brain structures) from the earliest stages of fetal development (American Academy of Pediatrics Committee on Environmental Health, 2003; Stiles & Jernigan, 2010). Children are also more vulnerable than adults to metal exposure due to their less developed blood–brain barrier; the blood–brain barrier, which protects the brain from many toxic chemicals, is not completely formed until about 6 months after birth (Grandjean & Landrigan, 2006; Jarup, 2003). Exposure to metals early in life can also lead to altered gene expression, increased risk of disease later in life, and a reduced capacity to recover from future neurological insults (e.g., strokes) (Pilsner et al., 2009; Schneider & Decamp, 2007). Children are also at increased risk for experiencing the detrimental effects of elevated metal exposure because they are more likely to have nutritional deficiencies that lead to the increased absorption of metals (Mahaffey, 1995), have a greater ratio of surface area to body mass than adults (Selevan, Kimmel, & Mendola, 2000), and breathe more contaminated air and ingest more contaminated water and food per unit of weight than adults (American Academy of Pediatrics Committee on Environmental Health, 2003; Moya, Bearer, & Etzel, 2004; Selevan et al., 2000).

Thus, children have a heightened vulnerability to heavy metal exposure and related detrimental effects; this vulnerability extends from the prenatal period through childhood, and early exposure can have long-lasting impacts on development. As previously noted, although the effects of particularly high levels of heavy metals concentration can result in severe medical consequences and even death (WHO, 2010), significantly lower concentrations (i.e., 1–20 μg/dl) can also affect child development outcomes in a variety of domains and can result in an elevated risk for the development of mental health disorders.

Intellectual Functioning

Most research on the effects of heavy metal exposure has focused on the association between lead exposure and intelligence. Overall, lead exposure has been inversely associated with intellectual functioning in all stages of childhood development (e.g., Bellinger, Stiles, & Needleman, 1992; Canfield, Kreher, Cornwell, & Henderson, 2003; Jusko et al., 2008; Lanphear et al., 2005; Schnaas et al., 2006). The association between BLLs and lower childhood intellectual functioning has been found whether lead exposure is measured by lifetime or infancy average measures, peak exposure, or on the same day that tests of intellectual functioning are administered (Jusko et al., 2008). Exposure to other types of metals has also been associated with intellectual functioning; exposure to manganese (Carvalho et al., 2014; Riojas-Rodríguez et al., 2010; Wasserman et al., 2011), methylmercury (Grandjean et al., 1997; Julvez, Debes, Weihe, Choi, & Grandjean, 2010), and cadmium (Kippler et al., 2012; Tian et al., 2009) have been associated with reduced cognitive functioning in children. Studies have largely established these associations even after adjusting for covariates (e.g., race, socioeconomic status, caregiver intelligence) that are posited to effect intellectual development (e.g., Jusko et al., 2008; Lanphear et al., 2005; Surkan et al., 2008).

The impact of heavy metal exposure on child intellectual functioning is significant. In the most severe cases, extremely high BLLs have been associated with intellectual disability (i.e., significant deficits in intellectual functioning [historically defined as performance at least two standard deviations below the mean on standardized tests of intelligence], along with deficits in adaptive functioning

[American Psychiatric Association, 2013]) (Fewtrell, Pruss-Ustun, Landrigan, & Ayuso-Mateos, 2004; Nevin, 2009). However, significant cognitive effects are also seen in children with lower BLLs. For example, multiple studies have found differences of 5–6 standard score points in the intelligence scores between children with elevated BLLs (10–30 μg/dl) and those with minimal BLLs (<10 μg/dl) (Jusko et al., 2008; Lanphear et al., 2005). Differences are primarily seen in full-scale or overall intelligence scores, but analyses have also suggested increased deficits in particular domains of intelligence, such as performance domains (Jusko et al., 2008). Notably, studies have established a dose–response relationship between BLLs and intellectual deficits. That is, children with higher BLLs exhibit worse performance on tests of intelligence. For example, Lanphear et al. (2005) estimated that intelligence test point decrements associated with an increase in blood lead from 2.4 to 10 μg/dL, 10 to 20 μg/dL, and 20 to 30 μg/dL were 3.9, 1.9, and 1.1, respectively. This finding also suggests a curvilinear relationship between BLLs and intellectual performance; most effects of BLL on intellectual functioning are seen in low increments of BLLs, with decreasing impact as BLLs continue to rise.

Neuropsychological Functioning

Although the majority of studies have examined effects of heavy metal exposure on general intelligence, lead exposure has also been associated with deficits in other aspects of cognitive functioning. Within this domain, deficits have been noted primarily in studies of the effects of lead on general executive functioning (e.g., Canfield et al., 2003; Canfield, Gendle, & Cory-Slechta, 2004); even though other areas of neuropsychological functioning are affected by BLL, it appears to be within the domain of executive functioning that children with elevated BLLs show their most consistent deficits (Chiodo et al., 2004; Surkan et al., 2007). Poorer performance on tests of executive function have been indicated as early as the preschool and early school-age years, even after adjusting for factors such as child intelligence test scores (Canfield et al., 2004; Surkan et al., 2007). Exposure to metals other than lead has also been associated with deficits in executive functioning (e.g., Carvalho et al., 2014). Elevated BLLs have also been inversely associated with working memory and spatial memory span (Canfield et al., 2004; Surkan et al., 2007), motor abilities (Chiodo et al., 2004; Ris, Dietrich, Succop, Berger, & Bornschein, 2004), and reaction time and attention (Chiodo et al., 2004, 2007; Minder, Das-Smaal, Brand, & Orlebeke, 1994; Plusquellec et al., 2007; Surkan et al., 2007).

Academic Functioning

As might be expected in a population characterized by diminished cognitive abilities, lower levels of academic achievement (e.g., lower reading and mathematics scores) and educational attainment have been found in children with high BLLs (e.g., Fergusson,

Horwood, & Lynskey, 1997; Kordas et al., 2006; McClaine et al., 2013; Miranda et al., 2007; Needleman, Schell, Bellinger, Leviton, & Allred, 1990; Wang et al., 2002). Notably, deficits have been found even after adjusting for common covariates (e.g., gender, race, SES, caregiver education level, and caregiver intelligence scores) (e.g., Amato et al., 2012; Lanphear, Dietrich, Auinger, & Cox, 2000; Surkan et al., 2007; Zhang et al., 2013) that are known to be associated with academic achievement.

Deficits in academic achievement have been found based on results of standardized, nationally normed tests of achievement. For example, in a sample of children aged 6–16 years using a standardized achievement test (the Wide Range Ability Test), results showed an inverse relationship between BLL and scores in areas of mathematics and reading (Lanphear et al., 2000). In other studies that utilized children with high BLLs and standardized achievement measures, differences on tests of achievement between those with and without elevated BLLs ranged from approximately 7–9 standard scores points, representing a different of approximately one-half of a standard deviation (Bellinger et al., 1992; Surkan et al., 2007). It is important to note that effects on academic achievement remained even after controlling for cognitive functioning. This implies that children's academic achievement was significantly lower than would be expected based on their intelligence. These findings are significant given that standardized tests are routinely used to diagnosis specific learning disorders in school and clinic settings, and they are used to inform special education eligibility decisions and educational planning and placement.

The inverse association between BLLs and academic achievement has also been reported in results of state-mandated tests of achievement and on end-of-grade tests (Amato et al., 2012; Miranda et al., 2007; Zhang et al., 2013). For example, a study consisting of children from Michigan found that detrimental effects were found for BLL on a standardized test taken by all public school students (Zhang et al., 2013). Specifically, high BLLs before age 6 years were strongly associated with poor academic achievement in math, reading, and science in grades 3, 5, and 8, and the likelihood of scoring "less than proficient" for those with BLLs > 10 μg/dl was more than twice the odds for those whose BLLs were < 1 μg/dl (Zhang et al., 2013). Another study that utilized scores from a state-mandated test from Wisconsin found similar deficits across a variety of academic achievement areas (Amato et al., 2012). Implications for lower scores on state-mandated tests are different than for lower scores on standardized, individually administered tests, as scores on state-mandated tests are not typically used to determine disability status. However, they have been widely implemented since the passage of the No Child Left Behind Act (2002) in the USA, and they are used in decision making regarding grade retention, school performance evaluations, and, more recently, teacher performance evaluations.

Behavioral Functioning

BLL has also been associated with a variety of behavior problems. This association was first described by Byers and Lord (1943) in a pioneering study of 20 cases of children who had "recovered" from lead poisoning but later exhibited serious behavior problems (e.g., attacking a teacher). Since then, studies of prenatal and postnatal lead poisoning have established associations between lead exposure and higher frequencies of delinquent behaviors, increased problem behavior, off-task behavior in school, conduct problems, and behavior associated with inattention and hyperactivity in children at all levels of child development (e.g., Dietrich, Douglas, Succop, Berger, & Bornschein, 2001; Marcus, Fulton, & Clarke, 2010; Ris et al., 2004; Sioen et al., 2013; Wasserman, Liu, Pine, & Graziano, 2001). Results of studies of the association between BLL and problem behaviors suggest that the association is dose-dependent (i.e., increased BLL was associated with increased risk for behavior problems) (Sioen et al., 2013); however, research also suggest that behavior problems are associated with lead exposure at levels as low as 3 μg/dl (Chiodo et al., 2004).

The effects of lead exposure on problem behavior have been seen in the earliest stages of development, during early childhood and the early school years. For example, in a study that included preschool children that were 3 years old, lead exposure was positively associated with destructive behaviors and withdrawal, even after adjusting for sociodemographic variables typically associated with behavior problems (Wasserman et al., 1998). Predictably, behavior problems persist into early the school years. In studies of 7-year-old children—commensurate with a typical grade level of 1 or 2—elevated BLLs were associated with increased social problems, withdrawal, delinquent behavior, inattention, off-task behavior, and hyperactivity (Chiodo et al., 2004, 2007). Behavior problems associated with high BLLs continue into adolescence. In a case–control study of youths aged 12–18 years, after adjusting for covariates such as race, parent education and occupation, presence of two parental figures in the home, and neighborhood crime rate, adjudicated delinquents were found to be four times more likely to have bone lead concentrations at higher levels (e.g., >25 μg/dl) than controls (Needleman et al., 2002). In a prospective longitudinal birth cohort study, prenatal exposure to lead was significantly associated with an increase in the frequency of parent-reported delinquent and antisocial behaviors, while prenatal and postnatal exposure to lead was significantly associated with an increase in frequency of self-reported delinquent and antisocial behaviors, including illegal substance use, in adolescence (Dietrich et al., 2001). Notably, the consequences of behavior problems are magnified as children transition from childhood to adolescence. Behavior problems in adolescence are more likely to involve aggression, the violation of others' rights, and substance use, leading to more severe disciplinary action and involvement with criminal justice systems. Thus, as behavior problems associated with exposure to lead persist into adolescence, the severity of consequent outcomes also increases.

Specific Diagnostic Outcomes

As exposure to heavy metals—especially lead—has been associated with detrimental effects in a variety of domains, it is unsurprising that metal exposure is also associated with multiple diagnosable mental health disorders and disabilities. These include disorders defined in the *Diagnostic and Statistical Manual of Mental Disorders* (DSM) (American Psychiatric Association, 2013) and the US Individuals with Disabilities Education Act (IDEA) (2004).

Attention-Deficit/Hyperactivity Disorder (ADHD)

Several studies have found a positive association between elevated BLLs and a formal diagnosis of ADHD (e.g., Braun et al., 2006; Froehlich et al., 2009; Kim et al., 2013; Nigg et al., 2008; Nigg, Nikolas, Knottnerus, Cavanagh, & Friderici, 2010; Silva, Hughes, Williams, & Faed, 1988; Thomson et al., 1989; Wang et al., 2008). Exposure to other heavy metals (e.g., manganese, methylmercury) has also been associated with ADHD symptoms in childhood (e.g., Boucher et al., 2012; Sagiv et al., 2012; Yousef et al., 2011). ADHD is defined in the DSM, and the disorder falls in the Other Health Impairment special education category of the IDEA. In the USA, children with ADHD may also access special education and related services through provisions in the Americans with Disabilities Act. Notably, comorbid disorders (e.g., conduct disorders, specific learning disorder) are frequently present in individuals with ADHD (American Psychiatric Association, 2013).

Specific Learning Disorder (SLD)

BLL has been inversely associated with academic achievement (Kordas et al., 2006; McClaine et al., 2013; Miranda et al., 2007; Wang et al., 2002), even after adjusting for intellectual functioning. This suggests that children with high BLLs have a greater likelihood of meeting criteria for a SLD. Notably, SLD is defined in both the DSM and the IDEA, and both allow for a diagnosis to be made when academic achievement scores are significantly lower than expected based on performance on tests of intellectual functioning. Although there are few studies that associate exposure to heavy metals directly with diagnosed SLDs instead of just academic difficulties, there is evidence of a link between exposure to lead and other metals (e.g., cadmium, mercury) and diagnosable SLDs (e.g., Koger, Schettler, & Weiss, 2005; Margai & Henry, 2003; Miranda, Maxson, & Kim, 2010). SLDs commonly co-occur with ADHD, communication disorders, and developmental disorders (American Psychiatric Association, 2013).

Oppositional Defiant Disorder (ODD) and Conduct Disorder (CD)

As lead exposure has been associated with a variety of behavior and social problems at multiple stages of development, it is unsurprising that it has also been associated with the diagnosis of ODD (e.g., Marcus et al., 2010; Nigg et al., 2008) and CD (e.g., Braun et al., 2008; Marcus et al., 2010). These disorders include conditions involving problems in self-control of emotions and behaviors, and age is one of the primary means of differentiating the two, with older children more likely to be diagnosed with CD. Although the IDEA does not include a special education category particularly for children with ODD or CD, the behavioral symptoms associated with these disorders (e.g., defiance, aggression to others, violations of rules) can have serious effects on school outcomes, as children with ODD and CD are likely to face disciplinary action that can include severe consequences such as suspension and expulsion.

Autism Spectrum Disorder (ASD)

Although there is a convincing relationship between exposure to heavy metals and the previously noted mental health disorders, the current state of research is inconclusive regarding the association between exposure to metals and the presence of ASDs. For example, some studies have found links between the release of heavy metal pollutants into the atmosphere and diagnoses of ASDs (Palmer, Blanchard, Stein, Mandell, & Miller, 2006; Palmer, Blanchard, & Wood, 2009; Windham, Zhang, Gunier, Croen, & Grether, 2006), but others have found that exposure to high levels of heavy metals does not differentiate children with ASDs from those without the disorder (Kalkbrenner et al., 2010). Investigations comparing heavy metal exposure using samples taken directly from children with and without ASDs, rather than examining environmental contamination, have also have produced mixed and inconclusive findings (Abdullah et al., 2012; Fido & Al-Saad, 2005; Hertz-Picciotto et al., 2010; Lakshmi Priya & Geetha, 2011; Soden, Lowry, Garrison, & Wasserman, 2007), and there is no evidence that thimerosal, a preservative containing ethyl mercury that was added to vaccines, is associated with increased risk of ASDs (Parker, Schwartz, Todd, & Pickering, 2004). More research is needed to confirm conclusions in this area.

Prognosis and Moderating Factors

Several studies suggest that the detrimental effects of high blood concentration of heavy metals are essentially irreversible. Results of medical treatments that remove lead from the body, as well as prospective studies that examine the effects of childhood lead exposure on adult outcomes, indicate no improvement in functioning across time. However, studies of children and adults suggest some moderating factors that may mitigate the effects of heavy metal exposure.

Prognosis

Lead and other metals accumulate in both soft and hard tissue. Once a person is removed from exposure, blood metal concentrations typically subside; however, lead can remain in soft tissue for 40 days and can stay in bony tissue for as long as 27 years (Markiewicz, 1993). Chelation therapy—involving injection of a solution into the body to which chemicals bind and then are eliminated—can be used to remove heavy metals from the body (Markiewicz, 1993). However, in the only randomized trial of the effects of chelation therapy on the child BLLs, chelation was effective in reducing BLLs in the short term, but the treatment did not result in any detectable improvement in a wide variety of measurements of cognitive or behavioral functioning, and the BLLs of treated children were similar to those of untreated children 1 year later (Dietrich et al., 2004). Overall, chelation therapy was ineffective in preventing or reversing cognitive deficits, suggesting that lead poisoning cannot be "cured."

The results of long-term prospective studies provide further evidence that the varied deficits associated with lead exposure do not resolve over time and that the damage caused by lead exposure may be irreversible (e.g., Bellinger et al., 1992; Fergusson et al., 1997; Needleman et al., 1990; Ris et al., 2004). For example, one study that measured BLLs at the age of 6–8 years found that early elevated BLL was associated with poorer reading abilities, lower level of success on school exams, and lower rates of completing school at age 18 years (Fergusson et al., 1997). In other studies of long-term academic outcomes, early childhood BLL was inversely associated with SAT scores during the high school years (Chandramouli, Steer, Ellis, & Emond, 2009; Nevin, 2009). Lead exposure during childhood has also predicted intellectual functioning in the young adult years (Mazumdar et al., 2011), and it has been associated with higher rates of criminality, violence, and arrests in adulthood (Nevin, 2000; Wright et al., 2008).

Moderating Factors

Although the effects of heavy metal exposure may be irreversible, evidence from adult and child studies indicates that certain factors can moderate the effects of exposure to heavy metals. For example, studies have shown that the physiological and psychological effects of stress can modify the adverse effects of exposure to lead; in particular, multiple studies have shown that psychological stress in adult participants modifies the relationship between lead exposure and cognitive performance and blood pressure. Adults with higher stress levels experienced greater deficits in cognitive performance and increased hypertension, even after adjusting for lead levels and other covariates (e.g., age, education, language, nutritional factors, physical activity, substance use) (Peters et al., 2010; Peters, Kubzansky, & McNeely, 2007). In a study involving children, a trend toward significance was found for a lead by SES interaction for intellectual functioning; that is, vulnerability to the cognitive effects of lead was influenced by SES, with children in lower SES households exhibiting increased cognitive deficits (Ris et al., 2004). Finally, in a study of mothers' self-esteem on children's cognitive outcomes that also explored the modifying effects of maternal self-esteem on the association between exposure to lead and neurodevelopment in children, there was evidence that maternal self-esteem attenuated the negative effects of lead exposure (Surkan et al., 2008).

There is also evidence that an enriched environment can mitigate the adverse neurological effects of lead. For example, studies using animal models of lead poisoning have examined the extent to which different environments may modify the effects of lead on the developing brain. In one study, young rats were raised in either enriched or impoverished environments; in this study, the impoverished environment did not allow rats to access any stimulus objects while those in the enriched environment had access to multiple toy objects that were rotated multiple time per week (Schneider, Lee, Anderson, Zuck, & Lidsky, 2001). Lead-exposed rats raised in the impoverished environment had spatial learning deficits; in contrast, those raised in the enriched environment were significantly protected against the behavioral and neurochemical toxicity of lead. These results demonstrate that impoverished environments may accentuate while enriched environments may limit effects of lead exposure (Schneider et al., 2001). In a similar study, environmental enrichment reversed the spatial learning deficits resulting from exposure to lead in rats during development. This showed not only prevention of deficits suggested in the previous study, but it also suggested reversal of the cognitive deficits resulting from developmental lead exposure (Guilarte, Toscano, McGlothan, & Weaver, 2003). Although these are animal studies, they have implications for intervention in lead and other heavy metal exposure in humans.

Considerations for Prevention and Intervention

Prevention

As previously noted, data suggests that chelation therapy is not effective at reversing the detrimental effects of lead exposure and that the problems of heavy metal exposure during childhood do not resolve with time. This indicates that primary prevention is the best strategy for limiting the effects of heavy metal exposure. Indeed, prevention activities are some of the key components presented by Hassanien and El Shahawy (2011) in their recommended actions for the mitigation of problems associated with heavy metal exposure. These include: (a) stricter regulations on heavy metals, (b) enhanced monitoring of levels of heavy metals, (c) wide scale screening of heavy metal levels in children and mothers, (d) health education programs, and (e) acceleration of decontamination efforts in known polluted areas (Hassanien & El Shahawy, 2011).

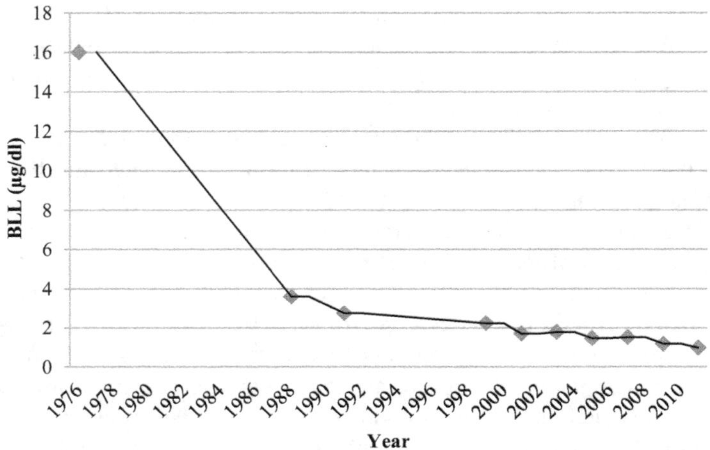

Fig. 8.1 Blood lead concentration for children ages 1–5 years in the US. BLL data were not available prior to 1976 or from 1981 to 1987. Data in this figure were reported by the CDC and are based on the National Health and Nutrition Examination Survey. *Note*: BLL data are not available for every year; data is reported based on multiyear averages. Thus, the trend line is only an estimate of yearly BLLs based on the actual multiyear averages

Prevention efforts, with an emphasis on limiting primary lead contamination and environmental metal concentrations, have been largely successful. For example, the phasing out of lead from gasoline has been a critical step in reducing lead exposure and BLLs. In the USA, initial stages of this process began in the 1970s, before leaded gasoline was banned in 1995. Data on BLLs from the 1970s to the present time show a dramatic decrease in lead exposure. The percentage of children in the USA ages 1–5 years with BLLs ≥ 10 µg/dl declined from 77.8 % in the late 1970s to 4.4 % in the early 1990s, and even further, to less than 1 %, in the late 2000s (CDC, 2005; Wheeler & Brown, 2013). Blood lead concentrations for children ages 1–5 years in the USA from 1976 to 2011 are represented in Fig. 8.1. Many other countries have reported similar outcomes after the removal of lead from gasoline (Lovei, 1998). Although effective primary prevention efforts are large scale operations that can be perceived as being expensive, benefits far outweigh the costs of creating programs for screening, monitoring, and treatment of the previously noted difficulties of lead poisoning (Gould, 2009; Grosse, Matte, Schwartz, & Jackson, 2002).

Intervention

Complete prevention of exposure to heavy metals by eliminating or significantly reducing contamination is ideal but not practical, and it does not represent a solution for professionals working directly with children and families. However, exposure can be minimized to a certain extent, and this can be accomplished via enhanced education programs (Hassanien & El Shahawy, 2011). Parents, as well as educators and mental health professionals (e.g., school psychologists), that will invariably interact with affected children should be made aware not only of the effects of heavy metal exposure, but also of the common methods of exposure.

If questions regarding exposure to lead sources (e.g., paint in older homes) are answered in the affirmative, it is appropriate to recommend regular blood testing to determine BLLs and relative risk for detrimental effects. Notably, since 1989, federal law has included the requirement that states provide blood lead assessment of young children (i.e., at 1 and 2 years of age, and at 3 and 6 years of age if they have not been previously tests) eligible for Medicaid (Wengrovitz & Brown, 2009). Some communities that have a history of elevated clusters of children with high BLLs have adopted more stringent testing policies. For example, the Department of Health and Wellness Promotion in Detroit, Michigan has a policy that children younger than 6 years should be tested for lead once a year by their primary care provider (Zhang et al., 2013).

If exposure to lead or other heavy metals is confirmed, professionals should be prepared to connect affected families with community agencies that can assist with physical health (e.g., nutrition services, safe housing, medical care) and mental health needs. Recommendations for treatment of children with confirmed elevated BLLs have been provided by the CDC (2002). Lead education and follow-up BLL monitoring are recommended for those with BLLs of 10–19 μg/dl. Completion of a complete history and physical exam—including lab work and an abdominal X-ray—are indicated for those with BLLs of 20–44 μg/dl; additionally, at this level, environmental investigation, lead hazard reduction, and neurodevelopmental monitoring are recommended. For children with BLLs of 45–69 μg/dl, the suggested treatment includes all previous actions as well as a complete neurological exam and chelation therapy. Finally, for those with BLLs ≥ 70 μg/dl, immediate hospitalization and commencement of chelation therapy are recommended, with previous actions undertaken after this initial treatment.

In addition to connecting affected children and families with community agencies, professionals can serve as advocates for children in schools, especially since the effects of lead exposure on multiple domains may not be known by school personnel but can cause significant school problems. This advocacy may be especially important for children with BLLs that have historically been deemed to be "safe" (i.e., <10 μg/dl) but that we now know are sufficient to affect functioning in a variety of domains and that create considerable disadvantage to exposed children (Amato et al., 2012). In the school setting, advocacy may include seeking additional educational supports to alleviate decrements in cognitive functioning and academic achievement, as well as behavior intervention support to address behavior problems common in children with elevated BLLs.

Finally, it is important to consider the implications to the family of confirmed cases of elevated BLLs in children. In addition to providing family support for education of heavy metal exposure and the effects of exposure, encouraging an enriching home environment, and providing assistance with behavior management strategies, it is also important to recognize that if children in a home are confirmed to have elevated BLLs, other family members can also be expected to have elevated BLLs (i.e., children and parents may all have elevated BLLs). If we consider the long-term effects of lead exposure (e.g., diminished cognitive functioning in young adulthood, lower levels of educational attainment, increased violence and criminality in adulthood), we can ostensibly presume that parents with elevated BLLs will also be at a disadvantage. Thus, prevention and intervention efforts that identify and serve at-risk families—not just children—are also recommended.

Conclusion

Although the prevalence of lead exposure and consequent lead poisoning, and that of other heavy metals, has decreased over the preceding decades, it is important to recognize that children are particularly susceptible to associated effects and that a growing body of research suggests that there is no "safe" level of lead exposure; effects on child development outcomes are seen at all BLLs. The examples discussed in this chapter demonstrate that exposure to lead and other heavy metals may increase risk for deficits in cognitive functioning, lower levels of academic achievement, and behavioral problems, all of which can have immediate and long-lasting impacts on child development and that may impossible to reverse. The effects can be severe enough to warrant diagnosis of multiple mental health disorders, and they are likely to be observed firsthand by those working closely with children, especially in education settings. Although the ability to influence the quantity of lead and other heavy metals in the environment is limited, interventions can focus on bringing awareness to the issue, supporting prevention efforts to continue to reduce instances of lead exposure, encouraging regular monitoring of children exposed to lead and other heavy metals, identifying families at-risk for exposure to lead, and intervening early with children suspected of lead poisoning by providing them with necessary services in multiple domains.

References

Abdullah, M. M., Ly, A. R., Goldberg, W. A., Clarke-Stewart, K. A., Dudgeon, J. V., Mull, C. G., … Ericson, J. E. (2012). Heavy metal in children's tooth enamel: Related to autism and disruptive behaviors? *Journal of Autism and Developmental Disorders, 42*(6), 929–936. doi:10.1007/s10803-011-1318-6.

Akkus, C., & Ozdenerol, E. (2014). Exploring childhood lead exposure through GIS: A review of the recent literature. *International Journal of Environmental Research and Public Health, 11*, 6314–6334. doi:10.3390/ijerph110606314.

Al-Saleh, I., Shinwari, N., Mashhour, A., Mohamed, G. E. D., & Rabah, A. (2011). Heavy metals (lead, cadmium and mercury) in maternal cord blood and placenta of healthy women. *International Journal of Hygiene and Environmental Health, 214*(2), 79–101. doi:10.1016/j.ijheh.2010.10.001.

Amato, M. S., Moore, C. F., Magzamenm S., Imm, P., Havlena, J. A., Anderson, H. A., & Kanarek, M. S. (2012). Lead exposure and educational proficiency: Moderate lead exposure and educational proficiency on end-of-grade examinations. *Annals of Epidemiology, 22*, 738–743. doi:10.1016/j.annepidem.2012.07.004.

American Academy of Pediatrics Committee on Environmental Health. (2003). *Pediatric environmental health* (2nd ed.). Elk Grove Village, IL: American Academy of Pediatrics.

American Psychiatric Association. (2013). *Diagnostic and statistical manual of mental disorders* (5th ed.). Washington, DC: Author.

Bellinger, D. (1994). Teratogen update: Lead. *Teratology, 50*(5), 367–373. doi:10.1002/tera.1420500508.

Bellinger, D., Stiles, K., & Needleman, H. (1992). Low-level lead exposure, intelligence and academic achievement: A long-term follow-up study. *Pediatrics, 90*(6), 855–861.

Bishop, N. J., Morley, R., Day, J. P., & Lucas, A. (1997). Aluminum neurotoxicity in preterm infants receiving intravenous-feeding solutions. *New England Journal of Medicine, 336*, 1557–1561. doi:10.1056/NEJM199705293362203.

Boucher, O., Jacobson, J. L., Jacobson, S. W., Plusquellec, P., Dewailly, É., Ayotte, P., … Muckle, G. (2012). Prenatal methylmercury, postnatal lead exposure, and evidence of attention deficit/hyperactivity disorder among Inuit children in Arctic Québec. *Environmental Health Perspectives, 120*(10), 1456–1461. doi:10.1289/ehp.1204976.

Braun, J. M., Froehlich, T. E., Daniels, J. L., Dietrich, K. N., Hornung, R., Auinger, P., & Lanphear, B. P. (2008). Association of environmental toxicants and conduct disorder in U.S. children: NHANES 2001–2004. *Environmental Health Perspectives, 116*(7), 956–962. doi:10.1289/ehp.11177.

Braun, M. U., Rauwolf, T., Bock, M., Kappert, U., Boscheri, A., Schnabel, A., & Strasser, R. H. (2006). Percutaneous lead implantation connected to an external device in stimulation-dependent patients with systemic infection: A prospective and controlled study. *Pacing Clinical Electrophysiology, 29*, 875–879. doi:10.1111/j.1540-8159.2006.00454.x.

Burns, J. M., Baghurt, P. A., Sawyer, M. G., McMichael, A. J., & Tong, S. (1999). Lifetime low-level exposure to environmental lead and children's emotional and behavioral development at ages 11–13 years. The Port Pirie cohort study. *American Journal of Epidemiology, 149*, 740–749. doi:10.1093/oxfordjournals.aje.a009883.

Byers, R. K., & Lord, E. E. (1943). Late effects of lead poisoning on mental development. *American Journal of Diseases of Children, 66*, 471–494. doi:10.1097/00005053-194410000-00009.

Caldwell, K. L., Mortensen, M. E., Jones, R. L., Caudill, S. P., & Osterloh, J. D. (2009). Total blood mercury concentrations in the U.S. population: 1999–2006. *International Journal of Hygiene and Environmental Health, 212*(6), 588–598. doi:10.1016/j.ijheh.2009.04.004.

Canfield, R. L., Gendle, M. H., & Cory-Slechta, D. A. (2004). Impaired neuropsychological functioning in lead-exposed children. *Developmental Neuropsychology, 26*, 513–540. doi:10.1207/s15326942dn2601_8.

Canfield, R. L., Kreher, D. A., Cornwell, C., & Henderson, C. R. (2003). Low-level lead exposure, executive functioning, and learning in early childhood. *Child Neuropsychology, 9*, 35–53. doi:10.1076/chin.9.1.35.14496.

Carvalho, C. F., Menezes-Filho, J. A., Matos, V. P. d., Bessa, J. R., Coelho-Santos, J., Viana, G. F. S., … Abreu, N. (2014). Elevated airborne manganese and low executive function in school-aged children in Brazil. *Neurotoxicology, 45*, 301–308. doi:10.1016/j.neuro.2013.11.006.

Centers for Disease Control and Prevention. (2002). *Managing elevated blood lead levels among young children: Recommendations from the Advisory Committee on Childhood Lead Poisoning Prevention*. Atlanta, GA: Author.

Centers for Disease Control and Prevention. (2005). Blood lead levels – United States, 1999–2002. *Morbidity and Mortality Weekly Report, 54*, 513–516.

Centers for Disease Control and Prevention (2012). Response to Advisory Committee on Childhood Lead Poisoning Prevention: Recommendations in low level lead exposure harms children: A renewed call of primary prevention. Retrieved from http://www.cdc.gov/nceh/lead/acclpp/cdc_response_lead_exposure_recs.pdf.

Chandramouli, K., Steer, C. D., Ellis, M., & Emond, A. M. (2009). Effects of early childhood lead exposure on academic performance and behavior of school age children. *Archives of Disease in Childhood, 94*, 844–848. doi:10.1136/adc.2008.149955.

Chiodo, L. M., Covington, C., Sokol, R. J., Hannigan, J. H., Jannise, J., Ager, J., … Delaney-Black, V. (2007). Blood lead levels and specific attention effects in young children. *Neurotoxicology and Teratology, 29*(5), 538–546. doi:10.1016/j.ntt.2007.04.001.

Chiodo, L. M., Jacobson, J. L., & Jacobson, S. W. (2004). Neurodevelopmental effects of postnatal lead exposure at very low levels. *Neurotoxicology and Teratology, 26*(3), 359–371. doi:10.1016/j.ntt.2004.01.010.

Cho, S., Kim, B., Hong, Y., Shin, M., Yoo, H. J., Kim, J., … Kim, H. (2010). Effect of environmental exposure to lead and tobacco smoke on inattentive and hyperactive symptoms and neurocognitive performance in children. *Journal of Child Psychology and Psychiatry, 51*(9), 1050–1057. doi:10.1111/j.1469-7610.2010.02250.x.

Costa, L. G., Aschner, M., Vitalone, A., Syversen, T., & Soldin, O. P. (2004). Developmental neuropathology of environmental agents. *Annual Review of Pharmacology and Toxicology, 44*, 87–110. doi:10.1146/annurev.pharmtox.44.101802.121424.

Davidson, P. W., Myers, G. J., Weiss, B., Shamlaye, C. F., & Cox, C. (2006). Prenatal methyl mercury exposure from fish consumption and child development: A review of evidence and perspectives from the Seychelles child development study. *Neurotoxicology, 27*(6), 1106–1109. doi:10.1016/j.neuro.2006.03.024.

Dietrich, K. N., Douglas, R. M., Succop, P. A., Berger, O. G., & Bornschein, R. L. (2001). Early exposure to lead and juvenile delinquency. *Neurotoxicology and Teratology, 23*(6), 511–518. doi:10.1016/S0892-0362(01)00184-2.

Dietrich, K. N., Ware, J. H., Salganik, M., Radcliffe, J., Rogan, W. J., Fay, M. E., … Jones, R. L. (2004). Treatment of lead-exposed children clinical trial group: Effect of chelation therapy on the neuropsychological and behavioral development of lead-exposed children after school entry. *Pediatrics, 114*, 19–26. doi:10.1542/peds.114.1.19.

Edwards, M. (2008). Lead poisoning: A public health issue. *Primary Health Care, 18*(3), 18.

Environmental Protection Agency (1998). Lead in your home: A parent's reference guide. Retrieved from http://www2.epa.gov/sites/production/files/documents/leadrev.pdf.

Environmental Protection Agency. (1995). Leaded gas phaseout. Retrieved from http://yosemite.epa.gov/R10/airpage.nsf/webpage/Leaded+Gas+Phaseout.

Fergusson, D. M., Horwood, L. J., & Lynskey, M. T. (1997). Early dentine lead levels and educational outcomes at 18 years. *Journal of Child Psychology and Psychiatry, and Allied Disciplines, 38*(4), 471–478. doi:10.1111/j.1469-7610.1997.tb01532.x.

Fewtrell, L. J., Pruss-Ustun, A., Landrigan, P., & Ayuso-Mateos, J. L. (2004). Estimating the global burden of disease of mild mental retardation and cardiovascular diseases from environmental lead exposure. *Environmental Research, 94*, 120–133. doi:10.1016/S0013-9351(03)00132-4.

Fido, A., & Al-Saad, S. (2005). Toxic trace elements in the hair of children with autism. *Autism, 9*(3), 290–298. doi:10.1177/1362361305053255.

Froehlich, T. E., Lanphear, B. P., Auinger, P., Hornung, R., Epstein, J. N., Braun, J., & Kahn, R. S. (2009). Association of tobacco and lead exposures with attention-deficit/hyperactivity disorder. *Pediatrics, 124*(6), e1054. doi:10.1542/peds.2009-0738.

Gilbert, S. G., & Weiss, B. (2006). A rationale for lowering the blood lead action level from 10 to 2 microg/dL. *Neurotoxicology, 27*(5), 693–701. doi:10.1016/j.neuro.2006.06.008.

Gould, E. (2009). Childhood lead poisoning: Conservative estimates of the social and economic benefits of lead hazard control. *Environmental Health Perspectives, 117*(7), 1162–1167. doi:10.1289/ehp.0800408.

Grandjean, P., & Landrigan, P. (2006). Developmental neurotoxicity of industrial chemicals. *The Lancet, 368*(9553), 2167–2178. doi:10.1016/S0140-6736(06)69665-7.

Grandjean, P., Weihe, P., White, R. F., Debes, F., Araki, S., Yokoyama, K., … Jorgensen, P. J. (1997). Cognitive deficit in 7-year-old children with prenatal exposure to methylmercury. *Neurotoxicology and Teratology, 19*(6), 417–428. doi:10.1016/S0892-0362(97)00097-4.

Grosse, S. D., Matte, T. D., Schwartz, J., & Jackson, R. J. (2002). Economic gains resulting from the reduction in children's exposure to lead in the United States. *Environmental Health Perspectives, 110*(6), 563–569. doi:10.1289/ehp.02110563.

Guilarte, T. R., Toscano, C. D., McGlothan, J. L., & Weaver, S. A. (2003). Environmental enrichment reverses cognitive and molecular deficits induced by developmental lead exposure. *Annals of Neurology, 53*(1), 50–56. doi:10.1002/ana.10399.

Hassanien, M. A., & El Shahawy, A. M. (2011). Environmental heavy metals and mental disorders of children in developing countries. In L. I. Simeonov, M. V. Kochubovski, & B. G. Simeonova (Eds.), *Environmental heavy metal pollution and effects on child mental development* (pp. 1–25). Dordrecht: Springer.

Hernberg, S. (2000). Lead poisoning in a historical perspective. *American Journal of Industrial Medicine, 38*(3), 244–254. doi:10.1002/1097-0274(200009)38:3<244::AID-AJIM3>3.0.CO;2-F.

Hertz-Picciotto, I., Green, P. G., Delwiche, L., Hansen, R., Walker, C., & Pessah, I. N. (2010). Blood mercury concentrations in CHARGE study children with and without autism. *Environmental Health Perspectives, 118*(1), 161–166. doi:10.1289/ehp.0900736.

Hinwood, A. L., Callan, A. C., Ramalingam, M., Boyce, M., Heyworth, J., McCafferty, P., & Odland, J. O. (2013). Cadmium, lead and mercury exposure in non smoking pregnant women. *Environmental Research, 126,* 118. doi:10.1016/j.envres.2013.07.005.

Individuals With Disabilities Education Act, 20 U.S.C. § 1400 (2004).

Jarup, L. (2003). Hazards of heavy metal contamination. *British Medical Bulletin, 68*(1), 167–182. doi:10.1093/bmb/ldg032.

Julvez, J., Debes, F., Weihe, P., Choi, A., & Grandjean, P. (2010). Sensitivity of continuous performance test (CPT) at age 14 years to developmental methylmercury exposure. *Neurotoxicology and Teratology, 32*(6), 627–632. doi:10.1016/j.ntt.2010.08.001.

Jusko, T. A., Henderson, C. R., Lanphear, B. P., Cory-Slechta, D. A., Parsons, P. J., & Canfield, R. L. (2008). Blood lead concentrations <10 microg/dL and child intelligence at 6 years of age. *Environmental Health Perspectives, 116*(2), 243. doi:10.1289/ehp.10424.

Kalkbrenner, A. E., Daniels, J. L., Chen, J., Poole, C., Emch, M., & Morrissey, J. (2010). Perinatal exposure to hazardous air pollutants and autism spectrum disorders at age 8. *Epidemiology, 21*(5), 631–641. doi:10.1097/EDE.0b013e3181e65d76.

Kim, S., Arora, M., Fernandez, C., Landero, J., Caruso, J., & Chen, A. (2013). Lead, mercury, and cadmium exposure and attention deficit hyperactivity disorder in children. *Environmental Research, 126*, 105. doi:10.1016/j.envres.2013.08.008.

Kim, B., Kim, Y., Kim, J., Cho, S., Hong, Y., Shin, M., … Bhang, S. (2010). Association between blood lead levels (<5 μg/dL) and inattention-hyperactivity and neurocognitive profiles in school-aged Korean children. *Science of the Total Environment, 408*(23), 5737–5743. doi:10.1016/j.scitotenv.2010.07.070.

Kippler, M., Tofail, F., Hamadani, J., Gardner, R., Grantham-McGregor, S., Bottai, M., & Vahter, M. (2012). Early-life cadmium exposure and child development in 5-year-old girls and boys: A cohort study in rural Bangladesh. *Environmental Health Perspectives, 120*(10), 1462–1468. doi:10.1289/ehp.1104431.

Koger, S. M., Schettler, T., & Weiss, B. (2005). Environmental toxicants and developmental disabilities: A challenge for psychologists. *American Psychologist, 60*(3), 243–255. doi:10.1037/0003-066X.60.3.243.

Kordas, K., Canfield, R. L., López, P., Rosado, J. L., Vargas, G. G., Cebrián, M. E., … Stoltzfus, R. J. (2006). Deficits in cognitive function and achievement in Mexican first-graders with low blood lead concentrations. *Environmental Research, 100*(3), 371–386. doi:10.1016/j.envres.2005.07.007.

Lakshmi Priya, M. D., & Geetha, A. (2011). Level of trace elements (copper, zinc, magnesium and selenium) and toxic elements (lead and mercury) in the hair and nail of children with autism. *Biological Trace Element Research, 142*(2), 148–158. doi:10.1007/s12011-010-8766-2.

Landrigan, P. J., Schechter, C. B., Lipton, J. M., Fahs, M. C., & Schwartz, J. (2002). Environmental pollutants and disease in American children: Estimates of morbidity, mortality, and costs for lead poisoning, asthma, cancer, and developmental disabilities. *Environmental Health Perspectives, 110*(7), 721–728. doi:10.1289/ehp.02110721.

Lanphear, B. P., Dietrich, K., Auinger, P., & Cox, C. (2000). Cognitive deficits associated with blood lead concentrations <10 μg/dL in U.S. children and adolescents. *Public Health Reports, 115*, 521–529. doi:10.1093/phr/115.6.521.

Lanphear, B. P., Hornung, R., Khoury, J., Yolton, K., Baghurst, P., Bellinger, D. C., … Roberts, R. (2005). Low-level environmental lead exposure and children's intellectual function: An international pooled analysis. *Environmental Health Perspectives, 113*(7), 894–899. doi:10.1289/ehp.7688.

Leviton, A., Bellinger, D., Allred, E. N., Rabinowitz, M., Needleman, H., & Schoenbaum, S. (1993). Pre- and postnatal low-level lead exposure and children's dysfunction in school. *Environmental Research, 60*(1), 30–43. doi:10.1006/enrs.1993.1003.

Lidsky, T. I., & Schneider, J. S. (2006). Adverse effects of childhood lead poisoning: The clinical neuropsychological perspective. *Environmental Research, 100*(2), 284–293. doi:10.1016/j.envres.2005.03.002.

Lovei, M. (1998). *Phasing out lead from gasoline: Worldwide experiences and policy implications*. Washington, DC: World Bank.

Mahaffey, K. R. (1995). Nutrition and lead: Strategies for public health. *Environmental Health Perspectives, 103*(6), 191–196. doi:10.1289/ehp.95103s6191.

Marcus, D., Fulton, J., & Clarke, E. (2010). Lead and conduct problems: A meta-analysis. *Journal of Clinical Child & Adolescent Psychology, 39*(2), 234–241. doi:10.1080/15374411003591455.

Margai, F., & Henry, N. (2003). A community-based assessment of learning disabilities using environmental and contextual risk factors. *Social Science & Medicine, 56*(5), 1073–1085. doi:10.1016/S0277-9536(02)00104-1.

Margai, F., & Oyana, T. (2010). Spatial patterns and health disparities in pediatric lead exposure in Chicago: Characteristics and profiles of high-risk neighborhoods. *The Professional Geographer, 62*(1), 46–65. doi:10.1080/00330120903375894.

Markiewicz, T. (1993). Clinical savvy: Recognizing, treating, and preventing lead poisoning. *The American Journal of Nursing, 93*(10), 59–64.

Markowitz, M. (2000). Lead poisoning. *Pediatrics in Review, 21*(10), 327–335. doi:10.1542/pir.21-10-327.

Mazumdar, M., Bellinger, D. C., Gregas, M., Abanilla, K., Bacic, J., & Needleman, H. L. (2011). Low-level environmental lead exposure in childhood and adult intellectual function: A follow-up study. *Environmental Health: A Global Access Science Source, 10*(1), 24. doi:10.1186/1476-069X-10-24.

McClaine, P., Navas-Acien, L., Lee, R., Simon, P., Diener-West, M., & Agnew, J. (2013). Elevated blood lead levels and reading readiness at the start of kindergarten. *Pediatrics, 131*(6), 1081–1089. doi:10.1542/peds.2012-2277.

Mielke, H. W., Laidlaw, M. A. S., & Gonzales, C. R. (2011). Estimation of leaded (Pb) gasoline's continuing material and health impacts on 90 U.S. urbanized areas. *Environment International, 37*(1), 248–257. doi:10.1016/j.envint.2010.08.006.

Minder, B., Das-Smaal, E. A., Brand, E. F., & Orlebeke, J. F. (1994). Exposure to lead and specific attentional problems in schoolchildren. *Journal of Learning Disabilities, 27*(6), 393–399. doi:10.1177/002221949402700606.

Miranda, M. L., Kim, D., Galeano, M. A., Paul, C. J., Hull, A. P., & Morgan, S. P. (2007). The relationship between early childhood blood lead levels and performance on end-of-grade tests. *Environmental Health Perspectives, 115*(8), 1242–1247. doi:10.1289/ehp.9994.

Miranda, M. L., Maxson, P., & Kim, D. (2010). Early childhood lead exposure and exceptionality designations for students. *International Journal of Child Health and Human Development, 3*(1), 77–84.

Moya, J., Bearer, C. F., & Etzel, R. A. (2004). Children's behavior and physiology and how it affects exposure to environmental contaminants. *Pediatrics, 113*(4), 996.

Needleman, H. L., McFarland, C., Ness, R. B., Fienberg, S. E., & Tobin, M. J. (2002). Bone lead levels in adjudicated delinquents: A case control study. *Neurotoxicology and Teratology, 24*(6), 711. doi:10.1016/S0892-0362(02)00269-6.

Needleman, H. L., Schell, A., Bellinger, D., Leviton, A., & Allred, E. N. (1990). The long-term effects of exposure to low doses of lead in childhood: An 11-year follow-up report. *The New England Journal of Medicine, 322*(2), 83–88. doi:10.1056/NEJM199001113220203.

Nevin, R. (2000). How lead exposure relates to temporal changes in IQ, violent crime, and unwed pregnancy. *Environmental Research, 83*(1), 1–22. doi:10.1006/enrs.1999.4045.

Nevin, R. (2009). Trends in preschool lead exposure, mental retardation, and scholastic achievement: Association or causation? *Environmental Research, 109*(3), 301–310. doi:10.1016/j.envres.2008.12.003.

Nigg, J. T., Knottnerus, G. M., Martel, M. M., Nikolas, M., Cavanagh, K., Karmaus, W., & Rappley, M. D. (2008). Low blood lead levels associated with clinically diagnosed attention-deficit/hyperactivity disorder and mediated by weak cognitive control. *Biological Psychiatry, 63*(3), 325–331. doi:10.1016/j.biopsych.2007.07.013.

Nigg, J. T., Nikolas, M., Knottnerus, G. M., Cavanagh, K., & Friderici, K. (2010). Confirmation and extension of association of blood lead with attention-deficit/hyperactivity disorder (ADHD) and ADHD symptom domains at population-typical exposure levels. *Journal of Child Psychology and Psychiatry, and Allied Disciplines, 51*(1), 58. doi:10.1111/j.1469-7610.2009.02135.x.

No Child Left Behind (NCLB) Act of 2001, Pub. L. No. 107–110, § 115, Stat. 1425 (2002).

Odland, J. O., Nieboer, E., Romanova, N., Thomassen, Y., & Lund, E. (1999). Blood lead and cadmium and birth weight among sub-arctic and arctic populations of Norway and Russia. *Acta Obstetricia Et Gynecologica Scandinavica, 78*(10), 852–860. doi:10.1034/j.1600-0412.1999.781004.x.

Palmer, R. F., Blanchard, S., Stein, Z., Mandell, D., & Miller, C. (2006). Environmental mercury release, special education rates, and autism disorder: An ecological study of Texas. *Health and Place, 12*(2), 203–209. doi:10.1016/j.healthplace.2004.11.005.

Palmer, R. F., Blanchard, S., & Wood, R. (2009). Proximity to point sources of environmental mercury release as a predictor of autism prevalence. *Health and Place, 15*(1), 18–24. doi:10.1016/j.healthplace.2008.02.001.

Parker, S. K., Schwartz, B., Todd, J., & Pickering, L. K. (2004). Thimerosal-containing vaccines and autistic spectrum disorder: A critical review of published original data. *Pediatrics, 114*, 793–804. doi:10.1542/peds.2004-0434.

Peters, J. L., Kubzansky, L., & McNeely, E. (2007). Stress as a potential modifier of the impact of lead levels on blood pressure: The normative aging study. *Environmental Health Perspectives, 115*(8), 1154. doi:10.1289/ehp.10002.

Peters, J. L., Weisskopf, M. G., Spiro, A., Schwartz, J., Sparrow, D., Nie, H., ... Wright, R. J. (2010). Interaction of stress, lead burden, and age on cognition in older men: The VA normative aging study. *Environmental Health Perspectives, 118*(4), 505–510. doi:10.1289/ehp.0901115.

Pilsner, J. R., Hu, H., Ettinger, A., Sánchez, B. N., Wright, R. O., Cantonwine, D., ... Hernández-Avila, M. (2009). Influence of prenatal lead exposure on genomic methylation of cord blood DNA. *Environmental Health Perspectives, 117*(9), 1466–1471. doi:10.1289/ehp.0800497.

Plusquellec, P., Muckle, G., Dewailly, E., Ayotte, P., Jacobson, S. S., & Jacobson, J. L. (2007). The relation between low-level prenatal lead exposure to behavioral indicators of attention in Inuit infants in Arctic Quebec. *Neurotoxicology and Teratology, 29*, 527–537. doi:10.1016/j.ntt.2007.07.002.

Rabin, R. (1989). Warnings unheeded: A history of child lead poisoning. *American Journal of Public Health, 79*, 1668–1674. doi:10.2105/AJPH.79.12.1668.

Reddy, A., & Braun, C. L. (2010). Lead and the Romans. *Journal of Chemical Education, 87*(10), 1052. doi:10.1021/ed100631y.

Riojas-Rodríguez, H., Solís-Vivanco, R., Schilmann, A., Montes, S., Rodríguez, S., Ríos, C., & Rodríguez-Agudelo, Y. (2010). Intellectual function in Mexican children living in a mining area and environmentally exposed to manganese. *Environmental Health Perspectives, 118*(10), 1465–1470. doi:10.1289/ehp.0901229.

Ris, M. D., Dietrich, K. N., Succop, P. A., Berger, O. G., & Bornschein, R. L. (2004). Early exposure to lead and neuropsychological outcome in adolescence. *Journal of the International Neuropsychological Society, 10*, 261–270. doi:10.1017/S1355617704102154.

Röllin, H. B., Sandanger, T. M., Hansen, L., Channa, K., & Odland, J. O. (2009). Concentration of selected persistent organic pollutants in blood from delivering women in South Africa. *Science of the Total Environment, 408*(1), 146–152. doi:10.1016/j.scitotenv.2009.08.049.

Sagiv, S. K., Thurston, S. W., Bellinger, D. C., Amarasiriwardena, C., & Korrick, S. A. (2012). Prenatal exposure to mercury and fish consumption during pregnancy and attention-deficit/hyperactivity disorder-related behavior in children. *Archives of Pediatrics & Adolescent Medicine, 166*(12), 1123. doi:10.1001/archpediatrics.2012.1286.

Salpietro, C. D., Gangemi, S., Minciullo, P. L., Briuglia, S., Merlino, M. V., Stelitano, A., ... Saija, A. (2002). Cadmium concentration in maternal and cord blood and infant birth weight: A study on healthy non-smoking women. *Journal of Perinatal Medicine, 30*(5), 395. doi:10.1515/JPM.2002.061.

Schnaas, L., Rothenberg, S. J., Flores, M., Martinez, S., Hernandez, C., Osorio, E., ... Perroni, E. (2006). Reduced intellectual development in children with prenatal lead exposure. *Environmental Health Perspectives, 114*(5), 791–797. doi:10.1289/ehp.8552.

Schneider, J. S., & Decamp, E. (2007). Postnatal lead poisoning impairs behavioral recovery following brain damage. *Neurotoxicology, 28*(6), 1153–1157. doi:10.1016/j.neuro.2007.06.007.

Schneider, J. S., Lee, M. H., Anderson, D. W., Zuck, L., & Lidsky, T. I. (2001). Enriched environment during development is protective against lead-induced neurotoxicity. *Brain Research, 896*(1), 48–55. doi:10.1016/S0006-8993(00)03249-2.

Selevan, S. G., Kimmel, C. A., & Mendola, P. (2000). Identifying critical windows of exposure for children's health. *Environmental Health Perspectives, 108*(3), 451–455. doi:10.1289/ehp.00108s3451.

Shannon, M. (2003). Severe lead poisoning in pregnancy. *Ambulatory Pediatrics, 3*(1), 37–39. doi:10.1367/1539-4409(2003)003<0037:SLPIP>2.0.CO;2.

Shirai, S., Suzuki, Y., Yoshinaga, J., & Mizumoto, Y. (2010). Maternal exposure to low-level heavy metals during pregnancy and birth size. *Journal of Environmental Science and Health, Part A: Toxic/Hazardous Substances & Environmental Engineering, 45*(11), 1468–1474. doi:10.1080/10934529.2010.500942.

Silbergeld, E. K. (1997). Preventing lead poisoning in children. *Annual Review of Public Health, 18*(1), 187–210. doi:10.1146/annurev.publhealth.18.1.187.

Silbernagel, S. M., Carpenter, D. O., Gilbert, S. G., Gochfeld, M., Groth III, E., Hightower, J. M., & Schiavone, F. M. (2011). Recognizing and preventing overexposure to methylmercury from fish and seafood consumption: Information for physicians. *Journal of Toxicology, 2011*, 983072. doi:10.1155/2011/983072.

Silva, P. A., Hughes, P., Williams, S., & Faed, J. M. (1988). Blood lead, intelligence, reading attainment, and behaviour in eleven year old children in Dunedin, New Zealand. *Journal of Child Psychology and Psychiatry, and Allied Disciplines, 29*(1), 43–52. doi:10.1111/j.1469-7610.1988.tb00687.x.

Sioen, I., Den Hond, E., Nelen, V., Van de Mieroop, E., Croes, K., Van Larebeke, N., ... Schoeters, G. (2013). Prenatal exposure to environmental contaminants and behavioural problems at age 7–8 years. *Environment International, 59*, 225–231. doi:10.1016/j.envint.2013.06.014.

Soden, S. E., Lowry, J. A., Garrison, C. B., & Wasserman, G. S. (2007). 24-hour provoked urine excretion test for heavy metals in children with autism and typically developing controls, a pilot study. *Clinical Toxicology, 45*(5), 476–481. doi:10.1080/15563650701338195.

Stiles, J., & Jernigan, T. L. (2010). The basics of brain development. *Neuropsychology Review, 20*, 327–348. doi:10.1007/s11065-010-9148-4.

Surkan, P. J., Schnaas, L., Wright, R. O., Wright, R. J., Téllez-Rojo, M. M., Lamadrid-Figueroa, H., ... Perroni, E. (2008). Maternal self-esteem, exposure to lead, and child neurodevelopment. *Neurotoxicology, 29*(2), 278–285. doi:10.1016/j.neuro.2007.11.006.

Surkan, P. J., Zhang, A., Trachtenberg, F., Daniel, D. B., McKinlay, S., & Bellinger, D. C. (2007). Neuropsychological function in children with blood lead levels <10 μg/dL. *Neurotoxicology, 28*(6), 1170–1177. doi:10.1016/j.neuro.2007.07.007.

Thomson, G. O., Raab, G. M., Hepburn, W. S., Hunter, R., Fulton, M., & Laxen, D. P. (1989). Blood-level levels and children's behavior results from the Edinburg Lead Study. *Journal of Child Psychology and Psychiatry, 30*, 515–528. doi:10.1111/j.1469-7610.1989.tb00265.x.

Tian, L., Zhaom Y., Wang, X., Gu, J., Sun, Z., Zhang, Y., & Wang, J. (2009). Effects of gestational cadmium exposure on pregnancy outcomes and development in the offspring at age 4.5 years. *Biological Trace Element Research, 132*, 51–59. doi:10.1007/s12011-009-8391-0.

United Nations Environment Programme. (1999). *Phasing lead out of gasoline: An examination of policy approaches in different countries*. Paris: Author.

United Nations Environment Programme. (2014). *Leaded petrol phase-out: Global status April 2014*. Retrieved from http://www.unep.org/Transport/PCFV/pdf/Maps_Matrices/world/lead/MapWorldLead_April2014.pdf.

Wang, C., Chuang, H., Ho, C., Yang, C., Tsai, J., Wu, T., & Wu, T. (2002). Relationship between blood lead concentrations and learning achievement among primary school children in Taiwan. *Environmental Research, 89*(1), 12–18. doi:10.1006/enrs.2002.4342.

Wang, H., Wang, S., Chen, X., Yang, B., Ma, F., Tang, M., … Ruan, D. (2008). Case-control study of blood lead levels and attention deficit hyperactivity disorder in Chinese children. *Environmental Health Perspectives, 116*(10), 1401–1406. doi:10.1289/ehp.11400.

Wasserman, G. A., Liu, X., Parvez, F., Factor-Litvak, P., Ahsan, H., Levy, D., … Graziano, J. H. (2011). Arsenic and manganese exposure and children's intellectual function. *Neurotoxicology, 32*(4), 450–457. doi:10.1016/j.neuro.2011.03.009.

Wasserman, G. A., Liu, X., Pine, D. S., & Graziano, J. H. (2001). Contribution of maternal smoking during pregnancy and lead exposure to early child behavior problems. *Neurotoxicology and Teratology, 23*, 13–21. doi:10.1016/S0892-0362(00)00116-1.

Wasserman, G. A., Staghezza-Jaramillo, B., Shrout, P., Popovac, D., & Graziano, J. (1998). The effect of lead exposure on behavior problems in preschool children. *American Journal of Public Health, 88*(3), 481–486. doi:10.2105/AJPH.88.3.481.

Wengrovitz, A. M., & Brown, M. J. (2009). Recommendations for blood screening of Medicaid-eligible children aged 1–5 years: An updated approach to targeting a group at high risk. *Morbidity and Mortality Weekly Report, 58*, 1–11.

Wheeler, W., & Brown, M. J. (2013). Blood lead levels in children aged 1–5 years-United states, 1999–2010. *Morbidity and Mortality Weekly Report, 62*(13), 245–248.

Windham, G. C., Zhang, L., Gunier, R., Croen, L. A., & Grether, J. K. (2006). Autism spectrum disorders in relation to distribution of hazardous air pollutants in the San Francisco Bay Area. *Environmental Health Perspectives, 114*(9), 1438–1444. doi:10.1289/ehp.9120.

World Health Organization. (2009). *Global health risks: Mortality and burden of disease attributable to selected major risks*. Geneva: World Health Organization.

World Health Organization. (2010). *Childhood lead poisoning*. Geneva: World Health Organization.

Wright, J. P., Dietrich, K. N., Ris, M. D., Hornung, R. W., Wessel, S. D., Lanphear, B. P., … Rae, M. N. (2008). Association of prenatal and childhood blood lead concentrations with criminal arrests in early adulthood. *PLoS Medicine, 5*(5), e101. doi:10.1371/journal.pmed.0050101.

Yousef, S., Adem, A., Zoubeidi, T., Kosanovic, M., Mabrouk, A. A., & Eapen, V. (2011). Attention deficit hyperactivity disorder and environmental toxic metal exposure in the United Arab Emirates. *Journal of Tropical Pediatrics, 57*(6), 457–460. doi:10.1093/tropej/fmq12.

Zhang, N., Baker, H. W., Tufts, M., Raymond, R. E., Salihu, H., & Elliott, M. R. (2013). Early childhood lead exposure and academic achievement: Evidence from Detroit public schools, 2008–2010. *American Journal of Public Health, 103*(3), e72–e77. doi:10.2105/AJPH.2012.301164.

Chapter 9
Academic and Psychosocial Impact of Air Pollution on Children

Natalie M. Johnson, Genny Carrillo, and Ranjana K. Mehta

Definitional Issues and Prevalence

There is mounting evidence of the impact of air pollution on childhood cognitive development. Exposure to outdoor and indoor air pollution is well recognized for causing adverse effects on the cardiopulmonary system. Specifically, early life exposures have been correlated with the etiology and exacerbation of childhood asthma. Air pollution has not yet been broadly accepted for its effects on the developing brain; however, biological plausibility evidenced through experimental models in conjunction with accumulating epidemiological studies support the overwhelming negative consequences of air pollution on neurodevelopment.

Air pollution is largely composed of aerosols and particles produced from combustion processes, i.e., vehicle emissions, burning of wood, coal, oil, and

N.M. Johnson, Ph.D. (✉)
Department of Environmental and Occupational Health, School of Public Health, Texas A&M Health Science Center, College Station, TX, USA

Faculty Member of the Texas A&M Interdisciplinary Faculty of Toxicology, College Station, TX, USA
e-mail: natalie.johnson@tamhsc.edu

G. Carrillo, M.D., Sc.D., M.P.H., M.S.P.H.
Department of Environmental and Occupational Health, School of Public Health, Texas A&M Health Science Center, College Station, TX, USA
e-mail: gcarrillo@tamhsc.edu

R.K. Mehta, Ph.D., M.S.
Department of Environmental and Occupational Health, School of Public Health, Texas A&M Health Science Center, College Station, TX, USA

Faculty of the Texas A&M Institute for Neuroscience, College Station, TX, USA
e-mail: rmehta@tamu.edu

C. Riccio, J. Sullivan (eds.), *Pediatric Neurotoxicology*, Specialty Topics in Pediatric Neuropsychology, DOI 10.1007/978-3-319-32358-9_9

other fossil fuels, and manufacturing processes. Millions of children live in areas where urban smog, very small particles, and toxic pollutants pose serious health concerns. In the USA, the Clean Air Act of 1970 required the Environmental Protection Agency (EPA) to set National Ambient Air Quality Standards for pollutants considered harmful to public health and the environment (EPA, 2011). Air quality standards are set for six common air pollutants. These air pollutants (also known as "criteria pollutants") are found in urban and non-urban settings and can be impacted by geography, season, and weather conditions. They include particulate matter, ground-level ozone, carbon monoxide, sulfur oxides, nitrogen oxides, and lead.

Particulate matter (PM) is believed to play a primary role in the systemic health effects caused by air pollution. PM is classified according to it aerodynamic diameter. Respirable particles less than 2.5 μm, known as fine particulate matter or $PM_{2.5}$, can penetrate deep into the lungs (Pope & Dockery, 2006). The chemical composition of these particles varies based on source and secondary atmospheric reactions. Metals and polycyclic aromatic hydrocarbons (PAHs), a large class of fused aromatic rings, are found adsorbed to these small particles. Many individual PAHs, commonly present in complex mixtures, are mutagenic and carcinogenic to humans (Kim, Jahan, Kabir, & Brown, 2013). Metals and hydrocarbons are also present in the nanoparticle size range. Ultrafine particulate, particles less than 100 nm, are of increasing concern due to the ability of these nano-sized particles to travel far into respiratory structures, as well as translocate to the brain (Nemmar et al., 2001).

In animal exposure models, ultrafine particles have been detected in the olfactory bulb, the cerebrum and cerebellum, demonstrating translocation across the blood–brain barrier (Donaldson et al., 2005; Elder et al., 2006). In addition, chronic inflammation in the respiratory tract, leading to systemic inflammation may provide the basis for structural and functional changes in the brain. Indeed, intranasal instillation of ultrafine black carbon in mice led to changes in brain cytokine and chemokine expression, altering normal immune processes (Tin-Tin-Win-Shwe et al., 2006). Calderón-Garcidueñas and colleagues (2008) have characterized clinical findings in children highly exposed to air pollution in the Mexico City metropolitan area, revealing ultrafine particle deposition, an altered immune response, disruption of the blood–brain barrier, and accumulation of amyloid beta-42 and alpha-synuclein, markers of neurodegeneration. Overall, their recent studies highlighting that children highly exposed to particle air pollution display significant neuroinflammation/degeneration, provides evidence for the biological basis of adverse effects of air pollution on the developing brain (Calderón-Garcidueñas, Cross, et al. 2013; Calderón-Garcidueñas, Franco-Lira, et al. 2013; Calderón-Garcidueñas, Solt, et al. 2008; Calderon-Garciduenas & Torres-Jardon, 2012). The increasing evidence of the effects on functional outcomes, i.e., impact on intellectual and academic functioning, neuropsychological functioning, emotional and behavioral outcomes, and other important sensory processes, described in detail below, indicate the growing need for awareness about the lasting effects of air pollution on the developing brain.

Impact on Neurodevelopment

Intellectual Functioning

An array of studies has shown children exposed prenatally to air pollution have lower IQ scores and perform worse on cognitive functioning tests. Perera et al. (2006) first reported high prenatal exposure to PAHs, assessed by personal air monitoring in the third trimester, was associated with a lower mental development index in African-American and Dominican children 3 years of age residing in New York City. Researchers adjusted for multiple confounders, including prenatal exposure to environmental tobacco smoke, the organophosphate insecticide chlorpyrifos, lead, and sociodemographic factors. No impairment was found at younger ages (1 or 2 years). Furthermore, prenatal PAH exposure was not associated with behavioral problems or adverse psychomotor development. In this same cohort, intellectual functioning was assessed in 249 children at 5 years of age using the Wechsler Preschool and Primary Scale of Intelligence-Revised (Perera et al., 2009). Children in the highest exposure group had significantly lower full-scale and verbal IQ scores, 4.31 and 4.67 points lower, respectively, compared to children in the lower exposure group. Research in additional cohorts has confirmed and extended these findings.

In Chongqing, a major city in Southwest China, PAH-DNA adduct levels measured in umbilical cord blood as a biomarker of prenatal PAH exposure were significantly lower in a 2005 prospective cohort compared to an identically recruited 2002 cohort following the closure of a coal-fired power plant in 2004 (Perera et al., 2008). Increased adduct levels in newborns enrolled in 2002 were associated with decreased developmental quotients in motor, adaptive, language, and social areas, as measured by the Gesell Developmental Schedules at 2 years of age (Tang et al., 2008). Again, potential confounders were accounted for, including blood lead level, environmental tobacco smoke and other sociodemographic factors. These associations were not observed in the 2005 cohort, indicating reducing prenatal PAH exposure may positively impact childhood neurodevelopment. In additional work published by this research group, prenatal PAH exposure, as measured by personal air monitoring, was associated with a reduction in childhood intelligence at 5 years of age in over 200 children in Krakow, Poland (Edwards et al., 2010). This diminution in nonverbal reasoning scores was estimated to be equivalent to an average decrease of 3.8 IQ points, confirming previous findings from the New York City cohort.

Other types of exposure assessment, amenable to large-scale epidemiological studies, have also provided evidence of cognitive impairment following early-life exposure to air pollution. Suglia, Gryparis, Wright, Schwartz, and Wright (2008) demonstrated black carbon levels, estimated using validated spatiotemporal land-use regression models, were positively associated with decreased cognitive function in a cohort of over 200 children approximately 9 years old living in Boston. In a birth cohort of similar size in Southern Spain, a negative effect on cognitive scores, albeit not significant, was found in children exposed to higher levels of nitrogen dioxide (NO_2), a marker of traffic-related air pollution (Freire et al., 2010).

In one of the largest studies to date, Guxens et al. recruited 2644 pregnant women from four Spanish regions in their first trimester and estimated average outdoor air pollution levels throughout pregnancy based on maternal address and data collected form ambient air monitors measuring NO_2 and benzene (Guxens et al., 2012). Results from 1889 children included in the analysis showed NO_2 and benzene exposure was inversely associated with mental development at an average of 14 months of age (range 11–23 months) after adjusting for potential confounders. Importantly, these associations were stronger in children whose mothers reported lower fruit and vegetable intake throughout pregnancy, born to mothers with lower maternal vitamin D levels, and in infants that were not breast-fed. These data offer important insight into modulating factors that may affect the impact of air pollution on childhood neurodevelopment. A recent study conducted in a prospective birth cohort of 520 mother-infant pairs in South Korea demonstrated maternal exposure to coarse particulate matter, PM_{10}, was associated with reduced mental and psychomotor development at 2 years of age (Kim et al., 2014). Maternal NO_2 exposure was associated with psychomotor development deficiencies but not cognitive function. While limitations have been addressed, overall, data from these diverse populations, which have utilized biomarker measurement and regression models to define exposure and employed a variety of cognitive tests, support the common conclusion that prenatal exposure to air pollutants adversely affects children's mental development.

Academic Functioning

A plethora of studies have shown children attending schools nearby major roadways are exposed to traffic-related air pollutants (Appatova, Ryan, LeMasters, & Grinshpun, 2008; Diapouli, Chaloulakou, & Spyrellis, 2007; Guo et al., 2010; Janssen, van Vliet, Aarts, Harssema, & Brunekreef, 2001; Van Roosbroeck et al., 2007). Ecological studies have established a link between air pollution levels at school locations and measures of academic performance. Pastor, Sadd, and Morello-Frosch (2004) previously reported a diminished academic performance index score for schools in the Los Angeles Unified School District was associated with ambient air toxics data in areas with higher respiratory hazards. The authors called attention to the disproportionate environmental health risks on low-income and minority children. While it is well established that sociodemographic factors affect school performance, results were striking after controlling for multiple variables, including parent education level, teacher quality, and so on. In another study conducted in 3880 Chilean schools, researchers found higher annual coarse particulate matter (PM_{10}) and ozone (O_3) levels were associated with reduced standardized test scores (Miller & Vela, 2013). Using the same unit of school standardized test scores, Mohai, Kweon, Lee, and Ard (2011) demonstrated schools located in highly polluted areas in Michigan had a higher proportion of students fail to meet state standards. In addition, the schools in areas with poorer air quality had the lowest attendance rates, which indicates poorer health, and may modulate performance. Other studies have clearly shown the effect of air pollution on school absenteeism (Currie, Hanushek, Kahn, Neidell, & Rivkin, 2009; Gilliland et al., 2001). Hence, the impact of air pollution on academic performance may be related to both the increase in respiratory illness-related absenteeism in addition to the direct effect on cognitive functioning.

Neuropsychological Functioning

The relationship between air pollution exposure and neuropsychological functioning in children has been investigated in numerous populations using a variety of neurobehavioral testing mechanisms. Wang, Zhang, Zeng, Zeng, and She (2009) conducted a cross-sectional study using manual and computer-assisted test batteries in second and third grade children from two different schools in Quanzhou, China. Concentrations of traffic-related air pollutants, NO_2 and PM_{10}, were monitored on two consecutive days. Results showed children attending school in the more polluted area performed worse on all tests and significantly worse on the following, visual simple reaction time, continuous performance, digit symbol, pursuit aiming, and sign register. Findings were significant after controlling for potential confounders; however, the authors warned design limitations required additional studies. Freire et al. (2010) also used NO_2 concentrations to study the neurotoxic effects of traffic-related air pollution on children's motor and cognitive abilities in a Spanish cohort of 4 year olds followed over 1 year. Based on the McCarthy Scales of Children's Abilities (MSCA), children exposed to NO_2 levels >24.75 $\mu g/m^3$ showed a decrease in general cognitive and quantitative scores, working memory and gross motor areas by 4.19, 6.71, 7.37, and 8.61 points, respectively. While only gross motor function deficits were statistically significant, the general negative effects even at this lower level of exposure signified an association between air pollution and adverse developmental effects. In a Dutch study of 553 children ages 9–11, researchers explored the dual effect of transportation noise and air pollution on motor and cognitive functioning. NO_2 exposure (based on school location) was independently associated with memory span length. Combined air pollution and noise exposure at school significantly affected reaction time. Interestingly, no effects were significant based on estimated home exposures.

Some of the strongest functional and mechanistic data has come from work by Calderón-Garcidueñas and colleagues. Healthy children residing in the polluted urban environment of Mexico City showed significant decreases in fluid and crystalized cognition tasks compared to children from a less polluted area (Calderón-Garcidueñas, Mora-Tiscareño, et al., 2008). A majority of Mexico City children exhibited structural brain changes evidenced by hypertensive MRI lesions in the prefrontal cortex. Similarly, healthy dogs in Mexico City showed frontal lesions in addition to neuroinflammation and deposited ultrafine particles in the brain. In further work, Calderón-Garcidueñas et al. (2011) demonstrated 20 children living in Mexico City had reduced cognitive abilities based on the Wechsler Intelligence Scale for Children Revised (WISC-R) digit span and vocabulary subtests versus matched controls. Children living in the urban area exhibited variation in white matter hyperintensities (ten children with and ten without); however, both groups performed poorly on cognitive test indicating this may be only part of the underlying pathology. Researchers determined that the complex modulation of pro-inflammatory and neuroprotective cytokines and chemokines overall influence the structural and volumetric responses associated with cognitive deficiencies due to air pollution exposure (Calderón-Garcidueñas et al., 2012).

Emotional and Behavioral Function

Studies have shown that psychological and toxic effects of air pollution can lead to psychiatric symptoms, such as anxiety, changes in mood and in behavior. Increased levels of some air pollutants are accompanied by an increase in psychiatric admissions and emergency visits for suicide attempts and, in some studies, by changes in behavior and a reduction in psychological well-being (Szyszkowicz, Willey, Grafstein, Rowe, & Colman, 2010). Specifically in children, recent studies have focused on the association between early life exposure to air pollution and the development of autism spectrum disorders (ASD) (Becerra, Wilhelm, Olsen, Cockburn, & Ritz, 2012; Larsson, Weiss, Janson, Sundell, & Bornehag, 2009; Roberts et al., 2013; Volk et al., 2014; Volk, Hertz-Picciotto, Delwiche, Lurmann, & McConnell, 2011; Volk, Lurmann, Penfold, Hertz-Picciotto, & McConnell, 2013; Windham, Zhang, Gunier, Croen, & Grether, 2006). ASD is defined as a group of developmental disabilities that can cause *significant social, communication and behavioral challenges* (Centers for Disease Control and Prevention (CDC), 2015b). A variety of factors, including genetic and environmental, contribute to the prevalence of ASD (Herbert, 2010). In initial work, Windham and colleagues suggested a potential association between hazardous air pollutant concentrations, including metals and possibly solvents in ambient air. Larsson et al. (2009) reported associations between indoor environmental factors, namely PVC flooring, which may generate airborne phthalates, and ASD diagnosis in a large Swedish cohort. Additionally, airway symptoms of wheezing and asthma diagnosis were associated with ASD at 5 years of age. Research from the Childhood Autism Risks from Genetics and the Environment (CHARGE) study in Southern California revealed autism was significantly associated with maternal residential proximity to a freeway during the third trimester (Volk et al., 2011).

Additional research from this group showed exposure during the prenatal period and first year of life to traffic-related pollutants, $PM_{2.5}$, PM_{10}, and NO_2, was associated with autism (Volk et al., 2013). Furthermore, having a functional promoter variant in the MET receptor tyrosine kinase gene interacted with air pollution exposure to increase the risk of ASD (Volk et al., 2014) exemplifying the complexity of genetic and environmental interactions involved in ASD. In another study carried out in California, Becerra et al. (2012) established a relationship between traffic-related air pollution exposure during pregnancy and ASD diagnosis using values from ambient air monitors for $PM_{2.5}$ and O_3 in combination with land use regression models. Roberts et al. (2013) also provided complimentary findings in a large cohort of Children of Nurses Study II participants indicating that perinatal exposure to diesel, lead, manganese, and cadmium, modeled from US EPA levels of hazardous air pollutants, was associated with ASD. Overall, this accumulating evidence suggests exposure to air pollution early in life may contribute to the etiology of ASD.

In addition, numerous studies have evaluated the link between exposure to air pollution and childhood attention deficit hyperactive disorder (ADHD). ADHD is one of the most *common neurodevelopmental disorders in children characterized by inattention, compulsive behaviors, and/or hyperactivity* (Centers for Disease Control and Prevention (CDC), 2015a). Siddique, Banerjee, Ray, & Lahiri, 2011 conducted a cross-sectional study in 996 middle school- and high school-aged children living in Delhi; another of 850 age- and sex-matched children were recruited from rural areas in northern India. ADHD was significantly more common in children living in the urban environment (11.0 %) versus rural (2.7 %). After adjusting for potential confounders, ambient PM_{10} levels were strongly correlated with ADHD. In the USA, children followed from birth as part of the Cincinnati Childhood Allergy and Air Pollution Study highly exposed to elemental carbon (a marker of traffic-related air pollution) were more likely to display ADHD-related symptoms at 7 years of age (Newman et al., 2013).

Traffic-related black carbon exposure has also been linked to decreased attention measures in 7–14 year olds from a Boston-based birth cohort (Chiu et al., 2013). Recent findings from Perera et al. (2014) illustrated prenatal exposure to air pollution, measured by levels of PAH-DNA adducts in maternal blood in a prospective birth cohort in New York City, was significantly associated with ADHD behavior problems in children at 9 years of age. Anxiety/depression were significantly correlated with ADHD behavior problems. These findings provide further confirmation of their previous results showing PAH-DNA adducts in maternal or umbilical cord blood coupled with personal air measurements of PAH exposure was positively associated with symptoms of anxiety/depression and attention problems at ages 6–7 (Perera et al., 2012).

Another area of similar research has linked ADHD symptoms with exposure to indoor air pollution from gas appliances. Morales et al. (2009) found indoor NO_2 concentrations during the early postnatal period (3 months) were associated with attention-hyperactivity behaviors and decreased cognitive function at age 4 years. The effect was strongest in children with genetic polymorphisms in the glutathione-S-transferase P1 gene (GSTP1), which codes for the protective enzyme expressed in the brain. These results were confirmed in additional birth cohorts in Spain where gas cooking was related to adverse mental development in children 11–22 months of age (Vrijheid et al., 2012). Because children with ADHD are at higher risk for substance abuse and mood disorders (Lee, Humphreys, Flory, Liu, & Glass, 2011; Shaw et al., 2012), the impact of air pollution exposure may be far reaching.

Impact on Other Areas of Functioning

Other important areas of functioning, such as hearing, balance, and smell, can be affected by air pollution exposure. Calderón-Garcidueñas et al. (2011b) measured brainstem auditory evoked potentials (BAEPs) and inflammatory markers in peripheral blood in children exposed to the highly polluted Mexico City urban air. They also determined brainstem neuropathology in nine children who had died by accidental death. Compared to controls, exposed children exhibited significant delays in central conduction time of brainstem neural transmission, signifying risk for auditory and vestibular disorders. In addition, exposed children showed evidence of systemic inflammation consistent with their previous findings (Calderón-Garcidueñas et al., 2007, 2009). The authors proposed that the abnormalities observed in auditory brainstem nuclei in highly exposed children, in particular, significantly smaller and rounder medial superior olive (MSO) neuronal cell bodies, may explain auditory dysfunction since the MSO plays a role in localization of sound sources, encoding temporal features of sound and encoding of speech. This same research group conducted another study in teens and young adults residing in Mexico City and a control population to assess the effect of air pollution on olfactory function (Calderón-Garcidueñas et al., 2010). The exposed group had significantly lower scores on the University of Pennsylvania Smell Identification Test, and olfaction deficits were observed in 35.5 % of Mexico City participants. These deficits were associated with olfactory bulb inflammation. Additionally, ultrafine particles were found deposited in olfactory bulb endothelial cytoplasm and basement membranes.

Overall, findings from these studies conducted in Mexico City have revealed the impact of air pollution on diverse neuronal functions and provided evidence of neuroinflammation and neurodegeneration. In fact, many of the observed cellular and molecular changes are reflected in the progression of neurodegenerative diseases like Alzheimer's Disease and Parkinson's Disease. Therefore, damage to the central nervous system by air pollution may directly impact functional outcomes in children and young adults as well as effect neurocognitive and neuropsychological functioning later in life.

Prognosis and Moderating Factors

Overall, the majority of studies have taken moderating factors such as gender, socioeconomic status, and occasionally nutritive status and genetics, into account. Other potential contributing factors like transportation noise and second-hand smoke exposures have also been addressed in many of the studies described. Since brain development hinges on a wide array of stimuli, the inclusion of possible confounders is absolutely critical for presenting a coherent argument for the independent effects of air pollution. However, an important environmental justice issue arises from these studies since it is often the most underserved communities, low-income and racial or ethnic minorities, which bear the disproportionate burden of high air pollution exposures (Mohai, Pellow, & Roberts, 2009). In a recent review, Calderón-Garcidueñas et al. (2014) recommended the identification of children at high risk for cognitive deficits should be prioritized in populations exposed to significant concentrations of air pollutants. Overall, this strategy could lead to better prognosis and hopefully prevention of adverse cognitive effects. Suggested approaches to identify early risk include more robust exposure assessment methods, e.g., land use regression modeling at schools and residences, speciation of particulate matter, for instance metal content, and improved cognitive screening for exposed children, including structural information that may be gleaned from BAEPs, MRI, fMRi, and so on. Our group also supports this strategy in addition to preventive strategies, including policy changes, educational intervention strategies, and early prevention during conception and throughout the prenatal and early postnatal period.

Considerations for Prevention and Intervention

Considerations for prevention and interventions may focus on decreasing air pollution exposure and increasing protection of vulnerable populations. In regards to decreasing exposure, data on the risk assessment at various exposure levels with neurotoxic effects as the endpoint remain to be determined. Notably, no current air quality standards address allowable levels of ultrafine particulate matter in ambient air. While standards are in place for PM_{10} and $PM_{2.5}$ particulate matter in many countries, the ultrafine nanoscale particles may ultimately play a predominant role in the neuroinflammatory/neurodegradative processes which underlie the adverse cognitive effects. Another major consideration for reducing exposure is awareness of school location to stationary sources of air pollution and proximity to major roadways (Amato et al., 2014; Amram, Abernethy, Brauer, Davies, & Allen, 2011). Numerous studies have shown that distance to major roadways is an important determinant of indoor air quality in schools and children's exposure. Currently in the USA, no regulations are set for existing or planned school locations in relation to major roadways or stationary sources of air pollution. This is also the case for early childcare centers, where infants and toddlers spend a majority of their day while their parents work. The ability to reduce exposure at the individual level may represent a viable option, in particular for populations that lack control of pollution sources in their communities. Previous research has shown increasing awareness through health education at the individual/family level by their health provider can help reduce respiratory health risks associated with outdoor air pollution.

Families and school officials should be advised how to monitor outdoor air quality, both ground level ozone and particulate matter advisories, as a way to know when to adjust children's outdoor activities, such as playing inside on air quality alert days (Suwanwaiphatthana, Ruangdej, & Turner-Henson, 2010). Air quality is reported by levels of health concern represented by a color scale indicative of air quality conditions as follows: *good* as green (no concerns for human health), *moderate* as yellow, *unhealthy for sensitive groups* (children, individuals with chronic respiratory conditions, older adults) as orange, *unhealthy* as red, *very unhealthy* as purple, and *hazardous* (for the entire population) as maroon. Another element crucial for effective air pollution prevention and intervention is the important role of diversity of cultures. The lack of understanding from the part of the health provider about the patient's culture can contribute to health disparities. Empowering families living in low income neighborhoods' with innovative ways to improve their own household conditions is imperative so that they may see the value of these changes in their children's health (Kueny, Berg, Chowdhury, & Anderson, 2011). Furthermore, relatively easy interventions, such as using extractor fans when cooking and employing the recirculation vent when driving, should be tested for efficacy and incorporated into educational materials.

Additionally, there are a variety of strategies to increase the protection of vulnerable subgroups, which include as mentioned before low-income minority or ethnic groups disproportionately exposed, and the biologically susceptible fetus and developing child, as well as children with asthma and other chronic health conditions. As supported by Calderón-Garcidueñas et al. (2014), neuropsychological and psychoeducational testing of children is a logical place to begin identifying those at highest risk. In addition, a diet rich in antioxidants may paly a role in protection since many studies propose inflammation is the underlying basis of neuropathology (Romieu, Castro-Giner, Kunzli, & Sunyer, 2008). In an experimental model of mice exposed to polluted urban air, Villarreal-Calderon et al. (2010) demonstrated intake of dark chocolate, which is rich in polyphenol antioxidants, protected against chronic inflammation in the dorsal vagal complex. Guxens et al. (2012) showed the neurocognitive effects of traffic-related air pollution were stronger in children whose mothers reported lower fruit and vegetable intake throughout pregnancy, had lower vitamin D levels, and were not breast-fed. Likewise, Jedrychowski et al. (2010) reported a greater reduction of birth weight among newborns exposed to particulate air pollution in mothers who reported low fish intake during pregnancy. In a follow-up study, researchers showed a reduction of the respiratory effects in the first 2 years of life in infants whose mothers consumed more fish in pregnancy Jedrychowski et al. (2008). Of course, the complexity of other potential exposures from fish (i.e., methyl mercury and PCBs) should be weighed.

Conclusion

In conclusion, the major objectives within this chapter illustrate the impact of air pollution on neurodevelopment. Accumulating evidence demonstrates a significant negative effect on a variety of cognitive and functional abilities in children. This may result in deficiencies in academic performance, emotional and behavioral changes, and in general may lead to deleterious societal outcomes. While it is required to call for additional research in larger populations to confirm recent studies, the existing data are quite compelling. As public health professionals, we must ask ourselves what can be done to spur change to reduce air pollution, protect vulnerable subgroups like children, and prevent these deleterious effects on the brain of future generations.

References

Amato, F., Rivas, I., Viana, M., Moreno, T., Bouso, L., Reche, C., … Querol, X. (2014). Sources of indoor and outdoor PM2. 5 concentrations in primary schools. *Science of the Total Environment, 490*, 757–765.

Amram, O., Abernethy, R., Brauer, M., Davies, H., & Allen, R. W. (2011). Proximity of public elementary schools to major roads in Canadian urban areas. *International Journal of Health Geographics, 10*(68), 1–11.

Appatova, A. S., Ryan, P. H., LeMasters, G. K., & Grinshpun, S. A. (2008). Proximal exposure of public schools and students to major roadways: a nationwide US survey. *Journal of Environmental Planning and Management, 51*(5), 631–646.

Becerra, T. A., Wilhelm, M., Olsen, J., Cockburn, M., & Ritz, B. (2012). Ambient air pollution and autism in Los Angeles County, California. *Environmental Health Perspectives, 121*(3), 380–386.

Calderón-Garcidueñas, L., Calderón-Garcidueñas, A., Torres-Jardón, R., Avila-Ramírez, J., Kulesza, R. J., & Angiulli, A. D. (2015). Air pollution and your brain: What do you need to know right now. *Primary Health Care Research & Development, 16*(4), 329–345.

Calderón-Garcidueñas, L., Cross, J. V., Franco-Lira, M., Aragón-Flores, M., Kavanaugh, M., Torres-Jardón, R., … Zhu, H. (2013). Brain immune interactions and air pollution: macrophage inhibitory factor (MIF), prion cellular protein (PrPC), Interleukin-6 (IL-6), interleukin 1 receptor antagonist (IL-1Ra), and interleukin-2 (IL-2) in cerebrospinal fluid and MIF in serum differentiate urban children exposed to severe vs. low air pollution. *Frontiers in Neuroscience, 7*(183). doi:10.3389/fnins.2013.00183

Calderón-Garcidueñas, L., Engle, R., Mora-Tiscareño, A., Styner, M., Gómez-Garza, G., Zhu, H., … Monroy-Acosta, M. E. (2011). Exposure to severe urban air pollution influences cognitive outcomes, brain volume and systemic inflammation in clinically healthy children. *Brain and Cognition, 77*(3), 345–355.

Calderón-Garcidueñas, L., Franco-Lira, M., Henríquez-Roldán, C., Osnaya, N., González-Maciel, A., Reynoso-Robles, R., … Keefe, S. (2010). Urban air pollution: influences on olfactory function and pathology in exposed children and young adults. *Experimental and Toxicologic Pathology, 62*(1), 91–102.

Calderón-Garcidueñas, L., Franco-Lira, M., Mora-Tiscareño, A., Medina-Cortina, H., Torres-Jardón, R., & Kavanaugh, M. (2013). Early Alzheimer's and Parkinson's disease pathology in urban children: Friend versus foe responses—It is time to face the evidence. *BioMed Research International, 2013*, 16. doi:10.1155/2013/161687.

Calderón-Garcidueñas, L., Franco-Lira, M., Torres-Jardón, R., Henriquez-Roldán, C., Barragán-Mejía, G., Valencia-Salazar, G., … Reed, W. (2007). Pediatric respiratory and systemic effects of chronic air pollution exposure: Nose, lung, heart, and brain pathology. *Toxicologic pathology, 35*(1), 154–162.

Calderón-Garcidueñas, L., Kavanaugh, M., Block, M., D'Angiulli, A., Delgado-Chávez, R., Torres-Jardón, R., … Villarreal-Calderon, R. (2012). Neuroinflammation, hyperphosphorylated tau, diffuse amyloid plaques, and down-regulation of the cellular prion protein in air pollution exposed children and young adults. *Journal of Alzheimer's Disease, 28*(1), 93–107.

Calderón-Garcidueñas, L., Macías-Parra, M., Hoffmann, H. J., Valencia-Salazar, G., Henríquez-Roldán, C., Osnaya, N., … Romero, L. (2009). Immunotoxicity and environment: Immunodysregulation and systemic inflammation in children. *Toxicologic Pathology, 37*(2), 161–169.

Calderón-Garcidueñas, L., Mora-Tiscareño, A., Ontiveros, E., Gómez-Garza, G., Barragán-Mejía, G., Broadway, J., … Maronpot, R. R. (2008). Air pollution, cognitive deficits and brain abnormalities: A pilot study with children and dogs. *Brain and Cognition, 68*(2), 117–127.

Calderón-Garcidueñas, L., Solt, A. C., Henríquez-Roldán, C., Torres-Jardón, R., Nuse, B., Herritt, L., … García, R. (2008). Long-term air pollution exposure is associated with neuroinflammation, an altered innate immune response, disruption of the blood-brain barrier, ultrafine particulate deposition, and accumulation of amyloid β-42 and α-synuclein in children and young adults. *Toxicologic Pathology, 36*(2), 289–310.

Calderon-Garciduenas, L., & Torres-Jardon, R. (2012). Air pollution, socioeconomic status, and children's cognition in megacities: The Mexico City scenario. *Frontiers in Psychology, 3*, 217. doi:10.3389/fpsyg.2012.00217.

Centers for Disease Control and Prevention (CDC). (2015a). Attention-deficit/hyperactivity disorder (ADHD). Retrieved February 20, 2015, from http://www.cdc.gov/ncbddd/adhd/index.html

Centers for Disease Control and Prevention (CDC). (2015b). Autism spectrum disorder (ASD). Retrieved February 20, 2015, from http://www.cdc.gov/ncbddd/autism/index.html

Chiu, Y.-H. M., Bellinger, D. C., Coull, B. A., Anderson, S., Barber, R., Wright, R. O., & Wright, R. J. (2013). Associations between traffic-related black carbon exposure and attention in a prospective birth cohort of urban children. *Environmental Health Perspectives, 121*(7), 859–864.

Currie, J., Hanushek, E. A., Kahn, E. M., Neidell, M., & Rivkin, S. G. (2009). Does pollution increase school absences? *The Review of Economics and Statistics, 91*(4), 682–694.

Diapouli, E., Chaloulakou, A., & Spyrellis, N. (2007). Levels of ultrafine particles in different microenvironments—Implications to children exposure. *Science of the Total Environment, 388*(1), 128–136.

Donaldson, K., Tran, L., Jimenez, L. A., Duffin, R., Newby, D. E., Mills, N., … Stone, V. (2005). Combustion-derived nanoparticles: A review of their toxicology following inhalation exposure. *Particle and Fibre Toxicology, 2*(1), 10. doi:0.1186/1743-8977-2-10

Edwards, S. C., Jedrychowski, W., Butscher, M., Camann, D., Kieltyka, A., Mroz, E., … Perera, F. (2010). Prenatal exposure to airborne polycyclic aromatic hydrocarbons and children's intelligence at 5 years of age in a prospective cohort study in Poland. *Environmental Health Perspectives, 118*(9), 1326–1331. doi:10.1289/ehp.0901070

Elder, A., Gelein, R., Silva, V., Feikert, T., Opanashuk, L., Carter, J., … Finkelstein, J. (2006). Translocation of inhaled ultrafine manganese oxide particles to the central nervous system. *Environmental Health Perspectives, 114*, 172–1178.

EPA, U. S. E. P. A. (2011, March 22). National ambient air quality standards. Retrieved September 21, 2011, from http://www.epa.gov/ttn/naaqs

Freire, C., Ramos, R., Puertas, R., Lopez-Espinosa, M. J., Julvez, J., Aguilera, I., … Olea, N. (2010). Association of traffic-related air pollution with cognitive development in children. *Journal of Epidemiology and Community Health, 64*(3), 223–228. doi:10.1136/jech.2008.084574.

Gilliland, F. D., Berhane, K., Rappaport, E. B., Thomas, D. C., Avol, E., Gauderman, W. J., … Islam, K. T. (2001). The effects of ambient air pollution on school absenteeism due to respiratory illnesses. *Epidemiology, 12*(1), 43–54.

Guo, H., Morawska, L., He, C., Zhang, Y. L., Ayoko, G., & Cao, M. (2010). Characterization of particle number concentrations and PM2. 5 in a school: influence of outdoor air pollution on indoor air. *Environmental Science and Pollution Research, 17*(6), 1268–1278.

Guxens, M., Aguilera, I., Ballester, F., Estarlich, M., Fernandez-Somoano, A., Lertxundi, A., … Project, I. (2012). Prenatal exposure to residential air pollution and infant mental development: modulation by antioxidants and detoxification factors. *Environmental Health Perspectives, 120*(1), 144–149. doi:10.1289/ehp.1103469

Herbert, M. R. (2010). Contributions of the environment and environmentally vulnerable physiology to autism spectrum disorders. *Current Opinion in Neurology, 23*(2), 103–110.

Janssen, N. A., van Vliet, P. H., Aarts, F., Harssema, H., & Brunekreef, B. (2001). Assessment of exposure to traffic related air pollution of children attending schools near motorways. *Atmospheric Environment, 35*(22), 3875–3884.

Jedrychowski, W., Flak, E., Mroz, E., Pac, A., Jacek, R., Sochacka-Tatara, E., … Perera, F. (2008). Modulating effects of maternal fish consumption on the occurrence of respiratory symptoms in early infancy attributed to prenatal exposure to fine particles. *Annals of Nutrition & Metabolism, 52*(1), 8–16.

Jedrychowski, W., Perera, F., Mrozek-Budzyn, D., Flak, E., Mroz, E., Sochacka-Tatara, E., … Spengler, J. D. (2010). Higher fish consumption in pregnancy may confer protection against the harmful effect of prenatal exposure to fine particulate matter. *Annals of Nutrition & Metabolism, 56*(2), 119.

Kim, K.-H., Jahan, S. A., Kabir, E., & Brown, R. J. (2013). A review of airborne polycyclic aromatic hydrocarbons (PAHs) and their human health effects. *Environment International, 60*, 71–80.

Kim, E., Park, H., Hong, Y.-C., Ha, M., Kim, Y., Kim, B.-N., … Ryu, J.-M. (2014). Prenatal exposure to PM 10 and NO 2 and children's neurodevelopment from birth to 24 months of age: Mothers and Children's Environmental Health (MOCEH) study. *Science of the Total Environment, 481*, 439–445.

Kueny, A., Berg, J., Chowdhury, Y., & Anderson, N. (2011). Poquito a poquito: How Latino families with children who have asthma make changes in their home. *Journal of Pediatric Health Care, 27*(1), e1–e11.

Larsson, M., Weiss, B., Janson, S., Sundell, J., & Bornehag, C.-G. (2009). Associations between indoor environmental factors and parental-reported autistic spectrum disorders in children 6–8 years of age. *Neurotoxicology, 30*(5), 822–831.

Lee, S. S., Humphreys, K. L., Flory, K., Liu, R., & Glass, K. (2011). Prospective association of childhood attention-deficit/hyperactivity disorder (ADHD) and substance use and abuse/dependence: A meta-analytic review. *Clinical Psychology Review, 31*(3), 328–341.

Miller S, Vela M (2013) The effects of air pollution on educational outcomes: Evidence from Chile *IDB Working Paper No. IDB-WP-468*. Washington, DC: Inter-American Development Bank, Research Department.

Mohai, P., Kweon, B. S., Lee, S., & Ard, K. (2011). Air pollution around schools is linked to poorer student health and academic performance. *Health Affairs (Project Hope), 30*(5), 852–862. doi:10.1377/hlthaff.2011.0077.

Mohai, P., Pellow, D., & Roberts, J. T. (2009). Environmental justice. *Annual Review of Environment and Resources, 34*, 405–430.

Morales, E., Julvez, J., Torrent, M., de Cid, R., Guxens, M., Bustamante, M., … Sunyer, J. (2009). Association of early-life exposure to household gas appliances and indoor nitrogen dioxide with cognition and attention behavior in preschoolers. *American Journal of Epidemiology, 169*(11), 1327–1336. doi:10.1093/aje/kwp067.

Nemmar, A., Vanbilloen, H., Hoylaerts, M., Hoet, P., Verbruggen, A., & Nemery, B. (2001). Passage of intratracheally instilled ultrafine particles from the lung into the systemic circulation in hamster. *American Journal of Respiratory and Critical Care Medicine, 164*(9), 1665–1668.

Newman, N. C., Ryan, P., LeMasters, G., Levin, L., Bernstein, D., Hershey, G. K., … Grinshpun, S. (2013). Traffic-related air pollution exposure in the first year of life and behavioral scores at 7 years of age. *Environmental Health Perspectives, 121*(6), 731–736.

Pastor, M., Sadd, J. L., & Morello-Frosch, R. (2004). Reading, writing, and toxics: children's health, academic performance, and environmental justice in Los Angeles. *Environment and Planning C, 22*(2), 271–290.

Perera, F. P., Chang, H.-w., Tang, D., Roen, E. L., Herbstman, J., Margolis, A., … Rauh, V. (2014). Early-life exposure to polycyclic aromatic hydrocarbons and ADHD behavior problems. *PLoS One, 9*(11). doi:10.1371/journal.pone.0111670.

Perera, F. P., Li, Z., Whyatt, R., Hoepner, L., Wang, S., Camann, D., & Rauh, V. (2009). Prenatal airborne polycyclic aromatic hydrocarbon exposure and child IQ at age 5 years. *Pediatrics, 124*(2), e195–e202. doi:10.1542/peds.2008-3506.

Perera, F. P., Li, T. Y., Zhou, Z. J., Yuan, T., Chen, Y. H., Qu, L., … Tang, D. (2008). Benefits of reducing prenatal exposure to coal-burning pollutants to children's neurodevelopment in China. *Environmental Health Perspectives, 116*(10), 1396–1400.

Perera, F. P., Rauh, V., Whyatt, R. M., Tsai, W.-Y., Tang, D., Diaz, D., … Camann, D. (2006). Effect of prenatal exposure to airborne polycyclic aromatic hydrocarbons on neurodevelopment in the first 3 years of life among inner-city children. *Environmental Health Perspectives, 114*, 1287–1292.

Perera, F. P., Tang, D., Wang, S., Vishnevetsky, J., Zhang, B., Diaz, D., … Rauh, V. (2012). Prenatal polycyclic aromatic hydrocarbon (PAH) exposure and child behavior at age 6–7 years. *Environmental Health Perspectives, 120*(6), 921–926.

Pope, C. A., & Dockery, D. W. (2006). Health effects of fine particulate air pollution: Lines that connect. *Journal of the Air & Waste Management Association, 56*(6), 709–742.

Roberts, A. L., Lyall, K., Hart, J. E., Laden, F., Just, A. C., Bobb, J. F., … Weisskopf, M. G. (2013). Perinatal air pollutant exposures and autism spectrum disorder in the children of Nurses' Health Study II participants. *Environmental Health Perspectives, 121*(8), 978–984.

Romieu, I., Castro-Giner, F., Kunzli, N., & Sunyer, J. (2008). Air pollution, oxidative stress and dietary supplementation: A review. *European Respiratory Journal, 31*(1), 179–197.

Shaw, M., Hodgkins, P., Caci, H., Young, S., Kahle, J., Woods, A. G., & Arnold, L. E. (2012). A systematic review and analysis of long-term outcomes in attention deficit hyperactivity disorder: Effects of treatment and non-treatment. *BMC Medicine, 10*, 99-7015-7010-7099. doi:10.1186/1741-7015-10-99.

Siddique, S., Banerjee, M., Ray, M. R., & Lahiri, T. (2011). Attention-deficit hyperactivity disorder in children chronically exposed to high level of vehicular pollution. *European Journal of Pediatrics, 170*(7), 923–929.

Suglia, S. F., Gryparis, A., Wright, R. O., Schwartz, J., & Wright, R. J. (2008). Association of black carbon with cognition among children in a prospective birth cohort study. *American Journal of Epidemiology, 167*(3), 280–286. doi:10.1093/aje/kwm308.

Suwanwaiphatthana, W., Ruangdej, K., & Turner-Henson, A. (2010). Outdoor air pollution and children's health. *Pediatric Nursing, 36*(1), 25–32.

Szyszkowicz, M., Willey, J. B., Grafstein, E., Rowe, B. H., & Colman, I. (2010). Air pollution and emergency department visits for suicide attempts in Vancouver, Canada. *Environmental Health Insights, 4*, 79–86. doi:10.4137/EHI.S5662.

Tang, D., Li, T. Y., Liu, J. J., Zhou, Z. J., Yuan, T., & Chen, Y. H. (2008). Effects of prenatal exposure to coal-burning pollutants on children's development in China. *Environmental Health Perspectives, 116*(5), 674–679.

Tin-Tin-Win-Shwe, Yamamoto, S., Ahmed, S., Kakeyama, M., Kobayashi, T., & Fujimaki, H. (2006). Brain cytokine and chemokine mRNA expression in mice induced by intranasal instillation with ultrafine carbon black. *Toxicology Letters, 163*(2), 153–160.

Van Roosbroeck, S., Jacobs, J., Janssen, N. A., Oldenwening, M., Hoek, G., & Brunekreef, B. (2007). Long-term personal exposure to PM 2.5, soot and NOx in children attending schools located near busy roads, a validation study. *Atmospheric Environment, 41*(16), 3381–3394.

Villarreal-Calderon, R., Torres-Jardon, R., Palacios-Moreno, J., Osnaya, N., Perez-Guille, B., Maronpot, R. R., … Calderon-Garciduenas, L. (2010). Urban air pollution targets the dorsal vagal complex and dark chocolate offers neuroprotection. *International Journal of Toxicology, 29*(6), 604–615.

Volk, H. E., Hertz-Picciotto, I., Delwiche, L., Lurmann, F., & McConnell, R. (2011). Residential proximity to freeways and autism in the CHARGE study. *Environmental Health Perspectives, 119*(6), 873–877.

Volk, H. E., Kerin, T., Lurmann, F., Hertz-Picciotto, I., McConnell, R., & Campbell, D. B. (2014). Autism spectrum disorder: Interaction of air pollution with the MET receptor tyrosine kinase gene. *Epidemiology (Cambridge, MA), 25*(1), 44–47.

Volk, H. E., Lurmann, F., Penfold, B., Hertz-Picciotto, I., & McConnell, R. (2013). Traffic-related air pollution, particulate matter, and autism. *JAMA Psychiatry, 70*(1), 71–77.

Vrijheid, M., Martinez, D., Aguilera, I., Bustamante, M., Ballester, F., Estarlich, M., … Project, I. (2012). Indoor air pollution from gas cooking and infant neurodevelopment. *Epidemiology (Cambridge, MA), 23*(1), 23–32. doi:10.1097/EDE.0b013e31823a4023.

Wang, S., Zhang, J., Zeng, X., Zeng, Y., & She, W. (2009). Association of traffic-related air pollution with children's neurobehavioral functions in Quanzhou, China. *Environmental Health Perspectives, 117*, 1612–1618.

Windham, G. C., Zhang, L., Gunier, R., Croen, L. A., & Grether, J. K. (2006). Autism spectrum disorders in relation to distribution of hazardous air pollutants in the San Francisco Bay area. *Environmental Health Perspectives, 114*, 1438–1444.

Chapter 10
Conclusion: Common Themes and Directions for Future Research

Jeremy R. Sullivan and Cynthia A. Riccio

Common Themes

Across the research on mechanisms of impact and effects of neurotoxins, there is a consistent pattern of heterogeneity of effects for children exposed. For some toxins with in utero effects, including many medications prescribed to address maternal health (Chaps. 5 and 6), there is minimal research of sufficient methodological rigor to allow for firm conclusions to be drawn. This limited research is also the case for in utero effects of opiate and marijuana use, especially with regard to specific academic outcomes among children exposed (Chap. 4). This is contrasted by the relative wealth of information available on FASD (Chap. 2) as well as research related to stimulants (particularly nicotine and cocaine; Chap. 3). Despite considerations for smog and pollution (Chap. 9), pesticides (Chap. 7), and lead exposure (Chap. 8), it is difficult to describe trends and patterns in the literature regarding neurodevelopmental effects due to inconsistent results across studies.

J.R. Sullivan, Ph.D. (✉)
Department of Educational Psychology, University of Texas at San Antonio, 501 W. Cesar E. Chavez Blvd., San Antonio, TX 78207, USA
e-mail: jeremy.sullivan@utsa.edu

C.A. Riccio, Ph.D.
Department of Educational Psychology and Institute of Neuroscience, Texas A&M University, 4225 TAMU, College Station, TX 77843-4225, USA
e-mail: criccio@tamu.edu

C. Riccio, J. Sullivan (eds.), *Pediatric Neurotoxicology*, Specialty Topics in Pediatric Neuropsychology, DOI 10.1007/978-3-319-32358-9_10

Moderating Factors

The inconsistency in research findings may be due to differences in specific substances, but also suggests the need to identify potential moderating factors that may help predict outcomes among individual children. These factors include timing of exposure and extent of exposure. For example, Loring et al. (Chap. 5) noted that exposure to valproate in the first trimester of pregnancy is associated with anatomical abnormalities, while exposure during the third trimester is associated with functional/behavioral deficits. Similar timing and extent of exposure effects have been demonstrated for alcohol and resulting severity of FASD (see Chap. 2), as well as lead (see Chap. 8) and air quality/pollution (see Chap. 9). With maternal use of recreational substances, the potential for exposure to multiple toxins at similar points in time adds yet an additional confound (see Chap. 4).

Additional risk and protective factors identified in the previous chapters are more systemic to the individual rather than the toxin. Genetic variations and differences in genetic vulnerability/predisposition may contribute to differences in manifestation. For example, the risk of a child developing FASD is influenced by the mother's ability to metabolize alcohol, which is genetically determined (Jones, 2011). As another example, effects of prenatal SSRI exposure on child behavior and mood may be influenced by genetic differences in a serotonin transporter gene (serotonin transporter promoter SLC6A4 genotype) within the exposed child (Oberlander et al., 2010; Chap. 6).

Socioeconomic status (SES) and resulting access (or lack of access) to resources and social supports, as well as exposure to (or lack thereof) an enriched environment also may impact outcome. For children with delayed or atypical developmental trajectories, early identification and early intervention efforts have been found to be critical. For example, among children with FASD, early identification is associated with significantly lower risk for adverse life experiences such as legal issues and substance abuse (Chap. 2). Further, early identification is necessary to prevent ongoing exposure to environmental neurotoxins (e.g., lead, pesticides, pollutants). As the child ages, parental involvement, parental psychopathology, parental substance use, maternal self-esteem, general nutrition, parent stress, and child abuse and neglect also can moderate outcome (Chaps. 2–4, and 8). Taken together, these moderating factors may explain the wide degree of variability in neuropsychological functioning among children who have been exposed to these toxins, such as the finding that effects on cognitive functioning may be long-lasting for some children, while others may "catch up" over time. Although it is difficult to account for all of these possible moderating factors when conducting a neuropsychological or psychoeducational evaluation or gathering developmental history information, this information will be important as part of the diagnostic process and for drawing inferences with regard to potential later difficulties.

Diagnostic Considerations

While there is variation in presentation, research suggests that neurotoxin exposure often results in referral for evaluation, often due to developmental delays or behavioral or academic concerns. Comprehensive assessment is necessary to identify individual strengths and weaknesses, and services must be individualized based on that profile of strengths and weaknesses. Knowing that a child has been exposed to a given toxin or toxins, and those functional systems likely affected, can help with tailoring the assessment and intervention to ensure that these areas are considered. For example, children with FASD, children who have a history of prenatal exposure to AEDs or stimulants such as nicotine or cocaine, and children with postnatal exposure to pesticides or lead often exhibit deficits in executive function. It would be important then for executive function to be assessed for children with those histories and monitored over time as classroom demands require more executive function skills. Conversely, children with learning disabilities, intellectual disabilities, and behavior disorders are at increased risk of abuse and neglect by parents (Sullivan & Knutson, 2000) in addition to bullying from peers (Blake, Lund, Zhou, Kwok, & Benz, 2012), so service providers should monitor closely for signs of maltreatment and bully victimization.

As indicated across chapters, neurotoxin exposure often results in deficits and possible diagnosis. For example, FASD and in utero exposure to stimulants are associated with high rates of externalizing issues such as attention-deficit/hyperactivity disorder (ADHD), oppositional defiant disorder (ODD), and conduct disorder (CD), which are often the reason for initial seeking of services (see Chaps. 2 and 3). In addition to deficits in intellectual functioning, FASD is associated with deficits in psychosocial functioning, motor skills, balance, language, executive function, vision, hearing, academic performance in math and reading, and internalizing issues such as depression, self-harm, and suicide. Valproate exposure is associated with lower cognitive ability and possible intellectual disability, as well as deficits in verbal skills, adaptive behaviors, social skills, memory, executive function, and increased risks of ADHD and ASD have been reported in the literature (see Chap. 5). Children exposed to cocaine in utero are more likely than their non-exposed peers to receive special education services and are at higher risk for problems with aggression, substance use, and language development (Chap. 3).

Similarly, recent studies suggest some of the neuropsychological domains impacted by pesticide exposure include motor skills, memory, and executive function (Chap. 7). Exposure to air pollution has been associated with deficits across a range of neuropsychological constructs and emotional/psychiatric symptoms, including overall intellectual functioning, motor skills, language, adaptive behavior, social functioning, and sensory abilities such as hearing and smell. There may be an association between early exposure to pollutants and symptoms of ADHD and ASD, and attending schools located in areas with high levels of air pollution has been associated with lower academic performance (in addition to increased absenteeism), even after controlling for sociodemographic variables (Chap. 9). Villarreal and Castro (Chap. 8) reviewed the literature on lead exposure and performance on tests of intellectual functioning, academic achievement, and executive function. Lead exposure is related to externalizing behaviors with diagnoses of ADHD, ODD, and CD common, all of which are related to problems with behavioral and emotional regulation. Although it is less direct, prenatal exposure to opioids is linked to low birth weight and other medical issues (Chap. 4), which in turn are associated with a multitude of neuropsychological difficulties (Riccio, Sullivan, & Cohen, 2010). Thus, despite variations in impact, children exposed to neurotoxins are more likely to need support and possible special education services in school than non-exposed children.

Prevention and Intervention

Major components of preventive efforts include psychoeducational approaches and the policies developed as a result of research. For example, it is critical that parents and other family members, as well as officials responsible for schools, daycare centers, and other settings be informed of the dangers of pesticides so they can help prevent exposure (Chap. 7). Prevention efforts based on reducing lead (e.g., in gasoline, in paint) have been largely effective in reducing exposure, but also may generate a false sense of security leading people to believe that lead exposure is no longer an issue. The effects of air pollutants on respiratory and cardiopulmonary function have been well documented, and increased attention is now being paid to the impact of air pollution on neurodevelopment, as extremely small particles are able to cross the blood–brain barrier and enter the brain via respiration. As with pesticides and lead, exposure to pollutants can occur prenatally as well as throughout the lifespan, so exposure may be ongoing. For example, studies of cohorts of children in certain geographic areas have found that they are impacted by pollutants in the air related to nearby factories, smog, power plants, and traffic-related air pollution (see Chap. 9). Thus, parent training and education are necessary to prevent both in utero and postnatal exposure to neurotoxins. For potential effects in utero, folate supplementation as an intervention is recommended for women who are pregnant and using AEDs; however, the supplementation has not been shown to completely prevent the teratogenic risks associated with AEDs (see Chap. 5).

Education and training programs targeting parents should also include training for physicians (e.g., obstetricians, gynecologists) in how to work effectively with mothers to eliminate exposure to harmful substances during pregnancy. Most doctors will advise against the use of alcohol or recreational drugs if pregnancy is anticipated or once the pregnancy has been confirmed (e.g., Carson et al., 2010; Centers for Disease Control and Prevention, National Center on Birth Defects and Developmental Disabilities, 2005). Since AEDs are used to control a legitimate medical issue (as opposed to used recreationally), their use presents an interesting dilemma. Sudden discontinuation of AEDs during pregnancy can be harmful to both mother and child, so professionals must work closely with the mother and the mother's physician when making decisions about continuing versus discontinuing treatment. Ideally, the physician will work to find the smallest effective dose to treat the symptoms of epilepsy while also minimizing risk to the fetus (see Chap. 5). Similarly, Power et al. (Chap. 6) addressed the use of antidepressants, antipsychotics, and lithium during pregnancy. Use of these medications during pregnancy is becoming more common with the prevalence of mental health issues among women who are pregnant. As with the continuation of AEDs, there is a difficult balance between the importance of treating mental illness among women who are pregnant and preventing harm to the developing fetus. For example, many physicians may recommend discontinuing the use of SSRIs during pregnancy due to potential teratogenic effects, but untreated maternal depression can also be harmful to the developing child (Hermansen & Melinder, 2015). Ideally, these issues would be articulated before pregnancy or early in the pregnancy.

Early Identification and Early Intervention

Early identification and early intervention make a significant contribution to reducing the effects of many risk factors (e.g., Kilgus, Riley-Tillman, Chafouleas, Christ, & Welsh, 2014; Oberklaid, Baird, Blair, Melhuish, & Hall, 2013; Stormont, Reinke, Herman, & Lembke, 2012). For example, research consistently supports the importance of early identification of children at risk for reading difficulties as a means of preventing more serious reading problems (Catts, Nielsen, Bridges, Liu, & Bontempo, 2015). Similarly, early intervention to address behavioral problems is a means of preventing more problematic behaviors (Greenwood, Kratochwill, & Clements, 2008; Stormont et al., 2012). Research suggests that children below 2 years of age receive fewer services than older children and children of high need parents are less likely to use the services available to them through the Individual Family Service Plan (Block, Rosenberg, Kellar-Guenther, Robinson, & Goetze, 2015). While family demographics have not consistently been found to be a factor in early intervention services, a necessary first step is that parents be referred to early intervention services. As the referral source for infants and toddlers is most often the pediatrician, it is important for medical personnel to be aware of prenatal and postnatal exposure, as well as the possible signs and symptoms of delayed development. It is critical for these professionals to identify the need for close follow-up, especially among children with additional biological risk factors (e.g., low birth weight). At the same time, the heterogeneity with which children exposed to neurotoxins often present points to the need for appropriate assessment methods that can identify these children with adequate reliability, sensitivity, and specificity.

Analogous to newborn screening for various medical conditions, some preschool programs and many school districts use brief universal screeners for academic and/or behavioral status in order to provide supportive services from a preventive perspective. The use of screeners for emerging and developmental problems is still controversial, in part because of the dynamic nature and individual variation in child development particularly prior to age 3, the limited focus of the screener used, or the length of the more comprehensive approaches (Stormont, Herman, Reinke, King, & Owens, 2015). The use of universal screeners in relation to potential academic problems, usually reading, has been supported in the literature, with provision of intervention services to those identified as at-risk (e.g., O'Connor & Jenkins, 1999). With regard to pollution, Johnson et al. (Chap. 9) speak to the need for screening protocols to identify exposed children, so continued exposure can be mitigated and interventions can be initiated. Similar protocols seem appropriate for other environmental toxins with risk for continued exposure, such as pesticides and lead. In conjunction with universal screening, the need to monitor progress and rate of development in response to intervention is important in determining next steps for support and the appropriateness of formal diagnosis.

Once difficulties have been identified, parent education will be necessary to teach parents how to manage their children's behavior and to advocate for services at school. Chapter 2 describes studies on the effectiveness of several parent education programs (e.g., CHOICES, Step-by-Step, Families Moving Forward), which may serve as useful models for similar program development. Similarly, pediatricians, psychologists, and education professionals (e.g., school counselors, school nurses) should receive continuing education to recognize children who may have been exposed to toxins, as well as methods to maximize positive outcomes for the child, rather than on blaming the child or parents for exposure-related deficits. Services may be provided in general education as a component of early intervention and response to intervention (Gresham, 2014). With continued difficulties, children with neurodevelopmental deficits may be eligible for special education services under the Individuals with Disabilities Education Act (IDEA; 2004). When deficits are apparent, but do not significantly impair educational functioning, support services (e.g., accommodations and modifications) may be provided through 504 services (Section 504 of the Rehabilitation Act of, 1973).

Since children with FASD are a more researched population as compared to children exposed to some of the other neurotoxins covered in this volume, it is not surprising that there are empirically evaluated prevention and intervention programs such as CHOICES, MILE, and other programs targeting academic, social, and adaptive behavioral variables. At the same time, there is still a long way to go in terms of investigating the generalizability and acceptability of these interventions when used with children with FASDs. With the exception of FASD, the research literature provides very few psychosocial or psychoeducational interventions with sufficient empirical support to be considered evidence-based, and this is especially true for school-based interventions. As a result, practitioners are left to apply construct-specific interventions (see Riccio et al., 2010, chapter 18) without empirically supported guidelines. It is important to note that although problems with attention, memory, executive function, motor skills, and so on may look similar across children exposed to different neurotoxins, the differing etiological, neurological, and environmental factors may lead to differential efficacy of interventions. Commonly used interventions for these deficits may need to be modified based on the child's level of cognitive functioning, which is often impacted by in utero exposure to alcohol or other substances. To be sure, there are excellent resources (e.g., Clay, 2004) that provide very helpful strategies for integrating children with medical issues into the school system. Finally, at least some individuals who experience exposure to neurotoxins will likely need long-term care, even into adulthood, due to impact on cognitive functioning and adaptive behaviors.

Limitations to Existing Research

Power et al. (Chap. 6) describe some of the difficulties with conducting research in pediatric neurotoxicology, including limitations to using the ideal experimental design, difficulty controlling for many variables, lack of random selection, and inability to control dosage or amount of exposure in relation to research on psychotropic medications. These research design challenges apply to all of the neurotoxin research reviewed in this volume. Although many chapters report a dose–response relationship, such that neuropsychological deficits are more pronounced with higher levels of exposure to neurotoxins, it is difficult to control or measure reliably and consistently dose response; the exposure is not likely a single instance, but variable over time. This applies to in utero exposure as well as exposure to environmental toxins postnatally. Further, research is also limited as the same child may be exposed to multiple toxins. For example, the research on the use of opiates, marijuana, and stimulants indicated that many studies involved women who reported using multiple substances during pregnancy (Chaps. 3 and 4). Similarly, a child exposed to pesticides in utero may experience continued exposure postnatally, which makes it difficult to determine when the greater impact occurred.

There also has been minimal control for other moderating factors in many studies. For instance, many studies examining differences due to maternal AED use in children's cognitive ability did not control for differences in maternal cognition. Maternal use of psychotropic medications adds a layer of complexity because it is extremely difficult to determine which developmental outcomes should be attributed to in utero medication exposure versus what should be attributed to the genetic predisposition to depression, anxiety, and other forms of psychopathology.

Research findings on developmental outcomes are extremely inconsistent, with some studies finding differences compared to control children, other studies finding differences that decrease over time (i.e., exposed children's functioning becomes more "normal" over time), and still other studies finding no differences. In addition to the moderating factors discussed earlier, some of these inconsistencies are likely due to a lack of uniform neuropsychological, academic, and psychosocial measures used across studies (Chap. 3). Further, most of the research focuses on young children. For example, studies of maternal psychotropic use have not followed children past 6 years of age so there is no indication of long-term effects (see Chap. 4). This is a significant gap in the literature, as many outcomes associated with exposure may become more conspicuous and more of a hindrance as children face the increased behavioral and academic demands of the school setting.

Professionals also lack a firm knowledge base regarding prognostic variables or factors that may impact or predict outcomes among exposed children. Although there have been advances in screening for school-age children, and for preschool, this screening does not occur until the child enters the school system. As yet, there is no practical, yet effective screener that could be used by pediatricians at well-child visits that might trigger referral and early identification. Finally, there has been very little research examining impact on specific academic skills or on school-based interventions or accommodations for children exposed to most of the toxins discussed in this volume.

Directions for Future Research in Pediatric Neurotoxicology

The general themes presented above point to important directions for future research. First, the field is in need of more research on the developmental trajectory and prognosis of children exposed to neurotoxins, so that we can begin to understand what these children look like as they transition to adolescence and young adulthood. As is the case for children with other neurodevelopmental and genetic disorders, children exposed to neurotoxins may exhibit changes in how their neuropsychological strengths and weaknesses are manifest over time. Most of the extant research has focused on short-term outcomes. More frequent and longer-term monitoring will be necessary to identify these developmental changes, and to more clearly understand the long-term impact of exposure. Similarly, some exposed children may appear to be typically developing upon initial assessment, with more subtle deficits becoming more conspicuous over time; these deficits may be missed without long-term follow-up.

Long-term studies must assess potential moderating factors beyond dose–response data, as these may account for differences in neuropsychological outcomes. The inconsistent findings reported throughout this volume may be partially explained by these moderating factors, and these variables must be studied more carefully and deliberately to better understand their relative influence on children's outcomes. Along with moderating factors, any intervention programs need to be accounted for in the long-term trajectory. At this time, there has been surprisingly little research on the efficacy of school-based intervention programs or accommodations for children exposed to neurotoxins even short-term. What is needed are resources for children exposed to the toxins covered in this book, to address such questions as: How well do interventions targeting certain constructs (e.g., memory, social skills) work with children who have been exposed to neurotoxins, and How do these interventions need to be adapted for exposed children with deficits in executive function and adaptive behaviors? Answering these questions will require developing programs (or modifying existing programs) specifically for children exposed to neurotoxins, and then evaluating their efficacy with this specific population. In addition to empirical studies with well-defined groups of exposed children, there is a need to develop and empirically investigate (a) parent education curricula for prevention and intervention efforts and (b) continuing education programs for professionals who work with children and families.

Current research suggests a lack of specificity in terms of means for early identification of resulting problems, common deficits, or outcomes. That is, exposure to a certain neurotoxin tends to result in deficits across several areas, and exposure to multiple neurotoxins may result in deficits in the same domain (e.g., deficits in executive function are described in multiple chapters in this volume, as are externalizing behaviors such as hyperactivity, impulsivity, aggression, and conduct problems). This lack of specificity suggests that certain domains of function may have a general vulnerability to the effects of neurotoxin exposure, but more research will be needed to evaluate this impression. It also may be the case that in many studies of children exposed to toxins, a narrow range of constructs was assessed, and more comprehensive assessment may reveal more widespread deficits across a range of constructs.

Lastly, without more research on many of these neurotoxins and how they impact child development, it is difficult to establish appropriate and reasonable prevention programs. For example, without more research on the use of AEDs, psychotropic medications, or other medications for maternal health, how can physicians adequately advise pregnant women? Professionals need empirically grounded guidelines to help them navigate the risk/benefit ratio associated with these substances when used by women who are pregnant and who need the medications to control symptoms of various disorders while minimizing risk to the developing fetus.

Conclusion

With advances in medicine, technology, and knowledge of vulnerability factors, more children who have been exposed to neurotoxins are being identified for intervention and are surviving at higher rates. At the same time, there are environmental changes and increases in the use of medication to treat maternal health that may be identified as having deleterious effects in the future. Given the increased survival rates, along with the movement for inclusive education, educational and health care professionals need to work collaboratively with these children to maximize their outcomes in public school settings. Thus, it is important to understand the academic and psychosocial outcomes associated with exposure to various neurotoxins.

This book reviews a great deal of data based on research with *groups* of infants and children. While this information is helpful in making predictions about psychosocial and academic outcomes, and in developing prevention/intervention programs, the most critical question from the perspective of the *individual* child is how programs can remediate areas of weakness while capitalizing on areas of strength. Clearly, this requires comprehensive assessment and developmental surveillance to monitor changes in functioning over time, similar to the frequent monitoring required for children who experience a traumatic brain injury (Riccio & Reynolds, 1999; Wetherington & Hooper, 2006). Finally, given the vulnerability of the developing central nervous system to toxins, practitioners are urged to consider neurotoxin exposure when gathering developmental history information from children and parents.

References

Blake, J. J., Lund, E. M., Zhou, Q., Kwok, O., & Benz, M. R. (2012). National prevalence rates of bully victimization among students with disabilities in the United States. *School Psychology Quarterly, 27*, 210–222. doi:10.1037/spq0000008.

Block, S. R., Rosenberg, S. A., Kellar-Guenther, Y., Robinson, C. C., & Goetze, L. (2015). Child and parent characteristics affecting the authorization and expenditure of funds for early intervention services. *Journal of Disability Policy Studies, 26*(1), 3–11. doi:10.1177/1044207313518070.

Carson, G., Cox, L. V., Crane, J., Croteau, P., Graves, L., Kluka, S., Koren, G., Martel, M. J., Midmer, D., Nulman, I., Poole, N., Senikas, V., & Wood, R. (2010). Alcohol use and pregnancy consensus clinical guidelines. *Journal of Obstetrics and Gynaecology Canada, 32*(8 Supplement 3), S1–S32.

Catts, H. W., Nielsen, D. C., Bridges, M. S., Liu, Y. S., & Bontempo, D. E. (2015). Early identification of reading disabilities within an RTI framework. *Journal of Learning Disabilities, 48*, 281–297. doi:10.1177/0022219413498115.

Centers for Disease Control and Prevention, National Center on Birth Defects and Developmental Disabilities. (2005). *Advisory on alcohol use in pregnancy: A 2005 message to women from the U.S. Surgeon General*. Washington, DC: U.S. Department of Health and Human Services.

Clay, D. L. (2004). *Helping schoolchildren with chronic health conditions: A practical guide*. New York, NY: Guilford.

Greenwood, C. R., Kratochwill, T. R., & Clements, M. (Eds.). (2008). *Schoolwide prevention models: Lessons learned in elementary schools*. New York, NY: Guilford.

Gresham, F. M. (2014). Best practices in diagnosis of mental health and academic difficulties in a multitier problem-solving approach. In P. L. Harrison & A. Thomas (Eds.), *Best practices in school psychology: Data-based and collaborative decision making* (pp. 147–158). Bethesda, MD: National Association of School Psychologists.

Hermansen, T. K., & Melinder, A. (2015). Prenatal SSRI exposure: Effects on later child development. *Child Neuropsychology, 21*, 543–569. doi:10.1080/09297049.2014.942727.

Individuals With Disabilities Education Act, 20 U.S.C. § 1400 (2004).

Jones, K. L. (2011). The effects of alcohol on fetal development. *Birth Defects Research Part C: Embryo Today: Reviews, 93*, 3–11. doi:10.1002/bdrc.20200.

Kilgus, S. P., Riley-Tillman, T. C., Chafouleas, S. M., Christ, T. J., & Welsh, M. E. (2014). Direct behavior rating as a school-based behavior universal screener: Replication across sites. *Journal of School Psychology, 52*, 63–82. doi:10.1016/j.jsp.2013.11.002.

O'Connor, R. E., & Jenkins, J. R. (1999). The prediction of reading disabilities in kindergarten and first grade. *Scientific Studies of Reading, 3*, 159–197.

Oberklaid, F., Baird, G., Blair, M., Melhuish, E., & Hall, D. (2013). Children's health and development: Approaches to early identification and intervention. *Archives of Diseases in Children, 98*, 1008–1011.

Oberlander, T. F., Papsdorf, M., Brain, U. M., Misri, S., Ross, C., & Grunau, R. E. (2010). Prenatal effects of selective serotonin reuptake inhibitor antidepressants, serotonin transporter promoter genotype (SLC6A4), and maternal mood on child behavior at 3 years of age. *Archives of Pediatric and Adolescent Medicine, 164*, 444–451.

Riccio, C. A., & Reynolds, C. R. (1999). Assessment of traumatic brain injury in children for neuropsychological rehabilitation. In M. Raymond, T. L. Bennett, L. Hartlage, & C. M. Cullum (Eds.), *Mild brain injury: A clinician's guide* (pp. 77–116). Austin, TX: Pro-Ed.

Riccio, C. A., Sullivan, J. R., & Cohen, M. J. (2010). *Neuropsychological assessment and intervention for childhood and adolescent disorders*. Hoboken, NJ: Wiley.

Section 504 of the Rehabilitation Act of 1973, 29 U.S.C. § 794; 34 C.F.R. Part 104.

Stormont, M., Herman, K. C., Reinke, W. M., King, K. R., & Owens, S. (2015). The kindergarten academic and behavior readiness screener: The utility of single item teacher ratings of kindergarten readiness. *School Psychology Quarterly, 30*, 212–228.

Stormont, M., Reinke, W., Herman, K., & Lembke, E. (2012). *Tier two interventions: Academic and behavior supports for children at risk for failure*. New York, NY: Guilford.

Sullivan, P. M., & Knutson, J. F. (2000). Maltreatment and disabilities: A population-based epidemiological study. *Child Abuse & Neglect, 24*, 1257–1273.

Wetherington, C. E., & Hooper, S. R. (2006). Preschool traumatic brain injury: A review for the early childhood special educator. *Exceptionality, 14*, 155–170.

Index

C. Riccio, J. Sullivan (eds.), *Pediatric Neurotoxicology*, Specialty Topics in Pediatric Neuropsychology, DOI 10.1007/978-3-319-32358-9

CPSIA information can be obtained
at www.ICGtesting.com
Printed in the USA
LVHW032346100520
655319LV00019B/676